D1563269

# TOXICANTS AND DRUGS

# Toxicants and Drugs:

## KINETICS AND DYNAMICS

ELLEN J. O'FLAHERTY

*University of Cincinnati Medical Center*
*Institute of Environmental Health*

A WILEY-INTERSCIENCE PUBLICATION

**JOHN WILEY & SONS**      New York   •   Chichester   •   Brisbane   •   Toronto

*Library of Congress Cataloging in Publication Data:*

O'Flaherty, Ellen J.    1936–
  Toxicants and drugs.

  "A Wiley-Interscience publication."
  Includes index.
    1.  Poisons—Metabolism—Mathematical models.
2.  Poisons—Dose-response relationship—Mathematical
models.  3.  Pharmacokinetics.  4.  Toxicology—
Mathematical models.  5.  Xenobiotic metabolism—
Mathematical models.  I.  Title.

RA1216.035    615.9′00724    80-24445
ISBN 0-471-06047-X

Printed in the United States of America

10 9 8 7 6 5 4 3 2 1

# Preface

It is unfortunate that our culture has permitted, and perhaps encouraged, the development of a dichotomy between the mathematical sciences and the life sciences. It is true that mathematics is written in a foreign language. It is also true that mathematical creativity requires discipline and rigorous logic of a degree unknown to most persons, even to most scientists. But the application of established mathematical principles to practical problems is within the reach of all scientists.

The strengths of mathematics lie in its generality, in the availability of a concise notation for the expression of an array of variables and the ways in which they interrelate, and in the existence of a body of rules for manipulating these variables. Once a physiological or biological problem has been expressed in terms of a mathematical model, all the powerful techniques of classical mathematics may be applied to it. If the model has utility, the resulting manipulations should not only facilitate organization, summary, comparison, and communication of experimental data, they should also provide insight into the workings of the physiological or biochemical system, lead to predictions about the behavior of the system under different experimental conditions, and facilitate the design of appropriate experiments to test these predictions.

This book focuses on modeling the behavior of compounds usually foreign to the human and animal body: namely, drugs and toxicants. The implications of observed relationships between measurable quantities such as concentration and time, effect and time, or dose and effect are explored with regard to the mechanisms of absorption, distribution, elimination, and action of toxicants and drugs.

No usable model can incorporate all the individual physical and biochemical steps that together make up the behavior of a compound. Only the features of the compound's absorption, distribution, and elimination that control its behavior—that is, the rate-determining mechanisms—are taken into account in designing a model. When the rate-determining mechanisms have been correctly identified and their kinetic nature understood, the model can be used with reasonable confidence (but also with reasonable care) to predict the behavior or effect of a drug or toxicant under conditions different from those under which the original observations of behavior were made. Accordingly the models that have proved to be most successful are those that are founded on established physical and biochemical principles.

For the life scientist, then, there are two challenges: to express the problem in terms of an appropriate model, and to be sufficiently knowledgeable to take advantage of the mathematical techniques and tools available to exploit the model.

The first chapter of this book provides a brief review of algebraic relationships and elementary calculus, presented at a level that would embarrass a mathematician but is designed to bring to nonmathematicians and antimathematicians the realization that they can perform the mathematical manipulations required of the kineticist, even though they may not be able to derive the applicable expressions or even to justify their application. It is assumed that students are familiar—or, more accurately, have been at some time in the past—with the simpler tools of algebra. It is further assumed that they have forgotten any calculus once learned. Most important, it is assumed that they have a reasonable degree of intellectual curiosity and do not underestimate their own capabilities.

Derivations of important expressions are given either in the text or in appendices. To students with a mathematical bent a derivation is often of use in understanding the applicability and limitations of a model. Students without a specific interest in mathematics can apply the relationships derived even though they may not fully understand the derivations themselves.

Chapters 2 through 5 cover the body of principles generally known as pharmacokinetics. The emphasis of this presentation, however, is different from that usually found in pharmacokinetics texts.

Pharmacokinetics is the application of the mathematical techniques of kinetics to the study of the absorption, distribution, and elimination of drugs. As a scientific discipline it is only 10 or 15 years old. Although many of the basic kinetics principles were outlined by Torsten Teorell in the mid-1930s, their utility was not at first generally recognized. Systematic application of kinetics principles to practical problems was undertaken during the 1960s primarily by pharmacologists, who had begun to recognize the potential utility of kinetic models in integrating plasma and urine concentration data into a coherent picture of drug disposition and action. This body of work is the origin of the word "pharmacokinetics."

However, the kinetics principles developed to deal with problems of drug delivery and effectiveness are equally applicable to toxicological problems. Throughout this book an effort has been made to illustrate the broad applicability of kinetics principles by selecting examples from both the pharmacology and toxicology literatures. Consequently the reader who has some familiarity with kinetics texts will find less emphasis than is usual on such specialized aspects of the discipline as dose regimen design and bioavailability of drugs from commercial preparations.

The last three chapters of the book deal with the relationships among dose, effect, and time, and with the incidence of effect in a population, or response.

Although the presentations begin with first principles, they are not simplistic. Sophisticated concepts are developed. Each chapter proceeds from a logical development of important principles to examples of how each new concept or principle has been applied to a real clinical or research problem. Simplified kinetic models are not applied to data they do not adequately describe. Deviations of real biological systems from predicted or ideal behavior are clearly illustrated.

Questions, the number depending on the variety and complexity of the material presented, follow each chapter. These fall into three groups: (1) simple derivations or questions about theory, mostly designed to give the student confidence; (2) literature data that conform well to a kinetic model and can be analyzed in accordance with that model; and (3) literature data whose deviations from expected behavior must be explained, or whose interpretation is open to discussion.

With the inclusion of the problems, this book is suitable for independent study. However, experience suggests that most of the problems are more valuable when they are used to stimulate group discussion. In the graduate level course for which this material was developed, students are encouraged to work together on homework assignments.

This material is suitable for graduate or advanced undergraduate students in pharmacy, pharmacology, toxicology, or industrial medicine. It can be covered in a survey fashion in one semester or even in one quarter, by dealing primarily with well-behaved systems and omitting consideration of nonlinear kinetics and specialized subject areas. Alternatively the material can be treated as fully as desired and in some depth in a year-long course. Since the choice of sections or chapters to be omitted for the purpose of a shorter course will depend on the academic context in which the course is offered, no single abbreviated course outline is suggested. However, some sections are more fundamental than others. This basic material includes all of Chapter 1 if needed, and Sections 3.1–3.11, 4.1–4.4.1, 5.1–5.3, 6.1–6.3 and 6.5, and 8.1–8.4.

The purpose of this book is to bridge the gap between pure mathematical theory, at the one extreme, and the indiscriminate application of simple standard models to data they may not adequately describe, at the other. If its users become educated in the proper application of a variety of kinetics techniques, it will have succeeded.

ELLEN J. O'FLAHERTY

*Cincinnati, Ohio*
*January 1981*

# Acknowledgments

I thank the several classes of toxicology and pharmacy graduate students who have responded generally favorably, sometimes critically, and always helpfully to this material during its development into a textbook.

Particular thanks are due to Dr. Edward R. Garrett, Graduate Research Professor of the University of Florida College of Pharmacy, for his encouragement and suggestions at the initiation of this project. The approach to the material in Chapter 1 and to some of the pharmacokinetics principles was inspired by the pharmacokinetics workshops taught by Ed Garrett.

I also thank Brenda Smith for careful and accurate typing of the manuscript, Lorraine Mercer and Elizabeth Taylor for their assistance with the very large task of obtaining copyright clearances for the many illustrations, and Wayne Adams for confirming the accuracy of all citations to published work.

E. J. O'F.

# Contents

Definitions of Symbols Used in the Text     xiii

1   The Mathematical Vocabulary and Grammatical Rules of Kinetics     1

2   Saturable Systems     31

3   Acute Exposure with First-Order Disposition     81

4   Acute Exposure with Nonlinear and Mixed Kinetics of Disposition     173

5   Chronic Exposure     222

6   Dose, Effect Relationships: Receptor Theory     278

7   Dynamics: The Time Course of Effect     322

8   Dose, Response Relationships     354

Index     391

# Definitions of Symbols Used in the Text

## 1 Dose and Dose Rate

| | |
|---|---|
| $D$ | Total acute dose. To avoid the need to designate "fraction absorbed" or "absorbed unchanged" in equations, $D$ represents either external or internal dose. Its significance in any particular application should be clear from the context. Most often $D$ represents internal dose. |
| $D_m$ | Maintenance drug dose. |
| $D_l$ | Loading drug dose. |
| $DR, A$ | Dose rate; $D/\Delta t$. |
| $TD$ | Total chronic dose, calculated as $(DR)$ (length of exposure). |

## 2 Time

| | |
|---|---|
| $t$ | Time. |
| $t_n$, $n = 0, 1, \ldots, \infty$ | Time points, from initial time $t_0$ to infinite time $t_\infty$. |
| $t_{max}$ | Time point at which the maximum concentration is achieved in a model compartment with first-order absorption and elimination. |
| $\Delta t$ | The time interval between repeated doses. |
| $t^*$ | Time point during the $n$th dose interval at which concentration, time curves for repeated exposure to dose $D$ at time intervals $\Delta t$ and for continuous exposure to dose rate $D/\Delta t$ cross each other. |

## 3 Concentration

| | |
|---|---|
| $C$ | Concentration |
| $C^A$ | Concentration of compound A. |

| | |
|---|---|
| $C_i$, $i = 1, 2, \ldots, n$ | Concentration in the $i$th compartment of a kinetic model with $n$ compartments. |
| $C_0$ | Initial concentration (at $t_0$). |
| $C_p$ | Concentration in plasma. |
| $C_u$ | Concentration in urine. |
| $\Delta C$ | Concentration increment or decrement, usually small. |
| $C_{max}$ | The maximum concentration achieved in a model compartment with first-order absorption and elimination. Also the plasma level at the beginning of the $\infty$th dose interval on repeated administration. |
| $C_{min}$ | The plasma level at the end of the $\infty$th dose interval on repeated administration. |
| $C(t)$ | Concentration as a function of time, especially on repeated administration or continuous exposure. |
| $C(t_\infty)$ | Plateau level; the concentration achieved after continuous exposure for an infinite length of time. Use of this form is restricted to continuous exposure. |
| $C(n)$ | Concentration at the beginning of the $n$th dose interval ($n$ discrete doses). |
| $C(n_\infty)$ | Plateau level; the concentration at the beginning of the $\infty$th dose interval. |
| $\overline{C}(n)$ | Average concentration within the $n$th dose interval. |
| $\overline{C}(n_\infty)$ | Average concentration within the $\infty$th dose interval. |
| $\overline{C}(\infty)$ | This form is equivalent to both $\overline{C}(n_\infty)$ and $C(t_\infty)$. |

## 4   Amount

| | |
|---|---|
| $B$ | Amount in blood. |
| $U$ | Amount in urine. |
| $B_0$ | Amount in blood at $t_0$. |
| $U_0$ | Amount in urine at $t_0$. |
| $U_\infty$ | Amount in urine at $t_\infty$. |
| $M_i$, $i = 1, 2, \ldots, n$ | Amount in the $i$th compartment of an $n$-compartment kinetic model. |
| $BB$ | Body burden. |

## 5  Rate Constants

| | |
|---|---|
| $k$ | First-order rate constant. |
| $k^A$ | Rate constant for compound A. |
| $k_e$ | Overall first-order elimination rate constant. |
| $k_{ij}$ | Rate constant for transfer from compartment $i$ to compartment $j$. If $j=0$, the rate constant represents transfer out of the system. |
| $k_m$ | Rate constant representing metabolite formation. |
| $k_u$ | Rate constant representing urinary excretion. |
| $k_b$ | Rate constant representing biliary excretion. |
| $k_a$ | Rate constant representing absorption. |
| $\alpha$ | Agglomerate rate constant representing net loss from the central compartment of a two-compartment model during the distributional phase. |
| $\beta$ | Agglomerate rate constant representing net elimination in a two-compartment model after the distributional phase is complete. |
| $k_u^M$ | Rate constant representing excretion of metabolite in urine. |
| $k_e^M$ | Overall elimination rate constant for metabolite. |
| $k_f^M$ | Formation rate constant for a particular metabolite; if only one metabolite is formed, $k_f^M = k_m$. |

## 6  Volume

| | |
|---|---|
| $V$ | Volume. |
| $V_D$ | Volume of distribution. |
| $V_D^A$ | Volume of distribution of compound A. |
| $V_i$, $i = 1, 2, \ldots, n$ | Volume of the $i$th compartment of an $n$-compartment kinetic model. |
| $V_{\text{extrap}}$ | Volume of distribution determined by back extrapolation of the terminal phase of a multicompartment model. |
| $V_{\text{ss}}$ | Volume of distribution determined either at infusion steady state or at the momentary steady state after acute administration when $dC_2/dt = 0$. |
| $V_\beta$ | Volume of distribution determined during the $\beta$ phase of dieaway after acute administration. |

## 7  Miscellaneous

| | |
|---|---|
| $K$ | Dissociation constant or half-saturation constant. |
| $K_m, K_t$ | Michaelis constants; half-saturation values for saturable processes. |
| $K_A, K_I$ | Michaelis constants; half-saturation values for A (activator) and for I (inhibitor). |
| $V_m, T_m$ | Maximum rates of saturable processes. |
| Cl | Clearance. |
| $Cl^A$ | Clearance of compound A. |
| $Cl^A_{total}$ | Total clearance of compound A. |
| $CL^A_{renal}$ | Renal clearance of compound A. |
| AUC | Area under the curve of plasma concentration versus time to time $t$. |
| $(AUC)_\infty$ | Area under the curve of plasma concentration versus time to the time when all of an acutely administered compound has been eliminated. |
| $\theta$ | Magnitude of effect. |
| $\theta_m$ | Maximum magnitude of effect. |

# TOXICANTS AND DRUGS

# *1*

# *The Mathematical Vocabulary and Grammatical Rules of Kinetics*

**1.1** Functional relationships

**1.2** The straight line function

**1.3** Linearization of common kinetic functions

**1.4** Linearization of exponential function; Definition and properties of logarithms

    1.4.1  Definition of a logarithm
    1.4.2  Properties of logarithms

**1.5** Graphing logarithmic relationships

**1.6** The derivative

**1.7** The integral

**1.8** Differentiating and integrating the exponential function

**1.9** Definitions used in kinetics

**1.10** Dimensionality of equations

**1.11** Recognition of kinetic forms by inspection

The purposes of this introductory chapter are to review the simple algebraic and calculus techniques required for manipulation of kinetic equations, and to define the basic kinetic terms. Thus fortified, the reader will be prepared to jump into the kinetic sea or, at any rate, to work his way into it by degrees, beginning with Chapter 2.

The reader who is certain of his mathematical competence may skip to Section 1.9.

## 1.1   FUNCTIONAL RELATIONSHIPS

The word "kinetic" implies motion or, more broadly, change. In principle change can occur either randomly or systematically. However, biological systems are governed by functional interrelationships at the molecular level having their ultimate expression in systematic, observable, and describable behaviors. The systematic nature of the behavior of biological systems is evident in the dependence of direction and magnitude of change on one or more independent variables.

When $y$ depends on $x$ we say that $y$ is a function of $x$:

$$y = f(x). \tag{1.1}$$

Equation 1.1 states that $y$ depends on $x$ in some unspecified fashion. The value of $x$ can be selected arbitrarily; the value of $y$ is then fixed. Therefore $x$ is called the *independent variable* and $y$ the *dependent variable*.

The dependent variable $y$ could be a function of more than one independent variable: $y = f(x, z, p, \ldots)$. The volume of a mole of oxygen, for example, is a function of the ambient temperature as well as of the pressure to which it is subjected. However, it will not be necessary for us to consider functions of more than one variable.

By writing an equation relating $y$ to $x$ explicitly, one specifies the form of the function $f(x)$. For example, the area $A$ of a circle is $\pi r^2$ and its circumference $C$ is $2\pi r$, where $r$ is the radius of the circle and $\pi$ is a constant whose value, rounded to five significant digits, is 3.1416. Expressed in the equivalent mathematical forms, $A = f(r) = \pi r^2$ and $C = g(r) = 2\pi r$, where $g$ is some function other than $f$. Thus $r$ is the independent variable; both area and circumference are functions of $r$.

The form of an equation does not of itself distinguish between the dependent and the independent variable. It simply specifies a relationship between two variables either of which, depending upon circumstances, may be the independent variable. We all know that

$$\text{distance} = \text{rate} \times \text{time}.$$

Assuming that we travel at a constant known rate, if we know the distance between our present location and our destination we can calculate the time at which we expect to arrive. On the other hand, if we do not know the distance (or if we got lost on the way), we can use the elapsed time determined on arrival to calculate the distance traveled. But we must know the value of one of the two variables to be able to calculate the value of the other.

In experimental situations the independent variable may be chosen by the experimenter, or it may be fixed by constraints beyond his control. For example, kinetic studies are usually conducted by monitoring plasma or tissue concentration as a function of time. The absurdity of considering time to be a function of concentration is obvious. But this relationship is an attribute of the system being studied. It is not inherent in the equation that describes the kinetic behavior of the system.

Use of single letters to designate the independent and dependent variables is purely a convenience (e.g., "*A*" was used above to designate "the area of a circle"). Sometimes it is desirable to preserve the full form of a variable to prevent obscuring the nature of the relationship being described. For example, Fick's first law,

$$\frac{dC_2}{dt} = DA(C_2 - C_1),$$

could equally well have been written

$$y = DAx;$$

but only the first form can be read, "the rate of change of $C_2$ is proportional to the difference between $C_2$ and $C_1$." Fick's first law is the foundation of a large part of kinetic theory. It appears again in Chapter 3.

## 1.2  THE STRAIGHT LINE FUNCTION

The equation

$$y = ax + b, \tag{1.2}$$

where $a$ and $b$ are constants, is the equation of a straight line. That is, if all the points $(x, y)$ that satisfy Equation 1.2 were graphed in a linear coordinate system, they would define a straight line. By convention, in a linear coordinate system the horizontal axis, or abscissa, is designated the $x$ axis, where $x$ represents the independent variable (Figure 1.1). The vertical axis, or ordinate,

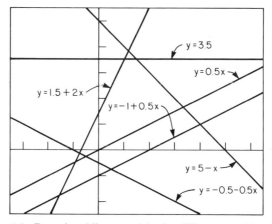

**Figure 1.1**  Examples of lines $ax + b$ having different $a$ and $b$ values.

is the $y$ axis, where $y$ represents the dependent variable. Then $b$ in Equation 1.2 is the ordinate intercept of the line defined by points $(x, y)$ and $a$ is its slope. Both $a$ and $b$ are general constants that may be any real numbers including zero and negative numbers. Their signs and magnitudes fix the position of the straight line in two-dimensional space. For example, if $b$ is negative the line intersects the $y$ axis below the origin. If $a$ is negative the line runs downhill rather than uphill. If $b$ is zero the line intersects the origin. Several straight lines having different $a$ and $b$ values are graphed in Figure 1.1.

Straight lines have distinct advantages over curves. The least squares line of best fit to experimental data can be found readily with desktop computer methods. Curves are more difficult to fit to data. Computer techniques have overcome some of the problems of curve fitting; however, different algorithms, or procedures for curve fitting, may give different best fits. Even with a single algorithm the researcher must specify an arbitrary "goodness of fit" that is acceptable to him. With a straight line this uncertainty does not arise. There is only one good fit, and it is the best one. Therefore many of the mathematical manipulations of kinetics have been directed at transforming kinetic equations into straight line, or linear, forms. There is nothing suspect about such manipulations. They do not violate scientific principle nor destroy the accuracy with which the kinetic equation describes the underlying biological system. Rather, they are a good illustration of one of the advantages of being able to describe biological behavior in mathematical language.

## 1.3   LINEARIZATION OF COMMON KINETIC FUNCTIONS

There are a number of kinetic functions whose forms occur over and over again. It will be instructive to use several of these forms to illustrate linear data plotting and some simple linear transformations.

$$\frac{dC}{dt} = -k_0.$$

(1.3)

This equation states that the rate of concentration decrease is $k_0$, a constant. It is the equation of a zero-order process (see Section 1.9), and would apply, for example, to the metabolism of a compound when the enzyme mediating the transformation is saturated. It represents a straight lie parallel to and below the abscissa and intersecting the ordinate at $-k_0$ (Figure 1.2a). The dependent and independent variables are identified and the values of the constants $a$ and $b$ are given for this and the subsequent examples in Table 1.1. Note that the notation $C(t)$ is shortened to $C$ when it is either obvious or understood that $C$ is a function of $t$.

$$C(t) = C_0 - k_0 t.$$

(1.4)

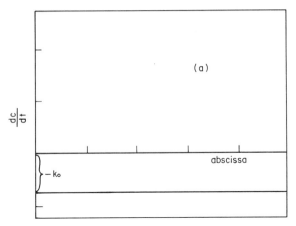

**Figure 1.2** Graphs of equations discussed in Section 1.3. ($a$) $dC/dt = -k_0$. ($b$) $C(t) = C_0 - k_0 t$. ($c$) $dC/dt = -kC(t)$. ($d$) $(AUC)\infty/D = D/2V_m V^2 + K_m/V_m V$. ($e$) $1/v(C) = 1/V_m + K_m/V_m C(t)$. (Graphs continued on pp. 6–8.)

This equation states that the concentration at time $t$ is $C_0 - k_0 t$, where $C_0$ is the concentration at time 0 and $k_0$ is a constant. It is the integral of Equation 1.3, with the boundary condition that $C = C_0$ at $t_0$. Integration is discussed in Section 1.7. Equation 1.4 represents a straight line (Table 1.1) with a downward slope, intersecting the ordinate at $C_0$ (Figure 1.2$b$).

$$\frac{dC}{dt} = -kC(t) \qquad (1.5)$$

This equation states that the rate of concentration change at time $t$ is

**Table 1.1** Breakdown of equations discussed in the text (Section 1.3)

| Function | | Independent Variable | Dependent Variable | $a$ | $b$ |
|---|---|---|---|---|---|
| 1.3 | $\dfrac{dC}{dt} = -k_0$ | $t$ | $\dfrac{dC}{dt}$ | $0$ | $-k_0$ |
| 1.4 | $C(t) = C_0 - k_0 t$ | $t$ | $C$ | $-k_0$ | $C_0$ |
| 1.5 | $\dfrac{dC}{dt} = -kC(t)$ | $C$ | $\dfrac{dC}{dt}$ | $-k$ | $0$ |
| 1.6 | $\dfrac{(AUC)_\infty}{D} = \dfrac{D}{2V_m V^2} + \dfrac{K_m}{V_m V}$ | $D$ | $\dfrac{(AUC)_\infty}{D}$ | $\dfrac{1}{2V_m V^2}$ | $\dfrac{K_m}{V_m V}$ |
| 1.7 | $\dfrac{1}{v(C)} = \dfrac{1}{V_m} + \dfrac{K_m}{V_m C(t)}$ | $\dfrac{1}{C(t)}$ | $\dfrac{1}{v(C)}$ | $\dfrac{K_m}{V_m}$ | $\dfrac{1}{V_m}$ |
| 1.8 | $\ln C = \ln C_0 - kt$ | $t$ | $\ln C$ | $-k$ | $\ln C_0$ |
| | or | | | | |
| | $\log C = \log C_0 - \dfrac{kt}{2.303}$ | $t$ | $\log C$ | $-\dfrac{k}{2.303}$ | $\log C_0$ |

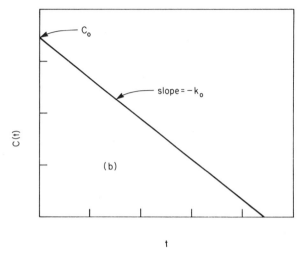

**Figure 1.2** (*continued*)

dependent on the concentration at time $t$. The proportionality constant is $-k$. It is the equation of a first-order process (see Section 1.9), and applies to both diffusion and filtration translocation mechanisms. It represents a straight line with negative slope, intersecting the origin (Figure 1.2c and Table 1.1).

$$(\text{AUC})_{\infty} = \frac{D^2}{2V_m V^2} + \frac{K_m D}{V_m V}. \tag{1.6}$$

Equation 1.6 states that the area under the concentration, time curve from time 0 to time $\infty$ for an acutely administered compound eliminated from the body by a saturated process, is a function of the dose $D$, the volume of

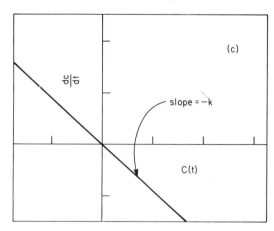

**Figure 1.2** (*continued*)

distribution $V$, and the Michaelis constant $K_m$ and maximum velocity $V_m$ of the elimination process. As written, it is not the equation of a straight line because the square of the independent variable $D$ occurs. It can be transformed into the equation of a straight line simply by dividing both sides of the equation by $D$, creating a new dependent variable:

$$\frac{(\text{AUC})_\infty}{D} = \frac{D}{2V_m V^2} + \frac{K_m}{V_m V}.$$

This is the equation of a straight line of positive slope $1/2V_m V^2$, which intersects the ordinate at $K_m/V_m V$ (Figure 1.2$d$ and Table 1.1).

$$v(C) = \frac{V_m C(t)}{K_m + C(t)}. \tag{1.7}$$

This is the equation describing the saturable elimination process itself. It states that the velocity $v(C)$ of elimination at time $t$ is a function of $C(t)$, the concentration at time $t$; and of $K_m$ and $V_m$, the constants that characterize the elimination process. Since $v(C) = dC/dt$, Equation 1.7 is a differential equation like Equations 1.3 and 1.5. To transform it into the equation of a straight line, we resort to a technique that is particularly useful in connection with rate equations describing saturable processes. When $x = y$, it is also true that $1/x = 1/y$; the second equation results from dividing both sides of the first equation by the quantity $xy$. Therefore

$$\frac{1}{v(C)} = \frac{K_m + C(t)}{V_m C(t)} = \frac{1}{V_m} + \frac{K_m}{V_m C(t)}.$$

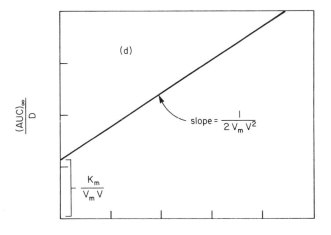

Figure 1.2   (*continued*)

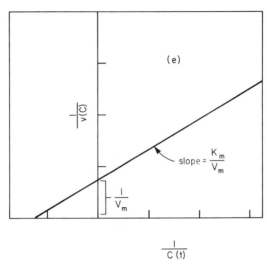

**Figure 1.2**　(*continued*)

When $1/v(C)$ is graphed as the dependent variable against $1/C(t)$ as the independent variable, the graph will be a straight line of positive slope $K_m/V_m$, intersecting the ordinate at $1/V_m$ (Figure 1.2e and Table 1.1). This transform is the well-known Lineweaver-Burk transform of the equation for the rate of a saturable process. There are two other possible linear transforms of Equation 1.7. Saturable processes are discussed in Chapter 2.

$$C(t) = C_0 e^{-kt}. \tag{1.8}$$

This is the integral of Equation 1.5, with the boundary condition that $C = C_0$ at $t_0$. It states that the concentration at time $t$ is $C_0 e^{-kt}$, where $C_0$ is the concentration at time 0, $k$ is a constant, and $e$ is the base of natural logarithms. It would be considered the equation of a straight line if the quantity $e^{-kt}$ were defined as the independent variable. But $e^{-kt}$ is an unwieldy and inconvenient independent variable. Equation 1.8, and forms related to it, occur very commonly in kinetics, and it would be very helpful to be able to graph concentration measurements against time in some simpler way. How can the exponential function $e^{-kt}$ be transformed so that the transform is linear with respect to time?

## 1.4  LINEARIZATION OF THE EXPONENTIAL FUNCTION; DEFINITION AND PROPERTIES OF LOGARITHMS

Logarithms aided in the performance of many complex computations prior to the advent of the calculator. Today they are less important in that regard but are still essential in dealing with the exponential functions that are regularly encountered in equations describing biological systems.

### 1.4.1 Definition of a Logarithm

The logarithm of a (real positive) number $x$ is the power to which a base must be raised to be equal to $x$. The bases in common use are 10 and $e$. The base of natural logarithms $e$ is approximately 2.718.

In mathematical notation,

$$\ln x = a \quad \text{if} \quad e^a = x; \quad \log x = b \quad \text{if} \quad 10^b = x.$$

Note that the logarithms of zero and of negative numbers are not defined. There are two special cases. These are:

**1** $e^1 = e$ and $10^1 = 10$.

**2** $e^0 = 10^0 = 1$.

The logarithm to the base $e$ of $e$ is 1; in alternative shorthand notation, $\ln e = 1$. The logarithm to the base 10 of 10 is also 1, or $\log 10 = 1$. But $\ln 1 = \log 1 = 0$. Therefore $\ln x = \log x = 0$ whenever $x = 1$. But remember that $x$ itself may not be 0. Only its logarithm may be 0.

A logarithm has no units, or dimensions. It is a pure number. Whatever the dimensions of $x$ may be, they are buried in $\ln x$. Section 1.10 shows that one consequence of the dimensionless nature of the logarithm is that the exponent in all exponential quantities can have no dimensions. For example, $e^{-kt}$ is a common exponential in kinetic equations. Since $t$ is time, $k$ must have the dimensions $1/\text{time}$, or $(\text{time})^{-1}$.

Logarithms either to the base 10 or to the base $e$ may be used, provided the same base is used throughout a series of related calculations. In general, it is easier to use natural logarithms whenever an equation has an exponential term. If $x = e^{-kt}$, it follows directly from the definition of the natural logarithm given above that

$$\ln x = -kt.$$

However, the semilog or log linear graph paper that is used in graphing equations of this form is always scaled to the base 10. Therefore we need to be able to convert $\ln x$ to $\log x$.

Values of $\ln x$ or $\log x$ for a given value of $x$ are obtainable from many pocket calculators. Alternatively, a table of natural logarithms may be consulted. Entering the table with the value $x = 10$, the reader will find that

$$\ln 10 = 2.303.$$

Since we know that

$$\log 10 = 1,$$

it follows directly that

$$\ln x = 2.303 \log x.$$

This is the rule for interconversion of natural logarithms and logarithms to the base 10.

### 1.4.2  Properties of Logarithms

**1**  $\log(ab) = \log a + \log b$
$\ln(ab) = \ln a + \ln b$

**2**  $\log(\frac{a}{b}) = \log a - \log b$
$\ln(\frac{a}{b}) = \ln a - \ln b$

**3**  $\log a^x = x \log a$
$\ln a^x = x \ln a$

A corollary of the second property is that

**4**  $\log(\frac{1}{b}) = \log 1 - \log b = -\log b;$

$\ln(\frac{1}{b}) = \ln 1 - \ln b = -\ln b,$

from which it follows that

**5**  $\log(\frac{1}{b}) = (-1)\log b = \log(b^{-1});$

$\ln(\frac{1}{b}) = (-1)\ln b = \ln(b^{-1}).$

Therefore logarithms of numbers lying between 0 and 1 are negative. The logarithm of 1 is, of course, 0; and the logarithms of numbers greater than 1 are positive.

Now we have the information we need to transform Equation 1.8 (Section 1.3) so that it is linear with respect to time:

$$C(t) = C_0 e^{-kt}.$$

By applying the first and third properties of logarithms, we find that

$$\ln C(t) = \ln C_0 - kt \ln e$$

$$= \ln C_0 - kt,$$

and
$$\log C(t) = \log C_0 - kt \log e.$$

But
$$\log e = \frac{\ln e}{2.303} = \frac{1}{2.303},$$

so
$$\log C(t) = \log C_0 - \frac{kt}{2.303}.$$

Note that the identity $\ln(e^{-kt}) = -kt$ can also be taken directly from the definition of a natural logarithm.

Each of the two logarithmic transforms of Equation 1.8 is the equation of a straight line. The dependent and independent variables are given together with the slopes and intercepts in Table 1.1.

## 1.5 GRAPHING LOGARITHMIC RELATIONSHIPS

In principle there are two ways to graph a logarithmic relationship such as Equation 1.8. One is to look up the values of the logarithms of the experimental concentration data and graph these logarithms against time on linear coordinate paper. This method is tedious, only slightly less inconvenient than calculating values of $e^{-kt}$, and it is subject to the errors that are likely to occur in reading a number of different values from a table. It is preferable to graph the data directly on semilog paper.

Semilog, or log linear, graph paper is designed with a linear abscissa but an ordinate that is *linear in logarithms*. The paper is scaled in logs to the base 10. It is available in configurations with one to six cycles; each cycle includes values that are 10 times greater than the values in the cycle below it. The result is a marked and accelerating compression of the ordinate scale as the values of the dependent variable increase. Because of this distortion of the ordinate, graphing numbers directly on semilog paper is the equivalent of graphing their logarithms on linear coordinate paper.

Consider the concentration, time data in Table 1.2. They are idealized data that fit Equation 1.8 with $C_0 = 10$ $\mu$g/ml and $k = 0.3$ hr$^{-1}$. Figure 1.3 is a graph of these data on semilog paper with two cycles. Graphing in this

**Table 1.2** $C(t)$, $t$ data generated from the equation $C(t) = C_0 e^{-kt}$ for $C_0 = 10$ $\mu$g/ml and $k = 0.3$ hr$^{-1}$

| $t$ (hr) | $C(t)$ ($\mu$g/ml) |
| --- | --- |
| 0 | 10.00 |
| 1 | 7.41 |
| 2 | 5.49 |
| 3 | 4.06 |
| 4 | 3.01 |
| 5 | 2.23 |
| 6 | 1.65 |
| 7 | 1.22 |
| 8 | 0.91 |
| 9 | 0.67 |
| 10 | 0.50 |

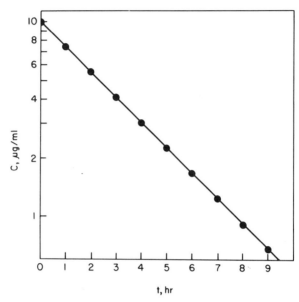

**Figure 1.3**  Semilogarithmic graph of data from Table 1.2.

coordinate system has linearized the entire set of data. The ordinate intercept is 10 $\mu$g/ml, or $C_0$; the slope should be $-k$. Let us verify this point by calculating the slope.

The slope of the line in Figure 1.3, like the slope of any straight line, is

$$\frac{y_2-y_1}{x_2-x_1};$$

in this case,

$$\frac{\ln C_2-\ln C_1}{t_2-t_1},$$

where the points $(t_1, \ln C_1)$ and $(t_2, \ln C_2)$ may be taken anywhere on the line, although of course the farther apart they are, the more accurate the slope estimate will be. Therefore we will take the points $(0, \ln 10)$ and $(10, \ln 0.50)$:

$$\text{slope} = \frac{\ln(0.50)-\ln(10)}{(10-0)\,\text{hr}}$$

$$= \left(\frac{-0.693-2.303}{10}\right)\text{hr}^{-1}$$

$$= -0.3\ \text{hr}^{-1}.$$

The slope of the line is equal to $-k$.

If the experimental range of data should extend over more than one cycle on semilog paper, as the line in Figure 1.3 does, there is a simple shortcut to use in estimating the slope. Remember that each cycle covers values 10 times larger than the values in the cycle below it. Since $\log 10 - \log 1 = \log 100 - \log 10 = \log 1000 - \log 100 = \log(10) = 2.303$, time points can be chosen that correspond to any two concentration values that are one cycle apart. Then

$$\text{slope} = \frac{-2.303}{t_2 - t_1}.$$

For the line in Figure 1.3, take the times corresponding to concentrations 1 $\mu g/ml$ and 10 $\mu g/ml$:

$$\text{slope} = \frac{-2.303}{(7.7-0) \text{ hr}} = -0.3 \text{ hr}^{-1}.$$

We could equally well have chosen any other concentrations separated by one cycle, say 0.5 $\mu g/ml$ and 5 $\mu g/ml$:

$$\text{slope} = \frac{-2.303}{(10-2.3) \text{ hr}} = -0.3 \text{ hr}^{-1}.$$

This shortcut is convenient not only because it is rapid, but also because it circumvents the need for logarithms altogether.


## 1.6 THE DERIVATIVE

It was noted in Section 1.3 that Equations 1.3, 1.5, and 1.7 are differential equations, or equations having derivatives in them. Derivatives express the way in which one variable changes relative to another. When the independent variable is time, the derivative expresses a rate of change. Frequently the rate of a biological process is dependent in some definable way on the concentration or amount of material present. Therefore differential equations are the foundation of kinetics.

If $y = f(x)$, how does $y$ change when $x$ changes a little bit?

First let us consider the simple function $y = 3x$ (Figure 1.4), and construct a table showing what happens to $y$ whenever $x$ changes by one unit (Table 1.3). The value of $y$ changes by 3 units every time $x$ changes by 1 unit; the rate of change of $y$ with respect to $x$ is 3. Note that this is also the slope of the line.

Now consider the slightly more complicated function $y = x + x^2$ (Figure 1.5 and Table 1.4). This time the change in $y$ as $x$ changes by one unit is dependent on the value of $x$. The rate of change of $y$ with respect to $x$ is a function of $x$.

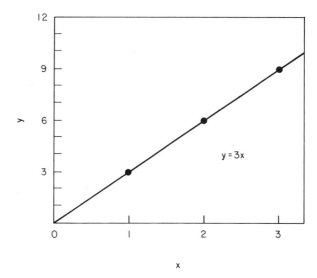

**Figure 1.4**  Graph of the equation $y = 3x$.

Let us look more closely at the quantity $\Delta y/\Delta x = f(x)$. In Figure 1.5 the values of the dependent variable $\Delta y/\Delta x$ are graphed at the corresponding midpoints, $x = 0.5$, 1.5, 2.5, 3.5, and 4.5 units, of the five intervals $\Delta x$. It appears that these five points define a straight line with slope 2 and ordinate intercept 1:

$$\frac{Y_n - Y_{n-1}}{X_n - X_{n-1}} = \frac{\Delta y}{\Delta x} = 1 + 2\frac{X_n + X_{n-1}}{2},$$

or

$$\frac{Y_n - Y_{n-1}}{X_n - X_{n-1}} = \frac{\Delta y}{\Delta x} = 1 + 2\left(X_{n-1} + \frac{\Delta x}{2}\right).$$

The first term on the left is also, by definition, the slope of a straight line through the points $(X_n, Y_n)$ and $(X_{n-1}, Y_{n-1})$. Therefore the function $1 + 2x$,

**Table 1.3**  $\Delta y$, $\Delta x$ Data generated from the equation $y = 3x$

|  | $y$ | $\Delta x$ | $\Delta y$ | $\dfrac{\Delta y}{\Delta x}$ |
|---|---|---|---|---|
| 1 | 3 |  |  |  |
| 2 | 6 | 1 | 3 | 3 |
| 3 | 9 | 1 | 3 | 3 |
| 4 | 12 | 1 | 3 | 3 |
| 5 | 15 | 1 | 3 | 3 |

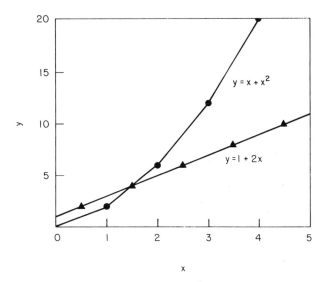

**Figure 1.5** Graphs of the equation $y = x + x^2$ and of its derivative, $y = 1 + 2x$.

when it is evaluated at the midpoint of the interval $(X_n - X_{n-1})$, is equal to the slope of a line drawn through the two points $(X_n, Y_n)$ and $(X_{n-1}, Y_{n-1})$ on the curve $y = x + x^2$.

Now if we choose successively smaller and smaller values of $\Delta x$, then, as $\Delta x$ approaches the infinitesimally small change $dx$, $\Delta y$ will approach the infinitesimally small change $dy$ and $\Delta y / \Delta x$ will approach the limiting value $dy/dx = 1 + 2x$. The relation $dy/dx = 1 + 2x$ is the derivative of the function $y = x + x^2$. Since it is equal to the "slope" of the curve $y = x + x^2$ within the infinitesimally small interval $dx$, it can be visualized as the tangent to the curve at any point $(x, y)$. It is the instantaneous rate of change of $y$ with respect to $x$ at any point $(x, y)$.

We saw in the first example that if $y = f(x)$ is a straight line, the derivative of $f(x)$ is a constant (the rate of change of $y$ with respect to $x$ is independent of the value of $x$). For all other $f(x)$, however, $dy/dx$ is not independent of $x$ and must be evaluated at each point $x$.

**Table 1.4** $\Delta y$, $\Delta x$ Data generated from the equation $y = x + x^2$

| $x$ | $y$ | $\Delta x$ | $\Delta y$ | $\dfrac{\Delta y}{\Delta x}$ |
|---|---|---|---|---|
| 0 | 0 | | | |
| 1 | 2 | 1 | 2 | 2 |
| 2 | 6 | 1 | 4 | 4 |
| 3 | 12 | 1 | 6 | 6 |
| 4 | 20 | 1 | 8 | 8 |
| 5 | 30 | 1 | 10 | 10 |

**Table 1.5** Common integral and derivative forms and rules for their use: $a$ is a constant; $f(x)$ and $g(x)$ are unspecified functions of $x$, and $f'(x)$ and $g'(x)$ are their derivatives

| When $y =$ | then $\dfrac{dy}{dx} =$ | and $\int y\,dx =$ |
|---|---|---|
| *Forms* | | |
| 1  $ax^n$ | $nax^{n-1}$ | $\dfrac{ax^{n+1}}{n+1}$ |
| Special case: $n=1$: $ax$ | $a$ | $\dfrac{ax^2}{2}$ |
| Special case: $n=0$: $a$ | $0$ | $ax$ |
| Special case: $ax^{-n}$ | $-nax^{-n-1}$ | $\dfrac{ax^{-n+1}}{1-n}$ |
| 2  $\ln g(x)$ | $\dfrac{g'(x)}{g(x)}$ | |
| Special case: $g(x)=x$: $\ln x$ | $\dfrac{1}{x}$ | |
| 3  $e^{g(x)}$ | $g'(x)e^{g(x)}$ | $\dfrac{e^{g(x)}}{g'(x)}$ |
| Special case: $g(x)=x$: $e^x$ | $e^x$ | $e^x$ |
| *Rules* | | |
| 1  $f(x)+g(x)$ | $f'(x)+g'(x)$ | $\int f(x)\,dx + \int g(x)\,dx$ |
| 2  $f(x)g(x)$ | $f'(x)g(x)+g'(x)f(x)$ | |
| 3  $af(x)$ | $af'(x)$ | $a\int f(x)\,dx$ |
| *Examples* | | |
| 2 | $0$ | $2x$ |
| $72x$ | $72$ | $36x^2$ |
| $3x^4$ | $12x^3$ | $\dfrac{3x^5}{5}$ |
| $17x^{-3}$ | $-51x^{-4}$ | $-\dfrac{17x^{-2}}{2}$ |
| $\dfrac{1}{x}$ | $-\dfrac{1}{x^2}$ | $\ln x$ |
| $\dfrac{2}{x}$ | $-\dfrac{2}{x^2}$ | $\ln(x^2)=2\ln x$ |
| $\ln(3x^2-4x)$ | $\dfrac{6x-4}{3x^2-4x}$ | |
| $e^{-kx}$ | $-ke^{-kx}$ | $-\dfrac{e^{-kx}}{k}$ |
| $C_0e^{-kx}$ | $-kC_0e^{-kx}$ | $-\dfrac{C_0e^{-kx}}{k}$ |
| $3xe^{-2x^2}$ | $3e^{-2x^2}-12x^2e^{-2x^2}$ $=e^{-2x^2}(3-12x^2)$ | |

Given any function $f(x)$, we could evaluate $\Delta y/\Delta x$ over a range of $x$ values and, with luck, we could use the observed relationship of $\Delta y/\Delta x$ to $x$ to infer the explicit form of the expression for $dy/dx$. This procedure would be both tedious and difficult, particularly since $dy/dx=f(x)$ is by no means always the equation of a straight line. Fortunately there is a body of rules accessible in any elementary calculus textbook that can be used in determining the derivative of a function. Some of these rules are given in Table 1.5. We will use almost exclusively the rule for differentiating the exponential function, which is discussed in Section 1.8.

Occasionally we will find it useful to take advantage of the fact that under certain conditions the rate of a reaction or of a transport process is zero. This means that the derivative of the function that describes the process is zero. The tangent to a curve has the value zero when it is, horizontal; remember that the slope of a horizontal line is zero (Section 1.3 and Table 1.1). Obviously the derivative of the equation of a horizontal straight line is zero. But the derivative of a curve also takes on the value zero at a maximum or a minimum in the curve or as the curve approaches a horizontal asymptote. This particular attribute of the derivative will be exploited in Section 3.10 when we will wish to determine the time at which the concentration of an acutely administered compound is at its maximum in a peripheral tissue.

## 1.7 THE INTEGRAL

Equations 1.4 and 1.8 are the definite integrals of Equations 1.3 and 1.5, respectively. This means that if we differentiate Equations 1.4 and 1.8 we will obtain Equations 1.3 and 1.5.

Integration is the reverse of differentiation. If

$$y=f(x),$$

then

$$\frac{dy}{dx}=f'(x) \qquad \text{and} \qquad dy=f'(x)\,dx,$$

where $f'(x)$ is shorthand for "the derivative of the function $y=f(x)$ with respect to $x$." The quantities $dy$, $dx$, and $f'(x)\,dx$ are *differentials*. We would like to be able to determine the form of $f(x)$ from the form of $f'(x)$; in other words, to integrate the function $f'(x)$. We denote this process by writing

$$\int dy = \int f'(x)\,dx,$$

where $\int dy=y$ and $\int f'(x)\,dx=f(x)$, and the sign "$\int$" symbolizes the process of integration.

Fortunately for the nonmathematician, the process of integration, like the process of differentiation, is expedited by using a table of integrals that provides the integral forms of a variety of commonly occurring differential equations. Some of these forms are given in Table 1.5. Unlike the process of differentiation, however, the process of integration involves an additional step after the indefinite integral has been found in the table. This step is application of the boundary conditions first mentioned in Section 1.3.

The process of differentiation results in a loss of information about the parent curve. For example, the derivative of $y = 3x$ is 3 (Section 1.6). But other straight lines also have slopes of 3: $y = 1 + 3x$, $y = 324 + 3x$, $y = e^6 + 3x$, $y = 17 + 3x$, $y = 2768 + 3x$, and so on. The derivative of each of these lines is 3. In other words, simply knowing the slope of the straight line does not enable us to fix its position in the coordinate system or, more specifically, to fix its ordinate intercept; nor does knowing the tangent to a curve at each point on it permit us to position the curve in two-dimensional space.

Therefore the integral form that is extracted from the table of integrals is called an *indefinite integral*. It is a general solution to the differential equation. The *definite integral* is a particular solution that has been evaluated, or positioned in two-dimensional space, by applying the known *boundary conditions* of measurement.

When a drug is given as a single intravenous injection, for example, its concentration in the blood declines continuously from time $t_0 = 0$, the instant of the injection, at a rate that is dependent on the way in which the drug is eliminated from the body. The maximum concentration, at $t_0$, can be designated $C_0$. Then (Equation 1.3), if the drug is eliminated by a zero-order mechanism (see Section 1.9),

$$\frac{dC}{dt} = f'(t) = -k_0, \quad \text{or} \quad dC = -k_0 dt; \tag{1.3'}$$

then

$$\int dC = \int (-k_0) \, dt.$$

From Table 1.5 we find that $\int dC = C$ and $\int (-k_0) \, dt = -k_0 \int dt = -k_0 t$. Both these quantities must now be evaluated between the particular boundary limits set by the conditions of measurement. In this case we are interested in the behavior of $C$ between $t = 0$, where $C = C_0$, and $t = t$, where $C = C$. Accordingly we write

$$C \Big|_{C_0}^{C} = \, t \Big|_{0}^{} - k_0 t,$$

which means "the integral of $dC$, evaluated from $C = C_0$ to $C = C$, is equal to the integral of $-k_0\,dt$ evaluated from $t=0$ to $t=t$." To evaluate an indefinite integral we apply the general rule

$$\left.f(x)\right|_{x_1}^{x_2}=f(x_2)-f(x_1),$$

so that

$$\left.C\right|_{C_0}^{C}=C-C_0 \quad \text{and} \quad \left.-k_0t\right|_0^t=-k_0t-(-0),$$

or finally

$$C=C_0-k_0t,$$

which is identical to Equation 1.4 in Section 1.3. Note that the negative sign in Equation 1.3 indicates that $C$ decreases with $t$. Equation 1.4 also states that $C$ decreases with $t$, since it represents a straight line with negative slope. $C$ is equal to $C_0$, its maximum value and the ordinate intercept of the straight line, when $t=0$.

Now suppose that the drug is eliminated from the body not by a zero-order mechanism but by a first-order mechanism (Section 1.9). Then (Equation 1.5),

$$\frac{dC}{dt}=f'(t)=-kC, \quad \text{or} \quad \frac{dC}{C}=-k\,dt; \tag{1.5'}$$

then

$$\int \frac{dC}{C} = \int(-k)\,dt.$$

From Table 1.5 we find that $\int dC/C = \ln C$ and $\int(-k)\,dt = -k\int dt = -kt$. Evaluating between the points 0, $C_0$ and $t, C$,

$$\left.\ln C\right|_{C_0}^{C}=\left.-kt\right|_0^t \quad \text{or} \quad \ln C-\ln C_0 = -kt;$$

$$C=C_0e^{-kt},$$

which is identical to Equation 1.8.

In all cases the process of evaluating the indefinite integral for a particular boundary condition involves specification of a point that is known to lie on the curve. Once any single point has been specified, the position of the curve in two-dimensional space is established. In both the examples above the known point was $(0, C_0)$.

The definite integral of a function from $(x_1, y_1)$ to $(x_2, y_2)$ may be visualized as the area under the curve of that function from $(x_1, y_1)$ to $(x_2, y_2)$. For example, the area under the curve $y = 1 + 2x$ from $(0,0)$ to $(x, y)$ (Section 1.6) is made up of a rectangle of area $1x$ and a triangle whose area is $\frac{1}{2}[x(y-1)]$. Therefore (area under $y = 1 + 2x) = x + \frac{1}{2}[x(y-1)]$. But $y = 1 + 2x$, so that $y - 1 = 2x$, and (area under $y = 1 + 2x) = x + \frac{1}{2}(2x^2) = x + x^2$, the equation for the parent curve used as an example in Section 1.6.

This relationship is particularly useful because under some conditions it allows total dose to be related to concentration, as the following section shows.

### 1.8   DIFFERENTIATING AND INTEGRATING THE EXPONENTIAL FUNCTION

Table 1.5 shows that differentiating and integrating the exponential function is straightforward and even especially easy. In fact, the simplest form of the exponential function $e^x$ is its own derivative; that is, it is unchanged on differentiation because $dx/dx = 1$. When the exponent is a function of $x$ other than $x$ itself, the processes become only slightly more complicated:

$$\frac{de^{f(x)}}{dx} = f'(x)e^{f(x)} \quad \text{and} \quad \int e^{f(x)}\,dx = \frac{e^{f(x)}}{f'(x)}.$$

This interesting property of the exponential function makes it particularly easy to manipulate and often facilitates the reduction of differential equations to conveniently simple forms. For example, if

$$C = C_0 e^{-kt}, \quad \text{then} \quad \frac{dC}{dt} = -kC_0 e^{-kt} = -kC.$$

Integration is equally easy. The following example has been selected not only to illustrate this point but also to demonstrate an application of the concept that the definite integral of a function is equal to the corresponding area under the function. The plasma concentration of a compound administered orally and eliminated by a first-order mechanism (Section 1.9) is given as a function of time by

$$C = \frac{aD}{V(a-b)}(e^{-bt} - e^{-at}) \tag{1.9}$$

where $a$ and $b$ are constants, $V$ is the volume within which the compound is distributed, and $D$ is the internal dose or the amount of the compound that was actually absorbed into the systemic circulation. We can use the area under an experimental plasma concentration, time curve to determine $D$.

Integrating Equation 1.9,

$$\int_{t=0}^{t=\infty} C\,dt = \frac{aD}{V(a-b)} \int_{t=0}^{t=\infty} (e^{-bt} - e^{-at})\,dt = \frac{aD}{V(a-b)}\Big|_{t=0}^{t=\infty} \frac{e^{-at}}{a} - \frac{e^{-bt}}{b}$$

$$= \frac{aD}{V(a-b)}\left(\frac{1}{b} - \frac{1}{a}\right) = \frac{aD}{V(a-b)}\,\frac{a-b}{ab} = \frac{D}{bV},$$

$$D = bV \int_{t=0}^{t=\infty} C\,dt.$$

Since $b$, $V$, and the area under the curve are all experimentally determinable quantities, $D$ may be estimated.

The area under the curve and its applications are discussed further in Section 3.12.

## 1.9  DEFINITIONS USED IN KINETICS

The several basic concepts and definitions that are fundamental to all kinetics are given here. Other definitions are given as needed in the appropriate chapters.

During the course of its passage through the body, a compound is *absorbed, distributed,* and *eliminated.* Distribution and elimination occur in parallel during at least a part of this time. Elimination consists of *metabolism, excretion,* or both occurring simultaneously.

Distribution takes place from a *central* compartment, of which the blood plasma is presumed to be a part, into one or more peripheral compartments. A kinetic *compartment* is the volume into, through, and out of which a given material moves with a particular degree of ease. It may or may not correspond to a physiological tissue or fluid volume; it may include functionally disparate tissues.

*Rate constants*, determined experimentally, relate the observed rate of a kinetic process to the variable, frequently concentration, that controls that process. Rate constants are microscopic rate constants, or *microconstants*, when they refer to a single clearly definable step, such as transformation by metabolism or excretion into the urine. Observed rate constants are nearly always combinations of microscopic rate constants.

A process is *first order* if the differential equation that describes it is of the form

$$\frac{dx}{dt} = kx^n$$

where $n = 1$. It is zero order when $n = 0$, in which case

$$\frac{dx}{dt} = k.$$

An overall first-order process is *linear*. A process that is zero order, or is a combination of first-order and zero-order steps proceeding simultaneously, is *nonlinear*. It is worthwhile to note that the terms "linear" and "first order" as they are used by kineticists are different from the same terms as they are used by mathematicians.

## 1.10   DIMENSIONALITY OF EQUATIONS

Dimensionality can be a very powerful tool. An equation expresses identity: identity of dimensions as well as identity of numerical values. The dimensions of an equation are independent of the numerical values of the independent and dependent variables and of any constants; an equation can be numerically correct but dimensionally incorrect, and vice versa.

For an equation to be dimensionally correct, its dimensions must meet two criteria: validity and consistency. For example, the equation

$$6 \text{ items} + 15 \text{ items} = 21 \text{ items} \tag{1.10}$$

is both numerically and dimensionally correct. But now consider another form of Equation 1.10 in which the kinds of items, or the units of measurement, are specified:

$$6 \text{ rats} + 15 \text{ mice} = 21 \text{ potatoes}. \tag{1.11}$$

Equation 1.11 is numerically correct but dimensionally incorrect because although dimensionally valid, it is dimensionally inconsistent. In fact it is absurd. Rats and mice cannot be added, at least not as long as they are distinguished from each other in this way; and neither of them is a potato. Once the unit of measurement of the dimension "item" has been specified, the unit must be used consistently. Three different units were used in Equation 1.11. One way to return Equation 1.11 to a dimensionally correct form would be to forget the potatoes entirely and write

$$6 \text{ laboratory animals} + 15 \text{ laboratory animals} = 21 \text{ laboratory animals}. \tag{1.12}$$

The criterion of dimensional validity can be a convenient and useful check on the validity of the form of a newly derived theoretical equation. Although students of kinetics will have little opportunity to use dimensional analysis in this way, it would be a useful discipline for readers of this book to confirm for their own satisfaction the dimensional validity of all equations presented.

The criterion of dimensional consistency will be, or at any rate should be, used frequently. The student will find it indispensable in working problems. To ensure that the correct answer is obtained, careful attention must be paid to the dimensions of the equations used in calculation. There are four basic rules of dimensional analysis:

**1** Quantities to be added to or subtracted from one another must have the same dimensions; their sum or difference will also have these dimensions.
**2** When quantities are multiplied or divided, their dimensions are also multiplied or divided.
**3** Dimensions on both sides of an equation must be the same.
**4** Logarithms have no dimensions.

Equation 1.12 is an example of the application of Rules 1 and 3. As an illustration of Rule 2, suppose that we want to house our rats and mice in standard cages that are designed to hold either two rats or five mice. How many cages will we need?

$$\frac{6 \text{ rats}}{2 \text{ rats/cage}} + \frac{15 \text{ mice}}{5 \text{ mice/cage}} = 3 \text{ cages} + 3 \text{ cages}. \qquad (1.13)$$

Since the cages are identical, the quantities may be added; we need six standard cages.

But suppose that instead of standard identical cages we have two kinds of cage: one designed for rats and the other for mice. Now the simple unit "cage" is misleading, since it suggests that there is no need to distinguish between rat cages and mouse cages, whereas in fact we must make this distinction. Equation 1.13 must be written

$$\frac{6 \text{ rats}}{2 \text{ rats/rat cage}} + \frac{15 \text{ mice}}{5 \text{ mice/mouse cage}} = 3 \text{ rat cages} + 3 \text{ mouse cages}. \quad (1.14)$$

Since the cages are not identical, these quantities may not be combined.

This deceptively simple example illustrates a common pitfall in working with dimensions: inaccurate or incomplete labeling of quantities. This problem can become acute when the researcher wishes to relate observations made on partial samples in such a way as to express an attribute of the whole sample. For example, suppose that the specific activity of an enzyme preparation is defined as

$$SA = \frac{\text{rate of substrate disappearance}}{\text{mass of protein}}.$$

Choosing the units $\mu$mole/min to express rate of disappearance of substrate and mg to represent protein mass, we can combine measurements of rate and quantity to obtain an estimate of *SA*. But, on second thought, can we? Was measurement of rate made using a sample of the same size and makeup as that used for measurement of protein content? *For calculation purposes only*, it would be preferable to write

$$SA = \frac{\text{rate of substrate disappearance catalyzed by a 10-}\mu\text{l aliquot of liver microsomal preparation}}{\text{quantity of protein contained in a 10-}\mu\text{l aliquot of liver microsomal preparation}},$$

thereby minimizing the likelihood of a scaling error in translation of the actual experimental observations to a statement about the value of *SA*.

The fundamental dimensions used in kinetics are mass, length, and time. Concentration is mass per unit of volume where volume is expressed as length$^3$. Units are likely to be micrograms ($\mu$g), milligrams (mg), microliters ($\mu$l), liters (l), minutes (min), hours (hr), and days. While working the problems in this book, the student should become facile at substituting minutes for hours, $\mu$g/ml for mg/ml, and so on, to achieve dimensional consistency. The simple but realistic kinetics problems that follow are examples of the technique.

*Example 1*   The equation for concentration decline in a single compartment when the elimination process is saturated is

$$\frac{D}{V} - C = kt,$$

where $D$ is the amount present initially, $V$ is the volume of the compartment, $k$ is a constant, and $t$ is time. If we are given the information that $D = 0.5$ g, $V = 50$ liters and $k = 0.03$ $\mu$g/ml/min, what is the predicted value of $C$ after 1 hr, when $t = 1$? Plugging values directly into the equation, we obtain

$$\left(\frac{0.5}{50}\right)\left(\frac{g}{1}\right) - C = (0.03)(1)\frac{\text{hr}\,\mu\text{g}}{\text{min}\,\text{ml}}.$$

Dimensionally this equation does not balance. Since [g/l] represents concentration and only like quantities can be subtracted, $C$ must be expressed in concentration units also. Since dimensions on both sides of an equation must be the same, our first step will be to eliminate the dimension (time) on the right-hand side of the equation. To do this we substitute the equality

$$1 \text{ hr} = 60 \text{ min,} \qquad \text{or hr/min} = 60:$$

$$0.01 \text{ g/liter} - C = (0.03)(1)(60)(\mu\text{g/ml})$$

This form is an improvement, but the equation still is not dimensionally consistent. Since

$$1 \text{ g/l} = 1000 \text{ mg/l} = 1000 \text{ } \mu\text{g/ml}, \qquad 0.01 \text{ g/l} = 10 \text{ } \mu\text{g/ml},$$

and

$$C = (10)(\mu\text{g/ml}) - (0.03)(1)(60)(\mu\text{g/ml}) = 8.2 \text{ } \mu\text{g/ml}.$$

**Example 2** The equation for the maximum concentration of a compound attained in the plasma after a very large number of equally spaced intravenous doses is (Section 5.2)

$$C_{max} = \frac{C_1}{1 - e^{-k \Delta t}},$$

where $C_1$ is the maximum concentration after the first dose, $k$ is a rate constant, and $\Delta t$ is the time interval between doses. Suppose that $\Delta t = 1$ day, $C_1 = 2$ $\mu$g/ml, and $k = 0.058$ hr$^{-1}$. What is $C_{max}$?

Rule 4 states that logarithms have no dimensions. This statement represents both an attribute of logarithms and a useful tool in dimensional analysis. Since the definition of a logarithm is

$$\ln x = a \qquad \text{if} \quad e^a = x,$$

it follows directly that all exponents must also be dimensionless, whatever their numerical value.

To work this problem, it is necessary to know that exponents can have no dimensions. Substitution of the equality 24 hr = 1 day, or days/hr = 24, eliminates all dimensions from the exponent:

$$C_{max} = \frac{2 \text{ } \mu\text{g/ml}}{1 - e^{-(.058 \text{ hr}^{-1})(1 \text{ day})(24 \text{ hr/day})}}$$

$$= \frac{2 \text{ } \mu\text{g/ml}}{1 - e^{-1.392}}.$$

Values of $e^x$ or $e^{-x}$ for a given value of $x$, like values of $\ln x$, can be obtained either from a pocket calculator or from a table of exponentials. The value of $e^{-1.392}$ is 0.248, so that

$$C_{max} = \frac{2 \text{ } \mu\text{g/ml}}{1 - 0.248} = \frac{2}{0.752} \frac{\mu\text{g}}{\text{ml}} = 2.66 \text{ } \mu\text{g/ml}.$$

The foregoing is a brief introduction to the uses of dimensions and units of measurement as they are required in this book. The reader who is interested in a more detailed discussion of the complexities of dimensional analysis is referred to an excellent chapter in the text by Riggs (1972).

## 1.11  RECOGNITION OF KINETIC FORMS BY INSPECTION

A number of forms occur so regularly in kinetic equations that it is useful to be able to recognize them by inspection. Some of them have already been introduced in this chapter.

The form

$$B = B_0 e^{-kt}$$

is a *decaying exponential*. It represents loss from a single compartment, or dieaway from the maximum achieved at the instant of introduction of an amount $B_0$. Its general shape is shown in Figure 1.6a.

The form

$$B = A e^{-k_1 t} + C e^{-k_2 t}$$

is the sum of two decaying exponentials. It represents net loss from the central compartment of a two-compartment model after instantaneous introduction into the central compartment. It is often found to be an adequate description of the behavior of an acutely administered compound in the human body. Its general shape is shown in Figure 1.6b.

$$U = U_\infty (1 - e^{-kt})$$

is an *inverted exponential*. It describes the cumulation of material being excreted via a single pathway, $U$ in this case designating the urine. Its shape is shown in Figure 1.6c.

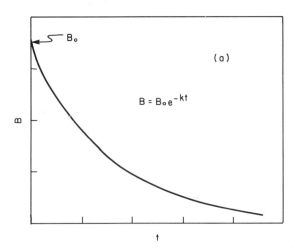

**Figure 1.6**  Graphs of common kinetic forms. (a) $B = B_0 e^{-kt}$. (b) $B = A e^{-k_1 t} + C e^{-k_2 t}$. (c) $U = U_\infty (1 - e^{-kt})$. (d) $B = A(e^{-k_e t} - e^{-k_a t})$.

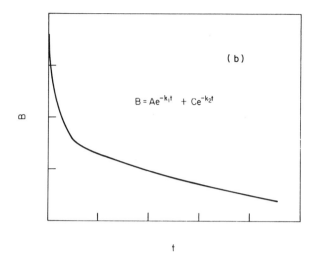

**Figure 1.6** (*continued*)

The form

$$B = A(e^{-k_e t} - e^{-k_a t})$$

represents absorption into and elimination from a single compartment by first-order processes, from a single depot. Its form is shown in Figure 1.6*d*. It is often used to describe the behavior of a compound administered orally or absorbed from a deposit on the surface of the skin, and eliminated by a first-order process.

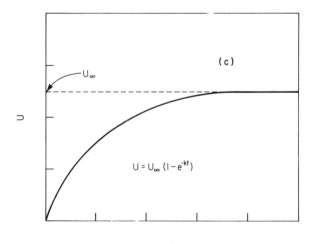

**Figure 1.6** (*continued*)

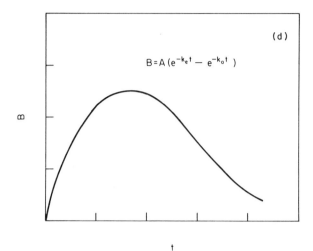

(d)

$$B = A(e^{-k_e t} - e^{-k_o t})$$

**Figure 1.6**  (*continued*)

These four forms, and combinations of them, are encountered regularly throughout this book. The reader would do well to practice recognition of form by inspection of the equation. Before any problem in this book is worked, it is important to ask, and answer, the question, "Is this equation of the proper form to describe the type of concentration behavior I expect in this system?"

### PROBLEMS

**1**  Given the equation

$$\frac{dC}{dt} = v(C) = \frac{V_m C}{K_m + C},$$

can you derive the two linear transforms that are distinct from the Lineweaver-Burk transform (Section 1.3)?

**2**  If $k_0 = 1.32$ $\mu$mole/l/min, $C_0 = 9.82$ nmole/ml, $k = 0.144$ min$^{-1}$, $k_t = 0.322$ $\mu$g/ml/min, $V_m = 1$ $\mu$mole/min and $K_m = 6 \times 10^{-3}$ mole/l, graph each of the following equations on appropriate axes in such a way as to give a straight line:

**(a)**  $\dfrac{dC}{dt} = k_0$

**(b)**  $C = C_0 - k_0 t$

**(c)**  $C = C_0 e^{-kt}$

**(d)**  $y = \dfrac{x^2}{k_t} - \dfrac{x}{2}$

If the dimensions of $y$ are $(\mu g)(min)(ml^{-1})$, what are the dimensions of $x$? What are the dimensions of the constant 2?

(e) $\dfrac{V_m C}{K_m + C} = v$

What are the dimensions of $v$?

3 Express each of the following relationships in terms of logarithms to the base $e$.

(a) $y = 3x^2$

(b) $y = \dfrac{5x\sqrt{3x}}{2}$

(c) $y = \dfrac{5x\sqrt{3x^2 - 4z}}{3z}$

(d) $C = C_0 e^{-kt}$

(e) $U = U_\infty(1 - e^{-k_e t})$

(f) $\dfrac{dU}{dt} = k_e C_0 e^{-k_e t}$

(g) $b = \dfrac{D_0 k_a}{V_f(k_e - k_a)}(e^{-k_a t} - e^{-k_e t})$

4 Express each of the relationships in Problem 3 in terms of logarithms to the base 10.

5 Can equations **e**, **f**, and **g** in Problem 3 be graphed so as to give a straight line? How? In answering this question, assume that the values of the rate constants $k_a$ and $k_e$ are not known and that the other quantities are measurable.

6 An expression that relates $v$, the velocity of an enzyme catalyzed reaction (note that $v$ is $dC/dt$), to the substrate concentration is $v = V_m C/(K_m + C)$. In an enzyme kinetic study the rates shown in Table 1.6 were measured.

**Table 1.6** The initial velocity of an enzyme reaction as a function of substrate concentration $C$

| $C(\mu \text{ mole}/l)$ | $v(\text{nmole}/\text{min})$ |
| --- | --- |
| 10 | 2.22 |
| 20 | 3.46 |
| 30 | 4.26 |
| 40 | 4.54 |
| 60 | 5.21 |
| 80 | 5.61 |
| 100 | 5.93 |

Graph these data in an appropriate linear form and estimate $V_m$, the maximum velocity of the catalyzed reaction at this enzyme concentration, and $K_m$, the Michaelis constant. Watch the dimensions of these constants!

7   The polysaccharide inulin is sometimes used to determine extracellular fluid volume (see Section 3.4). It is eliminated from the plasma in accordance with the first-order equation $C = C_0 e^{-k_e t}$, where $C$ is the concentration in the plasma at time $t$ and $C_0$ is the plasma concentration at time $t = 0$. $^3$H-Meoxyinulin was given intravenously to a 275-g rat and the plasma $^3$H concentration was measured at convenient intervals during the elimination phase. The results are given in Table 1.7. Graph these data appropriately and from your graph estimate $k_e$, the rate constant for elimination of inulin from the plasma.

**Table 1.7**   Plasma concentrations of $^3$H (cpm = counts per minute) after intravenous administration of $^3$H-methoxyinulin to a 275-g rat

| $t$ (min) | $^3$H Concentration (cpm/ml) |
|---|---|
| 0 | 23,575 |
| 13 | 17,070 |
| 22 | 18,420 |
| 37 | 11,795 |
| 50 | 11,710 |
| 60 | 9,390 |
| 71 | 8,610 |
| 84 | 6,150 |
| 92 | 4,960 |
| 101 | 5,810 |
| 113 | 4,290 |

## REFERENCES

Riggs, D. S. *The Mathematical Approach to Physiological Problems*, M.I.T. Press, Cambridge, Mass., 1973, Chapter 2, "Dimensions and Units, pp. 18–40.

# 2

## Saturable Systems

**2.1** Definition

**2.2** Historical development

**2.3** Kinetic behavior of a saturable system: Carrier-mediated transport

**2.4** The hyperbola and what determines its shape

**2.5** Estimation of $K_t$ and $T_m$ from experimental data

    2.5.1 Estimation by inspection

    2.5.2 Estimation from a linear transform

**2.6** Inhibition of a saturable system

    2.6.1 Competitive inhibition

    2.6.2 Noncompetitive inhibition

**2.7** The distinction between facilitated and active transport

**2.8** Examples illustrating the principles developed in this chapter

    2.8.1 Facilitated diffusion

    2.8.2 Active transport

    2.8.3 Saturable pinocytosis

    2.8.4 Enzyme catalysis

In a sense it is entering the discipline of kinetics by the back door to consider saturable processes first. Simple first-order processes are much more straightforward. But somewhere in every simple first-order model lurks at least one step that is potentially saturable. Its saturation, under the appropriate concentration conditions, will perturb the real system and cause it to deviate in one way or another from first-order behavior. Therefore, it is important to understand at the outset the kinetic behavior of capacity-limited processes and the consequences of their saturation.

There is a second reason for considering saturable processes first. A saturable process is a single unambiguously definable physical or biochemical step: the translocation of glucose across the erythrocyte membrane, for example, or the hydrolysis of cholesteryl oleate by cholesterol esterase. In such a relatively simple system the correspondence between the mechanism of action and the mathematical model that describes the behavior of that mechanism and translates it into a useful language is not difficult either to understand or to accept. Often the relationship of a more complex kinetic model to the individual mechanisms of which it is composed is obscured by the form and perhaps by the complexity of its mathematical expression. Such an expression may appear to have no basis in physiological reality. Its kinetic parameters, although they have the dimensions of rate constants and volumes, usually do not represent physiological volumes or the rate constants for individual processes. The expression may even appear to ignore summarily some activity that is known to be physiologically important but is not kinetically significant.

It is often difficult for the beginning student of kinetics to recognize that the mathematical representation of the kinetics of a complex system is a logical development based on reasonable assumptions about the kinetic nature of each of the individual processes making up the system. Accordingly, it is advisable to build an understanding of complex multiunit kinetic systems on a foundation of understanding of the kinetic behavior of single units. We begin by addressing the kinetics of saturable processes.

## 2.1 DEFINITION

Any process that requires that more than one component combine is potentially saturable or capacity limited.

Suppose that

$$A + B \underset{k_2}{\overset{k_1}{\rightleftharpoons}} AB \overset{k_3}{\rightarrow} products$$

Component B may be an enzyme, a nonenzymic protein adsorption site, a receptor site, a carrier transport molecule, or, simply, any reactive molecule; A is another molecule that combines with B to form a definable (although not necessarily physically isolatable) complex AB. AB is capable of breaking down either to regenerate A and B or to release the products of the reaction, whose character need not be specified. The rates at which AB will break down in these different directions are determined by the magnitudes of the rate constants $k_2$ and $k_3$, just as the rate of formation of AB depends on the rate constant $k_1$. At steady state the rate of formation of AB is exactly equal to its overall rate of breakdown. The application of this observation is considered in Section 2.3.

Whenever the amount of B is much smaller than the amount of A so that all B is combined with A, the amount of B is rate limiting and the rate of appearance of products will not increase even when the amount of A is increased. The system is said to be saturated with A.

Of course in principle there is nothing to prevent A from being saturated with B, and in a simple chemical reaction it is quite reasonable that either reactant can be rate limiting. But in most biological systems the concentration of one of the reactants can vary only over a very narrow range. The existence of maximum rates in biological systems is intuitively reasonable because it requires simply that there be a limited number of adsorption or receptor sites, or enzyme or carrier molecule binding sites. The number of such sites ordinarily does not vary widely. For example, the number of cadmium-binding sites in the kidney increases rapidly in response to cadmium exposure; but the maximum capacity of cadmium-binding protein in the kidney of the adult human is about 200 $\mu$g of cadmium per gram of kidney tissue, and the total amount of cadmium presented to the kidney following high level acute or long-term exposure is frequently in excess of the amount that can be accommodated by cadmium-binding protein. Hepatic microsomal mixed function oxidases are inducible by many of the drugs they metabolize; yet at least two such drugs, diphenylhydantoin and phenylbutazone, display elimination characteristics suggesting that the maximum capacity of the metabolizing enzyme system is still exceeded. Finally, perhaps the best known example of a compound displaying zero-order or capacity-limited elimination kinetics is ethanol, a powerful inducer of its own metabolism.

## 2.2 HISTORICAL DEVELOPMENT

The concept of a saturable process originated late in the nineteenth century with the idea that a substrate molecule might combine in some way with a molecule of enzyme. Quantitative studies of the hydrolysis of disaccharides by a variety of enzymes, such as yeast invertase and maltases and lactases from various sources, were initiated at about the same time. The results of these studies showed that as long as sugar was present in excess, the rate of its hydrolysis was independent of its concentration. It was recognized that in view of the relatively small quantity of enzyme present in a biological system, the requisite existence of an enzyme-substrate complex would impose a maximum on the reaction rate, and Brown (1902) outlined a new concept of enzyme action and applied it to laboratory data.

Mathematical formulation of the concept followed quickly. It was first published by Henri (1904), and 9 years later by Michaelis and Menten (1913). A more rigorous derivation, which gives an equation of the same general form, was subsequently developed and published by Briggs and Haldane (1925). It was not until 1937 that an enzyme-substrate complex was actually isolated and identified: the peroxide–horseradish peroxidase complex (Keilin and Mann, 1937).

Curiously, despite the relative sophistication of the art of enzyme kinetics by the 1930s, generalization of its fundamental concepts to other fields was slow. The peculiar concentration dependence of glucose uptake by the human erythrocyte had been a source of considerable experimental controversy for a number of years. Early studies of glucose uptake were performed by exposing erythrocytes to solutions containing different concentrations of glucose. As glucose diffused into the erythrocyte, water was expected to follow, to maintain an osmotic equilibrium across the cell membrane, If glucose transport were proportional to glucose concentration, the degree of erythrocyte swelling would be independent of the glucose concentration in the medium. Masing (1912), however, observed that when a glucose solution isosmotic with serum was added to human blood, erythrocyte swelling was limited and very slow, whereas at lower (physiologic) glucose concentrations the erythrocytes swelled rapidly and massively to the point of lysis. In two important articles, Ege (1920, 1921) proposed that this concentration dependence, as well as an observed species dependence of glucose uptake by erythrocytes, could be explained if each molecule of glucose were said to be bound or adsorbed to a specific site on the cell membrane. Little notice was taken of these papers, however; in 1935 Klinghoffer was still repeating the earlier studies of Ege and confirming the concentration dependence of sugar uptake by erythrocytes. Klinghoffer attributed concentration dependence to a "relative impermeability" or shutdown of the membrane, which was in some way related to an excessive level of glucose. In 1948 LeFevre proposed that a carrier mechanism might be responsible, and within the next few years Wilbrandt and Rosenberg (1951, 1956) and Widdas (1952, 1953) had published mathematical formulations of an active transport theory that Wilbrandt and Rosenberg termed "enzymic transport" by analogy with enzyme catalysis (1951). During the 1950s the theory was developed, confirmed, and applied to sugar transport in a number of laboratories (LeFevre, 1954; Wilbrandt et al., 1956; Wilbrandt and Rosenberg, 1961) and to amino acid transport largely by Christensen and his co-workers (Christensen, 1960). A brief review of trends in membrane transport research has been published (Wilbrandt, 1975).

## 2.3 KINETIC BEHAVIOR OF A SATURABLE SYSTEM: CARRIER–MEDIATED TRANSPORT

The two kinds of saturable biological mechanism commonly encountered are enzyme-mediated metabolism and carrier-mediated transmembrane transport. Note, however, that any group of binding sites or any volume can in principle be filled or saturated. Although sequestration is neither a transport nor an elimination mechanism, its saturation also alters observed kinetic behavior. Saturation of storage or sequestration sites is discussed in Chapter 4.

Since many readers probably are already familiar, if only superficially, with the Michaelis-Menten equation that describes the transformation of a single substrate by a single enzyme, it will be more illuminating to employ in this discussion the terminology of a different mechanism: carrier-mediated transport, the translocation of a substrate molecule by a carrier molecule. Kinetically the two mechanisms are exactly analogous. Indeed, a similar development is possible for any system within which one "reactant" (the term is used in a very general sense) is rate limiting. It is important to keep this point in mind at all times, and not to be diverted by the specificity of the terminology used in this chapter. To promote generality of thinking, examples of the principles developed are taken from the literature of both fields.

The cell membrane is composed of lipids and proteins. Essentially it consists of a bimolecular layer of phospholipid molecules aligned side by side, with their polar hydrophilic portions forming the relatively rigid membrane surfaces and their flexible hydrocarbon tails extending inward to form the rather fluid membrane interior. Globular proteins are embedded, to all appearances randomly, in this lipid bilayer. Contrary to earlier belief, membrane proteins are not simply structural but possess specific enzymic or transport functions. The quality and quantity of lipids and proteins in membranes of cells having different functions vary considerably, but all cell membranes conform to the basic fluid mosaic model outlined above (Fox, 1972).

There are two broad classes of membrane translocation: passive diffusion and carrier-mediated transport. A third mechanism of entry into the cell, pinocytosis, is saturable under some conditions.

Because of the nonpolar nature of the interior of the membrane, hydrophobic or lipid-soluble molecules of reasonable size can diffuse freely through the membrane down a concentration gradient. Passive diffusion is considered in Chapter 3. Water-soluble and very large molecules, however, are excluded from the membrane interior and must be translocated by specialized transport mechanisms. Macromolecules such as proteins enter the cell by pinocytosis, in which an invagination of the cell membrane first surrounds the macromolecule, then detaches itself, forming a vesicle that moves into the cell interior while the cell membrane closes. If the macromolecule must bind to a specific site on the cell membrane before invagination can occur, pinocytosis is saturable. An example of saturable pinocytosis is considered below. Kinetically pinocytosis is indistinguishable from carrier-mediated transport.

Carrier-mediated transport may be either facilitated diffusion or active transport; both mechanisms are included in the development given here. In a carrier-mediated translocation a complex is first formed at the membrane surface between the carrier molecule, B in the mechanism of Section 2.1, and the molecule to be transported, A. As a result of this association, A moves across the membrane and is discharged at the opposite membrane face.

Many membrane proteins surface at only one of the two membrane faces. However, all the membrane transport proteins that have been studied in any detail have been found to span the membrane. Until recently it was thought that transport proteins could rotate through the membrane, carrying the bound solute to the other membrane face. However, experimental evidence now available suggests that, instead of rotation, transport proteins undergo a conformational change associated with solute binding, which facilitates or promotes passage of the solute across the membrane (Guidotti, 1976). In the case of $Na^+$-$K^+$-ATPase, for example, there is evidence for the alternating appearance of two channel forms, one traversable only by sodium ion outward and the other only by potassium ion inward (Kyte, 1975).

To develop the equation that describes this process, we must first restate the description of the process in the form of five mathematically useful assumptions:

1. A complex is formed at one membrane surface between the molecule to be transported, A, and its carrier molecule B. For simplicity we will assume that there is only one molecule of A, but this is not a necessary restriction.

2. At the opposite surface of the membrane the complex dissociates to release A and return B to its former state.

3. The total amount of carrier molecule B does not change: $B_{total} = B + AB$. This restriction says that B is in a steady state; it is called a conservation equation, since it expresses the conservation of carrier molecules.

4. The amount of A in transit at any time, $A_2$, is insignificant compared with that waiting to be transported, $A_1$. This is a restatement of the requirement that A is much greater than B; that is, that B is rate limiting. If $B \ll A_1$, the amount of A bound to B, $A_2$, must also be much smaller than $A_1$. Note that we have not assumed that $A_1$ is constant, only that $A_1 \approx A_{total}$. Clearly $A_1$ is constantly decreasing.

5. An approximate steady state exists within the membrane with regard to the amount of AB. In other words, the number of B molecules occupied by A molecules is constant, or $d(AB)/dt = 0$.

Now the rate of change of the quantity of complex AB with time (Assumptions 1 and 2) is

$$\frac{d(AB)}{dt} = k_1(A_1)(B) - (k_2 + k_3)(AB). \qquad (2.1)$$

But (Assumption 5)

$$\frac{d(AB)}{dt} = 0,$$

so that

$$k_1(A_1)(B) = (k_2 + k_3)(AB),$$

and (Assumptions 3 and 4)

$$B = B_{total} - AB \qquad \text{and} \qquad A_1 \approx A_{total},$$

so that

$$k_1(A_{total})(B_{total} - AB) = (k_2 + k_3)(AB). \qquad (2.2)$$

Multiplying out the left-hand side of Equation 2.2 and collecting terms in AB, we have

$$(AB)\left[(k_2 + k_3) + k_1(A_{total})\right] = k_1(A_{total})(B_{total});$$

$$(AB) = \frac{(A_{total})(B_{total})}{\left[(k_2 + k_3)/k_1\right] + A_{total}}.$$

Define the quantity $(k_2 + k_3)/k_1$ as $K_t$, the transport constant. ($K_t$ has the dimensions of a dissociation constant, or [conc]. This is so because $k_2$ and $k_3$ are both first-order rate constants with dimensions [time$^{-1}$], whereas $k_1$ is a second-order rate constant with dimensions [conc$^{-1}$][time$^{-1}$].) Then

$$(AB) = \frac{(A_{total})(B_{total})}{K_t + A_{total}}. \qquad (2.3)$$

But we are interested in the transport rate, not in the concentration of complex AB. The transport rate is the velocity or rate at which A is discharged from the far side of the membrane, or

$$v = k_3(AB) = \frac{k_3(A_{total})(B_{total})}{K_t + A_{total}}.$$

But $k_3(B_{total})$ is the maximum possible transport rate $T_m$. It is the rate that would be achieved if all available carrier molecules B were occupied by molecules of A. Therefore

$$v = \frac{T_m A_{total}}{K_t + A_{total}}. \qquad (2.4)$$

It is interesting to compare the Michaelis-Menten and the Briggs-Haldane approaches to this expression. Michaelis and Menten defined $K_t$ as the dissociation constant of the complex AB. In other words, they assumed that AB is in true equilibrium with respect to the concentrations of free A and free B, so that $K_t = k_2/k_1$; $k_3$ was assumed to be not only rate determining but also negligible relative to $k_2$. Briggs and Haldane, on the other hand, simply assumed that during most of the course of the process AB is in a steady state. Although $k_3$ is still rate determining, it need not necessarily be negligible relative to $k_2$. Therefore $K_t$ is not truly a dissociation constant, although its reciprocal, while not truly an affinity constant, is often used to suggest the degree of affinity of A for B. Its real significance is made clearer in the next section.

## 2.4  THE HYPERBOLA AND WHAT DETERMINES ITS SHAPE

Equation 2.4 is the equation of a hyperbola, the general shape of which is shown in Figure 2.1$a$. Intuitively the hyperbolic relationship is reasonable. At very low $A_{total}$ the transport rate should be dependent on $A_{total}$ (first-order behavior) but at very high $A_{total}$, $B_{total}$ is saturated and the transport rate becomes independent of $A_{total}$ (zero-order behavior). Figure 2.1$b$ demonstrates that transport rate is indeed hyperbolically related to the concentration of the material being translocated.

The hyperbolic nature of the relationship between $A_{total}$ and $v$ follows directly from Assumptions 1, 2, 4, and 5. If any one of these restrictions is relaxed, the curve generated will not be a hyperbola. However, other changes may be made in the model without altering the hyperbolic form of the relationship. $B_{total}$ need not be constant. More than one molecule of A may combine with a single carrier molecule. There might also be more than one kind of carrier, or the participation of a third molecule in the transport process (intestinal transport of sodium ions, e.g., is closely associated with the absorption of amino acids and sugar). There may also be interference by inhibitors. In general, the impact of such changes is on either $K_t$ or $T_m$ or on both; and $K_t$ and $T_m$ fix the shape of the hyperbola. Let us see why this is so.

When $A_{total}$ is very large, so that $A_{total} \gg K_t$, $v \approx T_m$.
When $A_{total} = K_t$, $v = T_m/2$.

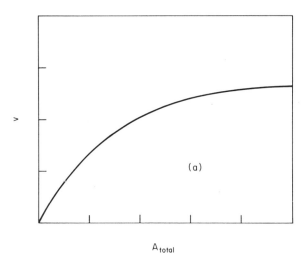

**Figure 2.1**  The dependence of initial velocity of a saturable mechanism on the amount of substrate present. ($a$) Predicted. ($b$) Observed uptake of 5-hydroxytryptamine (5-HT) by the myenteric plexus of the guinea pig small intestine. Values obtained at 37°C are corrected for a slight passive diffusion measurable at 0°C, at which temperature the carrier-mediated mechanism is not able to function. ($b$) Adapted with permission from Gershon and Altman, 1971, Figure 6, © 1971 by the Williams & Wilkins Co., Baltimore.

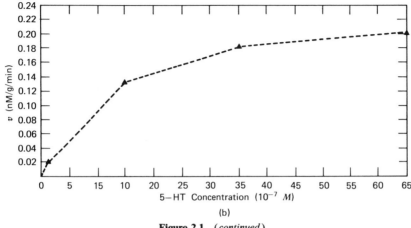

**Figure 2.1** (*continued*)

Therefore $T_m$ fixes the maximum height to which the hyperbola will rise and $K_t$ fixes the concentration range within which the curve will approach this maximum, as shown in Figure 2.2. Since $K_t$ represents the concentration of A at which the transport rate is half its maximum value, it also represents the concentration of A at which half the carrier molecules are occupied. $K_t$ is sometimes called the half-saturation value. It is a useful index to the substrate concentration range within which a transport process or enzyme-mediated transformation functions effectively. If that range includes the concentration of the substrate presented to the active site *in vivo*, the mechanism may be physiologically important.

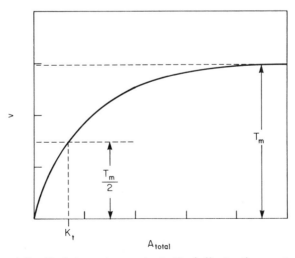

**Figure 2.2** The relationship between transport rate $T_m$, half-saturation constant $K_t$, and the shape of the curve for concentration dependence of saturable transport.

The relative magnitudes of $K_t$ and $T_m$ for two different compounds are important considerations in experimental rate comparisons. Suppose (Figure 2.3) that you wish to compare the rates of transport of glucose and galactose into human erythrocytes. Depending on whether the sugars were present in the experimental medium at 0.2, 0.4, or 0.8 concentration units, you might reach any one of three conflicting conclusions: that glucose is taken up faster than galactose, that the two are transported equally rapidly, or that galactose transport is faster than glucose transport. It is apparent that when two processes are saturable, the entire curves must be characterized ($K_t$ and $T_m$ found) before the rates of the two processes can be compared. Comparison is properly made by means of the $K_t$ and $T_m$ values that determine the shapes of the uptake curves. For glucose uptake into human erythrocytes, Miller (1965) found that $K_t$ and $T_m$ were 0.018 concentration units and 1.9 concentration units per minute respectively; for galactose uptake, $K_t$ and $T_m$ were 0.064 concentration units and 2.1 concentration units per minute respectively. It is interesting to consider briefly some of the factors that determine the magnitudes of $K_t$ and $T_m$.

$K_t$ is an inverse expression of the likelihood that a molecule of the substrate will be bound at the carrier site. The smaller $K_t$ is, the greater is the probability that any particular receptor site will be occupied by a substrate molecule. At a substrate concentration equal to $K_t$, half the carrier sites will usually be occupied.

Substrate size, structure, charge density and distribution, conformation, and surroundings are all determinants of $K_t$. The affinity of a substrate for its carrier site can vary from tissue to tissue, and the affinities of a homologous

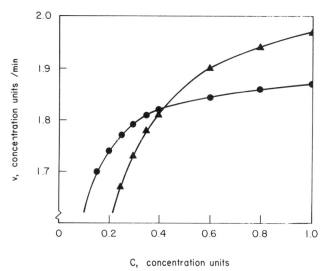

**Figure 2.3**  The concentration dependence of the uptake of galactose (▲) and glucose (●) by human erythrocytes. Idealized curves based on $T_m$ and $K_t$ data from Miller (1965).

**Table 2.1** Kinetic constants for several neutral amino acids

| Amino Acid | $K_t(\text{m}M)$ | $T_m$ (mmole/liter of cell water/min) |
|---|---|---|
| L-Leucine | 1.8 | 0.52 |
| L-Phenylalanine | 4.3 | 1.5 |
| L-Methionine | 5.2 | 0.56 |
| L-Valine | 7.0 | 1.0 |
| L-Alanine | 0.34 | 0.0068 |
| Glycine | 0.30 | 0.0012 |

Reproduced from Winter and Christensen, 1964, Table III.

series of substrates for a single carrier site can also very widely. Sometimes the behavior of a homologous series of substrates can be utilized to deduce which attributes of the substrate are critical to substrate-carrier complex formation.

For example, Table 2.1 lists a series of common amino acids together with the $K_t$ and $T_m$ values determined experimentally for their translocation across the erythrocyte membrane. For L-leucine, L-phenylalanine, L-methionine, and L-valine, the regularly increasing $K_t$ values can be interpreted to suggest that complexing is favored by a long nonpolar moiety. The small $K_t$ values associated with the small highly polar molecules L-alanine and glycine suggest that they may be bound to a site different from that to which the other four amino acids are bound.

In the case of sugars steric configuration has been shown to be one of the most important determinants of binding affinity. Monosaccharides can exist in two general steric configurations, descriptively named the chair and the boat forms. One of the two possible chair configurations is strongly preferred in binding to the erythrocyte membrane carrier site. Figure 2.4 shows that the conformational stability of a monosaccharide in the preferred chair configuration correlates well with its affinity for the red cell membrane.

By definition, $T_m$ is more complex than $K_t$. It is a function not only of rate constants but also of the total capacity of the carrier system. $B_{\text{total}}$, the capacity of the carrier system, depends on the tissue mass and on the concentration of transport molecules. There is no particular reason to suppose that it is influenced by the substrate. $k_3$ represents the net kinetic behavior of two distinguishable sequential steps: passage across the membrane, and release of substrate at the opposite membrane face. There is considerable experimental evidence that substrate translocation itself is rate determining (LeFevre, 1962; Miller, 1965); to what degree the rate of translocation may be influenced by the nature of the substrate has not been generally established.

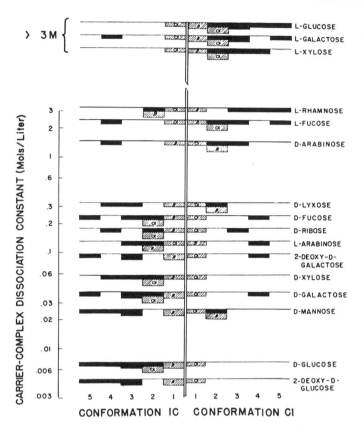

**Figure 2.4** Conformational stabilities of sugars in relation to their affinity for the human erythrocyte sugar transport system. Each block represents a range of "instability factors" estimated on the basis of structural and steric considerations. Cross-hatching marks instability factors shifting with mutarotation between isomers. Stability in the preferred C1 configuration increases from top to bottom. When the range of instability factors centers on zero, the sugar is about equally stable in either of the two possible chair configurations. Reproduced with permission from LeFevre, 1961, Figure 2, © 1961 by the Williams & Wilkins Co., Baltimore.

The amino acids listed in Table 2.1 can be divided into two different groups on the basis of their $T_m$ values. Despite substantial variation within each group, the distinctly lower $T_m$ values for L-alanine and glycine clearly reflect the existence of separate systems for their transport and for transport of the other four amino acids, as was already suggested by consideration of the $K_t$ values. There is not always as much variation in $T_m$ within a related group of substrates translocated by the same carrier. For example, a series of simple sugars that share a common carrier for which their $K_t$ values range over 3 orders of magnitude have a total range of $T_m$ values of only 28% of the mean maximum transport rate (LeFevre, 1962).

Ultimately, measurable kinetic parameters such as $T_m$ and $K_t$ all have their foundation in physical and chemical interactions at the molecular level.

When isolated processes can be studied directly, as membrane transport has been, it is possible to see how specific molecular level mechanisms are reflected in the microconstants that themselves determine kinetic parameters. Even when processes cannot be isolated for study, it is essential to remember that kinetic parameters always have a basis in biochemical and physiological reality.

## 2.5  ESTIMATION OF $K_t$ AND $T_m$ FROM EXPERIMENTAL DATA

### 2.5.1  Estimation by Inspection

If $v$ is graphed against $A_{total}$ over a wide range of $A_{total}$ values until the initial rate approaches constancy (zero-order behavior), an experimental curve similar to the idealized curve in Figure 2.2 will be obtained. $T_m$ is the maximum this curve approaches, and $K_t$ is equal to the concentration of $A_{total}$ at which $v = T_m/2$. This method is cumbersome, requires a large number of experimental points, and is subject to the serious and nonquantifiable biases that always accompany subjective estimates. In particular, $T_m$ is nearly always underestimated. Therefore one of the three possible linear transforms of Equation 2.4 is usually used for the estimation of $K_t$ and $T_m$.

### 2.5.2  Estimation from a Linear Transform

If both sides of Equation 2.4 are inverted,

$$\frac{1}{v} = \frac{K_t + A_{total}}{T_m A_{total}} = \frac{1}{T_m} + \left(\frac{K_t}{T_m}\right)\left(\frac{1}{A_{total}}\right). \tag{2.5}$$

When $1/v$ is graphed against $1/A_{total}$, as in Figure 2.5a, the result is a straight line whose intercept is $1/T_m$ and whose slope is $K_t/T_m$. This is the Lineweaver-Burk or double reciprocal transform of the rate equation (Lineweaver and Burk, 1934); it is the most commonly used of the three possible linear transforms.

Note that the intercept of the Lineweaver-Burk line on the $1/A_{total}$ axis occurs at $-1/K_t$.

Figure 2.5b is a Lineweaver-Burk plot of the uptake into slices of rat brain of tritium-labeled γ-aminobutyric acid, which is thought to have an inhibitory function in the central nervous system (Iversen and Neal, 1968). $K_t$ for this process was estimated from the experimental data to be $2.2 \times 10^{-5}$ $M$ and $T_m$ to be 0.115 $\mu$ mole/min/g of cortex.

If both sides of Equation 2.4 are multiplied by $(K_t + A_{total})/A_{total}$, the result can be rearranged to

$$v = T_m - \frac{v K_t}{A_{total}}. \tag{2.6}$$

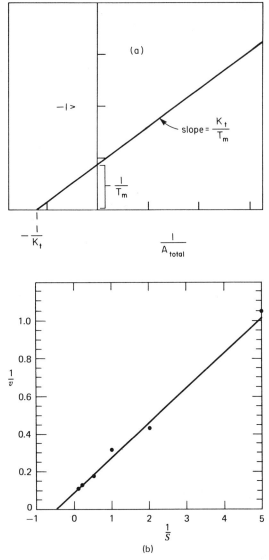

**Figure 2.5** The Lineweaver-Burk or double reciprocal transform. (*a*) Predicted. (*b*) Observed uptake of γ-aminobutyric acid (GABA) by slices of rat brain. $v$ = rate of GABA uptake ($10^{-7}$ mole/min/g cortex), $S$ = GABA concentration ($10^{-5}M$). (*b*) Reproduced, with permission, from Iversen and Neal, 1968, Figure 3.

When $v$ is graphed against $v/A_{total}$ as shown in Figure 2.6a, the graph will be a straight line whose slope is $-K_t$ and whose ordinate intercept is $T_m$. This type of graph is variously referred to as an Eadie or Hofstee plot (Eadie, 1942; Hofstee, 1952), depending on the type of data being graphed and the school from which the researcher came.

Figure 2.6b is an Eadie (Hofstee) plot for the uptake of 5-hydroxy-tryptamine by the myenteric plexus of the guinea pig small intestine *in vitro*. (Compare Figure 2.6b with Figure 2.1b.)

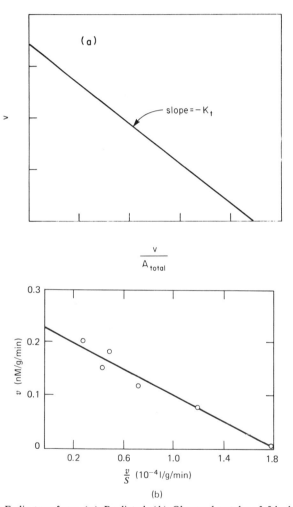

**Figure 2.6** The Eadie transform. (a) Predicted. (b) Observed uptake of 5-hydroxytryptamine (5-HT) by the myenteric plexus of the guinea pig small intestine. $v$ = rate of 5-HT uptake, $S$ = 5-HT concentration. (b) Reproduced with permission from Gershon and Altman, 1971, Figure 7, © 1971 by The Williams & Wilkins Co., Baltimore.

The Eadie plot distributes experimental data of the form usually gathered (constant increments in $A_{total}$) more or less uniformly along the experimental line, whereas the double reciprocal plot clusters such experimental points low on the line. When fitting double reciprocal plots by hand the researcher tends to give greater weight to the more widely spaced points high on the line. Unfortunately these are the observations made at the lowest substrate concentrations and are, therefore, presumably the least reliable. With the advent of computer fitting of such lines and the introduction of proper weighting techniques to compensate for the differences in reliability, however, this objection to the double reciprocal plot is no longer relevant. Furthermore, detailed analysis of the often much more complex reactions characteristic of saturable systems such as enzyme-mediated transformations has been developed entirely around the double reciprocal plot. For these reasons the double reciprocal plot is to be preferred today; however, the reader should be able to recognize and to interpret the other two forms as well.

The third linear transform of Equation 2.4 is developed by multiplying the double reciprocal form by $A_{total}$ to obtain

$$\frac{A_{total}}{v} = \frac{K_t + A_{total}}{T_m} = \frac{K_t}{T_m} + \frac{A_{total}}{T_m}. \tag{2.7}$$

When $A_{total}/v$ is graphed against $A_{total}$ as in Figure 2.7a, the graph is a straight line with intercept $K_t/T_m$ and slope $1/T_m$. This is a Hanes plot (1932), also referred to as a Woolf plot.

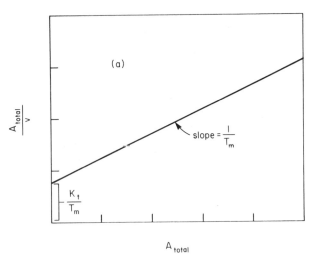

**Figure 2.7** The Hanes transform. (*a*) Predicted. (*b*) Observed dependence of the urinary excretion rate of salicyluric acid (SU) on the body burden of its parent salicylic acid (SA). (*b*) Reproduced with permission from Garrettson et al., 1975, Figure 3.

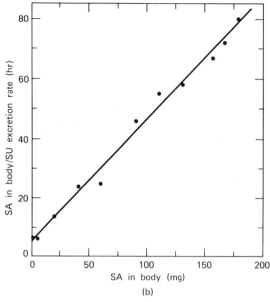

**Figure 2.7** (*continued*)

It is not usual to find data graphed in this fashion, perhaps because it offers no specific advantages over either of the other two forms; but Figure 2.7*b* shows one such graph, for the rate of excretion of salicylic acid as its metabolite salicyluric acid. Presumably the metabolic transformation of salicylic acid is the saturable and rate-determining step in the transformation and translocation sequence from salicylic acid in the blood plasma to salicyluric acid in the urine.

## 2.6 INHIBITION OF A SATURABLE SYSTEM

Every saturable system is subject to inhibition by molecules that are capable of interacting with and altering the system in some critical way. In general, for a single-substrate process, whenever A and inhibitor I compete for the same or closely associated sites on B, the inhibition will be competitive; when they occupy different sites it will be noncompetitive unless there is interaction between the sites, in which case the inhibition will be mixed. The meaning of these terms will become clear as mathematical development of the relationships progresses.

Excluding inhibition by combination of I with A, there are two possible kinds of inhibitor binding to the system. I may combine with B or I may combine with AB. Pictured in the shorthand notation adopted by Cleland

(1963) to describe enzyme-mediated reactions, these possibilities are shown below.

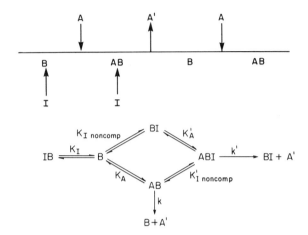

If I combines with B it may do so either at the active site to form IB and inhibit competitively, or at a different site to form BI and inhibit noncompetitively. In the latter case $V_m$ is altered but $K_A$ may or may not be.

If I combines with AB it can do so only to form ABI and inhibit noncompetitively. In this case the kinetic behavior of the system is dependent on whether I can combine with both B and AB, or only with AB. In both cases $V_m$ is altered; $K_A$, however, may or may not be changed in the presence of a noncompetitive inhibitor.

To see why interaction with inhibitors causes such alterations in the kinetic behavior of the system, consider a generalized two-substrate enzyme model. One substrate is the preferred substrate, A; the other is in this case the inhibitor I, although it could equally well be an activator or a coenzyme.

To simplify the development of the associated rate equations, we will assume equilibrium rather than steady state conditions: that is, that true equilibrium rather than steady state applies, and that the $K$'s are, therefore, equilibrium constants. A more proper treatment assuming only pseudo–steady state is too complex for inclusion here. As long as $k$ is rate limiting a pseudo–steady state derivation will generate the same form of relationship as an equilibrium derivation; but the $K$'s will be agglomerates of rate constants rather than equilibrium constants.

Depending on where and when I combines, whether $k'$ is $\geqslant 0$, and whether $K'_A = K_A$, there are different possibilities for inhibition. We will assume that inhibition is complete; that is, that $k' = 0$. Then

$$\frac{dA'}{dt} = v = k(\text{AB}).$$

The conservation equation is

$$B_{total} = B + AB + IB + BI + ABI. \qquad (2.8)$$

Since the $K$'s are by assumption equilibrium constants,

$$K_{I\,noncomp} = \frac{(B)(I)}{(BI)} \quad \text{and} \quad (BI) = \frac{(B)(I)}{K_{I\,noncomp}}$$

$$K_{I\,comp} = \frac{(B)(I)}{(IB)} \quad \text{and} \quad (IB) = \frac{(B)(I)}{K_{I\,comp}}$$

$$K_A = \frac{(B)(A)}{(AB)} \quad \text{and} \quad (AB) = \frac{(B)(A)}{K_A}$$

$$K'_{I\,noncomp} = \frac{(AB)(I)}{(ABI)} \quad \text{and} \quad (ABI) = \frac{(AB)(I)}{K'_{I\,noncomp}}$$

$$= \frac{(A)(B)(I)}{K'_{I\,noncomp} K_A}$$

$$K'_A = \frac{(BI)(A)}{(ABI)} \quad \text{and} \quad (ABI) = \frac{(BI)(A)}{K'_A}$$

$$= \frac{(B)(I)(A)}{K'_A K_{I\,noncomp}}.$$

Note that $K_{I\,noncomp} K'_A = K'_{I\,noncomp} K_A$, so that if $K_A = K'_A$, then $K_{I\,noncomp} = K'_{I\,noncomp}$.

Substituting into Equation 2.8,

$$B_{total} = B\left(1 + \frac{I}{K_{I\,comp}} + \frac{I}{K_{I\,noncomp}} + \frac{(I)(A)}{K_A K'_{I\,noncomp}} + \frac{A_{total}}{K_A}\right)$$

and therefore

$$v = \frac{k\,B_{total}\,A_{total}}{K_A\left(1 + \dfrac{I}{K_{I\,comp}} + \dfrac{I}{K_{I\,noncomp}} + \dfrac{A_{total}}{K_A} + \dfrac{IA_{total}}{K_A K'_{I\,noncomp}}\right)}$$

$$= \frac{V_m A_{total}}{K_A + A_{total} + \dfrac{K_A I}{K_{I\,comp}} + \dfrac{K_A I}{K_{I\,noncomp}} + \dfrac{IA_{total}}{K'_{I\,noncomp}}}. \qquad (2.9)$$

The maximum velocity of an enzyme-catalyzed reaction is usually denoted by $V_m$, and the Michaelis constants for the various substrates are identified by subscripts. $V_m$, of course, is analogous to $T_m$ and is defined in the same way.

### 2.6.2  Competitive Inhibition

In exclusively competitive inhibition, $K_{I noncomp}$ and $K'_{I noncomp}$ are both infinitely large, and the complete rate equation (2.9) reduces to

$$v = \frac{V_m A_{total}}{A_{total} + K_A(1 + I/K_{I comp})}.$$  (2.10)

Its reciprocal is

$$\frac{1}{v} = \frac{1}{V_m} + \left(\frac{K_A}{V_m}\right)\left(1 + \frac{I}{K_{I comp}}\right)\left(\frac{I}{A_{total}}\right),$$  (2.11)

so that the slope of a Lineweaver-Burk plot increases with the addition of a competitive inhibitor to the system while the ordinate intercept remains the same. $V_m$ is unchanged, but $K_A$ appears to be larger, as shown in Figure 2.8a.

Intuitively it is reasonable that $K_A$ should appear to be larger in the presence of a competitive inhibitor. Since A and I are competing for the same (or very nearly the same) site on B, additional A is required in the presence of I to overcome the competition by I and to half-saturate B. The more I present, the larger the quantity

$$K_A\left(1 + \frac{I}{K_{I comp}}\right),$$

which is the apparent $K_A$.

Figure 2.8b is a double reciprocal plot of data showing the competitive inhibition by heme of δ-aminolevulinic acid dehydrase, one of the enzymes of the heme synthetic pathway. Feedback inhibitions such as this one are often competitive, since product is likely to resemble its precursors in one or more critical respects and, therefore, to be able to compete with precursors for enzyme-binding sites. Feedback inhibitions are important and often essential homeostatic mechanisms. In this particular case, feedback inhibition by heme of heme synthetase, the terminal enzyme of the heme synthetic pathway, is of greater homeostatic importance than the inhibition shown in Figure 2.8b.

The Eadie transform of the rate equation describing competitive inhibition is obtained as before, by multiplying both sides of the equation by

$$\frac{A_{total} + K_A(1 + I/K_{I comp})}{A_{total}}$$

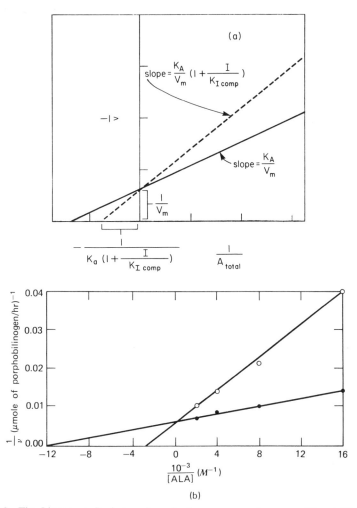

**Figure 2.8** The Lineweaver-Burk transform in the presence of a competitive inhibitor. (*a*) Predicted. (*b*) Observed inhibition of δ-aminolevulinic acid (ALA) metabolism by heme. O, heme present; ●, heme absent. (*b*) Reproduced with permission from Calissano et al., 1966, Figure 2.

and rearranging it to

$$v = V_m - K_A \left( 1 + \frac{I}{K_{I\,comp}} \right) \frac{v}{A_{total}}. \qquad (2.12)$$

As with a double reciprocal plot, the slope of an Eadie plot increases but the ordinate intercept is unchanged when a competitive inhibitor is added to the system. Figure 2.9*a* demonstrates the effect of competitive inhibition on an Eadie plot.

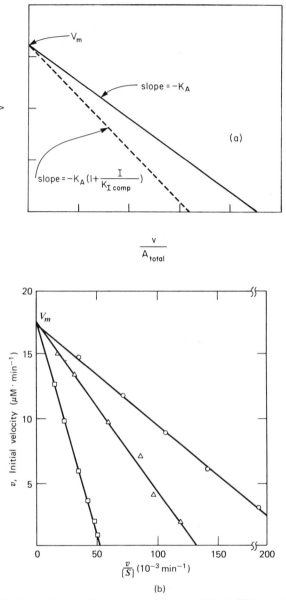

**Figure 2.9** The Eadie transform in the presence of a competitive inhibitor. (*a*) Predicted. (*b*) Observed inhibition of rabbit muscle phosphoglucose isomerase by 5-phosphoarabinonate. O, uninhibited line; △, □, with different concentrations of 5-phosphoarabinonate added. (*b*) Reproduced with permission from Chirgwin and Noltman, 1975, Figure 2A.

Figure 2.9*b* is an Eadie plot of data showing the competitive inhibition of phosphoglucose isomerase from rabbit muscle by 5-phosphoarabinonate present at two different concentrations. 5-Phosphoarabinonate is a structural analogue of the natural substrate phosphoglucose. In this system $K_A$ is 0.1 m$M$ but $K_I$ is only 0.46 $\mu M$, suggesting that in spite of the competitive nature of 5-phosphoarabinonate inhibition, inhibitor is bound to the active site of the enzyme in a manner quite different from that of the natural substrate.

### 2.6.2 Noncompetitive Inhibition

In exclusively noncompetitive inhibition, $K_{I\,comp}$ is infinitely large and the complete rate equation (2.9) reduces to

$$v = \frac{V_m A_{total}}{A_{total} + K_A + \dfrac{K_A I}{K_{I\,noncomp}} + \dfrac{I\,A_{total}}{K'_{I\,noncomp}}} .$$

Substituting $K'_A / K'_{I\,noncomp}$ for its equivalent $K_A / K_{I\,noncomp}$,

$$v = \frac{V_m A_{total}}{A_{total} + K_A + \dfrac{K'_A I}{K'_{I\,noncomp}} + \dfrac{I A_{total}}{K'_{I\,noncomp}}}$$

$$= \frac{V_m A_{total}}{(A_{total} + K_A) + \dfrac{I}{K'_{I\,noncomp}}(A_{total} + K'_A)} .$$

In Lineweaver-Burk form the rate equation for noncompetitive inhibition is therefore

$$\frac{1}{v} = \frac{1}{V_m}\left(1 + \frac{I}{K'_{I\,noncomp}}\right) + \left(\frac{1}{A_{total}}\right)\left[\frac{K_A}{V_m} + \left(\frac{K'_A}{V_m}\right)\left(\frac{I}{K'_{I\,noncomp}}\right)\right]. (2.13)$$

Clearly both the slope and the ordinate intercept of a reciprocal plot are increased in the presence of a noncompetitive inhibitor. What happens to the abscissa intercept? When $1/v = 0$,

$$\frac{1}{A_{total}} = -\frac{1 + \dfrac{I}{K'_{I\,noncomp}}}{K_A\left(1 + \dfrac{I}{K_{I\,noncomp}}\right)} .$$

Therefore the abscissa intercept is also altered by I unless $K_{\text{I noncomp}}$ is equal to $K'_{\text{I noncomp}}$. (Remember that if $K_{\text{I noncomp}} = K'_{\text{I noncomp}}$ then $K_A = K'_A$). When this restriction applies, then and then only

$$\frac{1}{A_{\text{total}}} = -\frac{1}{K_A} \qquad \text{when} \qquad \frac{1}{v} = 0.$$

Therefore the abscissa intercept of a double reciprocal plot is unchanged by noncompetitive inhibition only when $K_A = K'_A$. What is the physical significance of this mathematical observation? $K'_A$ is equal to $K_A$ when the presence of I on B does not hinder the binding of A to B; in this case also the presence of A on B does not hinder the binding of I. In other words, there is no interaction between the binding sites for A and I. A priori there is usually no reason to reject the possibility of interaction unless something else is known about the system to suggests that there should be none. Therefore reciprocal plots of data that conform to a noncompetitive inhibition pattern should never be forced to intersect on the abscissa. In fact, it is more reasonable to expect that interaction between sites will occur in most cases than that it will not; since any alteration in the binding site for A, even a conformational alteration mediated from some distance through a macro-molecule, is likely to alter the affinity of A for B. This point is particularly important because there are so many examples in the scientific literature of double reciprocal lines unjustifiably forced to intersect on the abscissa. Fortunately the rate of appearance of such examples has fallen off recently as more and more data sets are fit by objective regression techniques that define lines in accordance with the experimental data points, not necessarily in accordance with expectation.

Figure 2.10$a$ illustrates the appearance of double reciprocal plots for noncompetitive inhibition with and without an alteration in $K_A$.

Figure 2.10$b$ is a Lineweaver-Burk plot of data showing the effect of the microsomal mixed function oxidase inhibitor piperonyl butoxide on two different metabolic transformations of the insecticide parathion. Piperonyl butoxide inhibits both transformations noncompetitively and without altering $K_A$, which is $1.71 \times 10^{-4}$ $M$ for parathion oxidative activation and $1.23 \times 10^{-4}$ $M$ for parathion oxidative cleavage (deactivation). The $K_I$'s are $2.38 \times 10^{-4}$ $M$ for the activation and $2.00 \times 10^{-4}$ $M$ for the deactivation, so that both activities are inhibited by piperonyl butoxide to about the same extent.

The anesthetic ketamine has certain pharmacologic effects that resemble the manifestations associated with elevated acetylcholine levels. Cohen et al. (1974) found that in preparations of mammalian brain, ketamine inhibits acetylcholinesterase, the enzyme responsible for acetylcholine breakdown. The inhibition is mixed noncompetitive, as shown in the double reciprocal plot in Figure 2.10$c$. Both $V_m$ and $K_A$ are altered by the presence of ketamine.

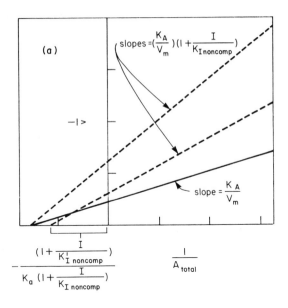

$$\text{slopes} = \left(\frac{K_A}{V_m}\right)\left(1 + \frac{I}{K_{I\,noncomp}}\right)$$

(a)

$-I >$

$$\text{slope} = \frac{K_A}{V_m}$$

$$-\frac{\left(1 + \dfrac{I}{K'_{I\,noncomp}}\right)}{K_a\left(1 + \dfrac{I}{K_{I\,noncomp}}\right)}$$

$$\frac{1}{A_{total}}$$

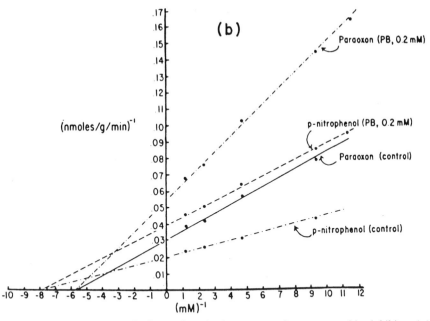

(b)

$(nmoles/g/min)^{-1}$

Paraoxon (PB, 0.2 mM)

p-nitrophenol (PB, 0.2 mM)

Paraoxon (control)

p-nitrophenol (control)

$(mM)^{-1}$

**Figure 2.10** The Lineweaver-Burk transform in the presence of a noncompetitive inhibitor. (*a*) Predicted. (*b*) Observed inhibition by piperonyl butoxide (PB) *in vitro* on the oxidative activation (paraoxon formation) and oxidative cleavage (*p*-nitrophenol formation) of parathion by mouse liver homogenates. (*c*) Observed inhibition by ketamine of purified acetylcholinesterase (AChE) activity. S = concentration of substrate acetylthiocholine. (*b*) Reproduced with permission from Levine and Murphy, 1977, Figure 2. (*c*) Reproduced with permission from Cohen et al., 1974, Figure 2.

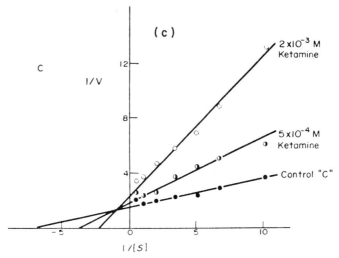

**Figure 2.10**  (*continued*)

The corresponding Eadie transform for noncompetitive inhibition is

$$v = \frac{V_m}{1 + \dfrac{I}{K'_{I\,noncomp}}} - \left(\frac{v}{A}\right)(K_A)\,\frac{1 + \dfrac{I}{K_{I\,noncomp}}}{1 + \dfrac{I}{K'_{I\,noncomp}}}. \qquad (2.14)$$

Both the slope and the ordinate intercept are altered by the presence of inhibitor. If, however, $K_A = K'_A$, then

$$v = \frac{V_m}{1 + \dfrac{I}{K'_{I\,noncomp}}} - (K_A)\left(\frac{v}{A}\right)$$

and the ordinate intercept but not the slope is affected by inhibitor. Figure 2.11*a* illustrates these relationships.

Figure 2.11*b* is an Eadie plot of the noncompetitive inhibition by galactose of valine transport into sacs of rat intestine. Since $K_A$ is unchanged, there is no interaction between the binding site for galactose, a monosaccharide, and that for valine, an amino acid. Apparently the membrane conformational changes associated with galactose transport affect only the rate of valine translocation, not the affinity of valine for its binding site on the membrane.

Figure 2.11*c* is an Eadie plot demonstrating noncompetitive inhibition by two different inhibitors of serotonin uptake into the guinea pig myenteric plexus where serotonin (5-hydroxytryptamine, 5-HT) may act as a neurotransmitter. Methamphetamine, an amphetamine, and chlorimipramine, a

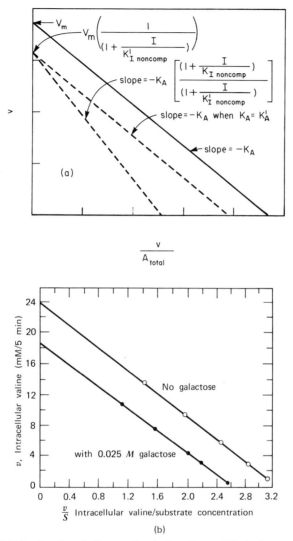

Figure 2.21 Inhibition by ethanol of tryptophan hydroxylase activity in the supernatant fraction of rat midbrain homogenates. (a) With tryptophan concentration variable, 10–100 $\mu M$. DMPH$_4$ concentration, 1 m$M$. Units of $v$ are picomoles of 5-HT formed per 0.2 ml of enzyme preparation per 45 min incubation. (b) With DMPH$_4$ concentration variable, 50 $\mu M$–1 m$M$. Tryptophan concentration, 10 $\mu M$. Units of $v$ as in (a). Reproduced with permission from Rogawski et al., 1974, Figure 3 and Figure 4.

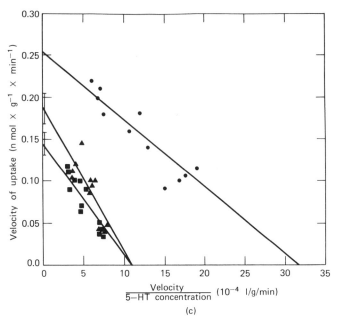

**Figure 2.11**  (*continued*)

tricyclic antidepressant, each exhibited the inhibitory behavior characteristic of other drugs in its respective class; but as Figure 2.11*c* shows, the two classes of drugs behaved quite differently. $K_T$ and $V_m$ in the absence of any inhibitor were $7.9 \times 10^{-7}$ *M* and 0.25 nmole/min/g, respectively. In the presence of methamphetamine $V_m$ was 0.19 nmole/min/g while in the presence of chlorimipramine it was only 0.14 nmole/min/g. $K_I$ values were $9.3 \times 10^{-7}$ *M* for methamphetamine and $4.0 \times 10^{-5}$ *M* for chlorimipramine. Note that the affinity of methamphetamine for its membrane binding site is about the same as that of the substrate 5-HT, whereas chlorimipramine is a considerably less potent inhibitor. Furthermore, even within its range of inhibiting concentrations, it can be seen that chlorimipramine does not alter the affinity of 5-HT for its binding site as radically as methamphetamine does, since the slope of the chlorimipramine line is not as markedly different from the uninhibited slope as that of the methamphetamine line. The apparent $K_m$ in the presence of $10^{-4}$ *M* chlorimipramine was $13 \times 10^{-7}$ *M*; in the presence of $5 \times 10^{-6}$ *M* methamphetamine it was $17 \times 10^{-7}$ *M*.

Noncompetitive inhibitors are most often not structurally related to the natural substrate. Heavy metals such as mercury, cadmium, and silver are noncompetitive enzyme inhibitors; so are trivalent arsenic, derivatives of iodoacetate, and organophosphorus compounds. Metal complexing agents such as cyanide, sulfide, fluoride, and carbon monoxide may form complexes with metalloenzymes. They may also remove the metal from a metal-activated enzyme, as do chelating agents such as ethylenediamine tetraacetate and diethyldithiocarbamate. One effect of all these activities is to alter $V_m$. As we have seen from several of the examples given in this section, drugs may also alter $V_m$ with or without altering $K_m$.

## 2.7  THE DISTINCTION BETWEEN FACILITATED AND ACTIVE TRANSPORT

Until now we have not distinguished between facilitated diffusion and active, or concentrative, transport. Both mechanisms require a carrier. What distinguishes them kinetically?

We have considered transport occurring in only one direction. In fact, of course, transport takes place in both directions across the membrane. If $K_A$ and $V_m$ are the same for transport in either direction, then at equilibrium $A = A'$ and the mechanism is facilitated diffusion:

$$v = \frac{V_m A_{total}}{K_A + A_{total}} ; \qquad v' = \frac{V_m A'_{total}}{K_A + A'_{total}}.$$

At equilibrium $v = v'$ so that

$$\frac{V_m A_{total}}{K_A + A_{total}} = \frac{V_m A'_{total}}{K_A + A'_{total}}$$

and $A_{total}$ must equal $A'_{total}$.

The transport of essential nutrients such as sugars and amino acids across the plasma membrane of most cells is a facilitated diffusion.

If, however, $K_A$ or $V_m$ is not the same for transport in one direction as it is for transport in the other, A will not be equal to A' at equilibrium and active transport will take place against a chemical gradient. Since $V_m$ seems to be determined principally by the rate of passage across the membrane, not by the rate of dissociation, and is therefore relatively constant, and since measured values of $K_A$ have been shown to be widely variable as discussed in Section 2.4, it seems probable that in most cases differences in $K_A$'s are responsible for concentration differences existing across biological membranes at steady state (Skou, 1964). If $V_m = V'_m$ and $K'_A > K_A$, then at steady state

$$\frac{A'_{total}}{A_{total}} = \frac{K'_A}{K_A}.$$

Conformational changes that would result in asymmetry of the membrane either with respect to $V_m$ or with respect to $K_A$ must be mediated by controlled energy input. Many of the active transport systems that have been studied appear to be coupled to the $Na^+$-$K^+$-ATPase pump.

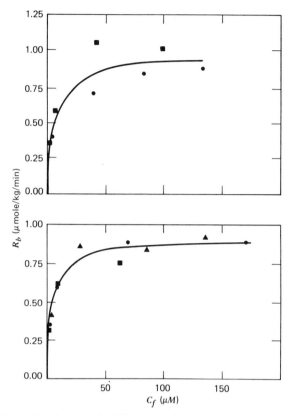

**Figure 2.12** Relationship between the biliary excretion rate $R_b$ and the concentration $C_f$ of iodipamide in two dogs. Reproduced with permission from Lin et al., 1977, Figure 3.

The absorption of sugars and amino acids across the intestinal wall and their reabsorption in the kidney in healthy individuals are active transport mechanisms. In addition, the kidney secretes and reabsorbs many other compounds, both endogenous and foreign, by active or concentrative mechanisms. Secretion from the liver into the bile is also an active transport process for many compounds. An example of saturable biliary excretion is shown in Figure 2.12.

## 2.8   EXAMPLES ILLUSTRATING THE PRINCIPLES DEVELOPED IN THIS CHAPTER

### 2.8.1   Facilitated Diffusion

Carbon dioxide is a terminal product of metabolism in all animal tissues. It diffuses into erythrocytes, where it is hydrated by carbonic anhydrase to carbonic acid, most of which dissociates to bicarbonate ion in the buffered erythrocyte interior. Much of this bicarbonate then leaves the cell in exchange for plasma chloride, a process called the chloride shift. The exchange is readily reversible. In the lung the reverse exchange does in fact take place, returning bicarbonate to the erythrocyte interior, where carbon dioxide is freed for diffusion into the expired air.

Gunn and his co-workers (1973) studied the rate of movement of radio-labeled chloride out of isolated human erythrocytes as a function of total intracellular chloride concentration. The cells containing labeled chloride were suspended in a medium whose total chloride concentration was adjusted to be equal to the intracellular concentration. The authors called the subsequent movement of radiolabeled chloride out of the cell a "chloride self-exchange flux," since no net shift of chloride occurred. Their results (Figure 2.13) show clearly that the rate of transfer is dependent on chloride concentration at low concentrations. Above concentrations of about 20 meq per liter of cell water, however, the transport system begins to show the effect of approaching saturation. At concentrations above 120 meq/l the transport system is saturated.

Since chloride transport is saturable it is mediated by a carrier. Since chloride is in equilibrium across the erythrocyte membrane when its intracellular and extracellular concentrations are equal, chloride is transported across the erythrocyte membrane by facilitated diffusion.

It is interesting to see what effect bicarbonate has on chloride transport. Gunn and his co-workers found that bicarbonate was a competitive inhibitor of chloride self-exchange. Figure 2.14 presents their inhibition data in a commonly used form called a Dixon plot (Dixon, 1953), which is different from the linear plots discussed earlier in this chapter. Instead of determining chloride transport over a range of chloride concentrations in the presence and in the absence of a fixed bicarbonate concentration, the investigators chose to measure chloride transport over a range of bicarbonate concentrations at two different fixed chloride concentrations. The general reciprocal rate equation for competitive transport inhibition, when terms in I rather than terms in A

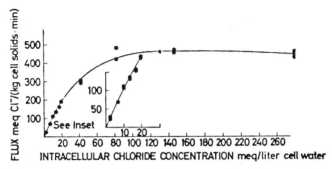

**Figure 2.13** Dependence on intracellular chloride concentration of the rate of chloride transfer (flux) out of the human erythrocyte. Reproduced with permission from Gunn et al., Figure 5 (*J. Gen. Physiol.*, 1973, **61**, 185–206) by copyright permission of the Rockefeller University Press.

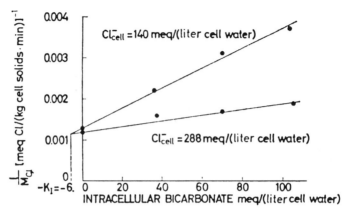

**Figure 2.14** Dixon plot of the inhibition by bicarbonate of chloride transport out of the human erythrocyte at two different intracellular chloride concentrations. Reproduced with permission from Gunn et al., Figure 9 (*J. Gen. Physiol.*, 1973, **61**, 185–206) by copyright permission of the Rockefeller University Press.

are collected, takes the form

$$\frac{1}{v} = \left(\frac{1}{T_m}\right)\left(1 + \frac{K_A}{A}\right) + \left(\frac{K_A}{T_m A}\right)\left(\frac{I}{K_I}\right).$$

Therefore a graph of $1/v$ against I, as in Figure 2.14, should be a straight line whose slope is $K_A / T_m K_I A$ and whose ordinate intercept is $(1/T_m)(1 + K_A/A)$. Note that the ordinate intercept is dependent on the concentration of A. At the point at which lines determined at different fixed substrate concentrations A and A′ intersect,

$$\left(\frac{1}{T_m}\right)\left(1 + \frac{K_A}{A}\right) + \left(\frac{K_A}{T_m A}\right)\left(\frac{I}{K_I}\right) = \left(\frac{K_A}{T_m A'}\right)\left(\frac{I}{K_I}\right) + \left(\frac{1}{T_m}\right)\left(1 + \frac{K_A}{A'}\right),$$

$$\left(\frac{I}{K_I}\right)\left(\frac{K_A}{T_m A} - \frac{K_A}{T_m A'}\right) = -\left(\frac{K_A}{T_m A} - \frac{K_A}{T_m A'}\right),$$

and

$$I = -K_I.$$

Therefore graphs of this form can be used to estimate $K_I$ directly and very simply. As shown in Figure 2.14, $K_I$ for bicarbonate in this transport system is about 6 meq per liter of cell water, or about one-fourth the $K_{Cl}$ value of 25 meq/l. Bicarbonate binds 4 times as strongly to the carrier molecule as chloride does.

It is hardly surprising that bicarbonate and chloride compete for, and therefore share, the same reversible transport system in the erythrocyte membrane, since in this way transport equivalence can be assured.

### 2.8.2 Active Transport

Sugars are absorbed from the intestinal lumen by an active transport process linked with the enzyme $Na^+$-$K^+$-ATPase, which in turn is responsible for the maintenance of transcellular membrane gradients of sodium and potassium. Having evidence that the phenylglycoside phlorizin was a particularly potent inhibitor of sugar uptake, Alvarado and Crane (1964) became interested in the use of phlorizin as a probe to assist in defining the nature of the sugar-binding site on the cell surface. Their initial objective was to characterize the transport of the phenylglycosides themselves.

First they determined that the simple phenylglycoside arbutin is actively transported into cells of the hamster intestinal wall *in vitro* because it continues to enter the intestinal wall against a concentration gradient after equimolar concentrations have been achieved in the incubation medium and tissue water (Figure 2.15). In addition, arbutin uptake is inhibited by dinitrophenol, one of the classic uncouplers of the oxidative phosphorylation required by energy-dependent processes; and by restriction of the partial pressure of oxygen in the incubation systems, as shown in Table 2.2.

Second, they demonstrated that arbutin transport, like sugar transport, is dependent on $Na^+$-$K^+$-ATPase activity. Substitution of potassium ion for the sodium ion of the medium (Table 2.2 and Figure 2.15), which abolishes $Na^+$-$K^+$-ATPase activity, greatly restricts arbutin uptake.

Third, arbutin uptake is competitively inhibited by phlorizin (Figure 2.16), just as sugar uptake had been shown to be.

Fourth, both sugar uptake and arbutin uptake were found to be limited to the small intestine. Neither process takes place in the large intestine.

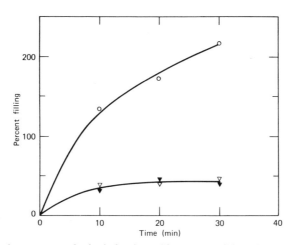

**Figure 2.15** Active transport of arbutin by rings of hamster small intestine. O, uninhibited line; ▼, with $K^+$ replacing $Na^+$ in the medium; ▽, with 0.1 *M* phlorizin added. Adapted with permission from Alvarado and Crane, 1964, Figure 1.

**Table 2.2**  Active transport of arbutin by rat small intestine. Initial arbutin concentration 2 m$M$

| Condition[a] | Percentage Filling[b] | $\nu$($\mu$mole/ml of tissue water)[c] | Inhibition (%)[d] |
|---|---|---|---|
| No additions | 188 | 3.20 | — |
| | 210 | 3.62 | |
| 0.25 m$M$ Dinitrophenol | 81 | 1.54 | 52 |
| | 91 | 1.74 | |
| K$^+$ Medium | 44.5 | 0.89 | 80 |
| | 26.6 | 0.51 | |
| No additions | 254 | 4.80 | — |
| | 243 | 4.45 | |
| 0.062 m$M$ Dinitrophenol | 175 | 3.25 | 35 |
| | 135 | 2.72 | |
| 0.25 m$M$ Dinitrophenol | 80 | 1.61 | 70 |
| | 60 | 1.25 | |
| $O_2$-$CO_2$(95:5, v/v) | 166 | 2.59 | — |
| | 160 | 2.73 | |
| Air-$CO_2$ (95:5, v/v) | 70 | 1.41 | 50 |
| | 63.5 | 1.27 | |

Reproduced from Alvarado and Crane, 1964, Table I.
[a]Incubations were for 10 min in Krebs-Henseleit bicarbonate buffer except where K$^+$ is indicated.
[b]100 $\nu$/final medium concentration.
[c]Uncorrected for 2-deoxygalactose space.
[d]Calculated from control values of $\nu$.

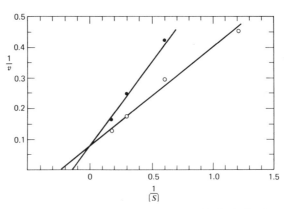

**Figure 2.16**  Inhibition by phlorizin of the active transport of arbutin by rings of hamster small intestine. ○, uninhibited line; ●, with $2.5 \times 10^{-6}$ $M$ phlorizin added. Reproduced with permission from Alvarado and Crane, 1964, Figure 6.

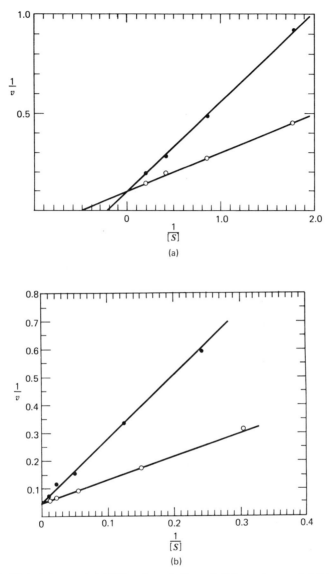

**Figure 2.17** Mutual transport inhibition by arbutin and 6-deoxyglucose. (*a*) Inhibition by 6-deoxyglucose of the active transport of arbutin by rings of hamster small intestine. O, uninhibited line; ●, with $2.5 \times 10^{-3}$ *M* 6-deoxyglucose added. (*b*) Inhibition by arbutin of 6-deoxyglucose transport. O, uninhibited line; ●, with $2.5 \times 10^{-3}$ *M* arbutin added. Reproduced with permission from Alvarado and Crane, 1964, Figure 4 and Figure 5 (adapted).

Finally, Alvarado and Crane demonstrated that arbutin and the sugar 6-deoxyglucose each competitively inhibits the uptake of the other (Figure 2.17a and b). Furthermore, the $K_A$ value for each compound is about equal to the $K_I$ value. (Although the two $K_A$ values are also about equal, about 2 m$M$, this observation did not bear on the authors' conclusion.)

Alvarado and Crane concluded that arbutin uptake into cells of the hamster small intestinal wall utilizes the same transport pathway as active sugar transport.

### 2.8.3  Saturable Pinocytosis

Mucopolysaccharidoses are a group of clinically related storage disorders in which genetic deficiency of a catabolic enzyme results in accumulation of a mucopolysaccharide within the lysosomes of cells throughout the body. Cells cultured from tissues of patients with mucopolysaccharidoses are capable of extracting the missing enzyme from the culture medium, thereby eliminating their excess mucopolysaccharide load. Uptake of the enzyme is by pinocytosis, but binding to a specific membrane site is an obligatory first step in the pinocytosis process, as shown in Figure 2.18 for the uptake of $N$-acetyl-$\alpha$-D-glucosaminidase, the missing enzyme in Sanfilippo B syndrome, a form of mucopolysaccharidosis. The existence of an enzyme-membrane site complex is implicit in the demonstration of saturability in Figure 2.18.

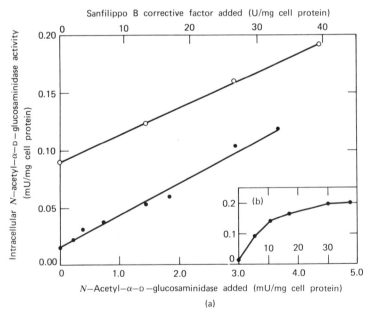

**Figure 2.18**  Uptake of $N$-acetyl-$\alpha$-D-glucosaminidase by normal (○) and Sanfilippo B (●) fibroblasts after 3-hr incubations. (*a*) Uptake at concentrations up to 5 m U/mg cell protein. (*b*) (inset) Uptake by Sanfilippo B fibroblasts at higher concentrations. Reproduced with permission from von Figura and Kresse, 1974, Figure 1.

It has been suggested that pinocytosis is a physiological mechanism for cellular internalization of lysosomal enzymes (Neufeld, 1977). The exceptionally small half-saturation constant for $N$-acetyl-$\alpha$-D-glucosaminidase transport supports this concept. $K_T$ is of the order of magnitude of half-saturation constants for the binding of steroid hormones and glucose regulatory harmones to their receptor sites (Cuatrecasas, 1974; Nelson, 1974), essential mechanisms whose sensitivity and effectiveness depend on high receptor specificity for the natural hormone. The correspondingly high specificity for binding and uptake of $N$-acetyl-$\alpha$-D-glucosaminidase suggests that this mechanism may be equally important physiologically.

### 2.8.4  Enzyme Catalysis

The discovery of insect juvenile hormones and the availability of juvenile hormone analogues (JHA) have provoked much interest in the potential of these substances for insect control. An interesting and important question in connection with the mechanism of action of JHA is whether they increase the effectiveness of the natural hormone in some way or whether they possess intrinsic hormonal qualities themselves. Mayer and Prough (1976) investigated the possibility that JHA act as synergists of the natural hormone by inhibiting the microsomal mixed function oxidase system, thereby preventing inactivation of juvenile hormone (JH) by metabolism. They were able to demonstrate by means of absorption measurements in the wavelength range 400–490 nm that the JHA RO-20-3600 was rapidly metabolized by the rat liver mixed function oxidase system. The metabolite produced formed a complex with cytochrome P450, a heme-containing enzyme that is an essential constituent of the mixed function oxidase system. Once formed, the metabolite–cytochrome P450 complex was quite stable and, although it underwent spectral changes on oxidative treatment, it did not release active cytochrome P450.

From a Lineweaver-Burk plot of the initial rate of metabolite–cytochrome P450 complex formation (measured as spectral change) as a function of RO-20-3600 concentration, Mayer and Prough estimated that the $K_A$ for this process was about 86 $\mu M$. They reasoned that if JH is metabolized by the same cytochrome P450 system, then JH should competitively inhibit formation of the metabolite–cytochrome P450 complex. Figure 2.19 shows that JH does inhibit complex formation competitively. $K_I$ for JH was determined to be about 95 $\mu M$, suggesting that the JHA RO-20-3600 can interfere with JH metabolism effectively at concentrations about equal to normal JH concentrations. Mayer and Prough concluded that one mechanism of RO-20-3600 action is the inhibition of JH metabolism, which increases the effectiveness of JH by prolonging its residence time in the body, therefore prolonging its opportunity to act. Note that this conclusion in no way rules out the possibility that RO-20-3600 (or its metabolite) binds to JH receptor sites as well as to JH metabolic sites, thereby mimicking the activity of the natural hormone.

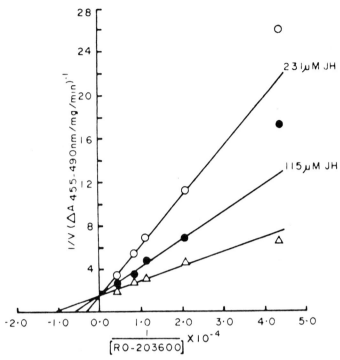

**Figure 2.19** Competitive inhibition by juvenile hormone (JH) of formation from juvenile hormone analogue (RO-20-3600) of a hormone analogue metabolite–cytochrome P450 complex. Reproduced with permission from Mayer and Prough, 1976, Figure 9.


## PROBLEMS

1   In an *in vitro* study of the influence of sugars on the uptake of amino acids into the intestinal mucosal cell, Reiser and Christiansen (1969) obtained the data in Table 2.3.


**Table 2.3**   Rate of valine uptake into mucosal cell of intestine as a function of valine concentration

| Valine Concentration in Incubation Medium (m$M$) | Intracellular Valine Concentration at End of 5-min Incubation (m$M$) |
|:---:|:---:|
| 0.5 | 1.57 |
| 1.0 | 2.82 |
| 2.0 | 4.89 |
| 5.0 | 9.71 |
| 10.0 | 13.94 |

Adapted from Reiser and Christensen, 1969, Table 7.

Graph these data both directly (as a hyperbola) and in Lineweaver-Burk form. Estimate $K_t$ and $V_m$ from *each* graph. In which set of estimates do you have greater confidence? Why?

2 Matthews et al. (1974) presented evidence for active transport of the dipeptide carnosine by hamster jejunum *in vitro*. Two of their graphs are reproduced in Figure 2.20.

(a) Estimate (to one significant figure) the maximum velocity, $V_m$, and Michaelis constant, $K_t$, from each graph.

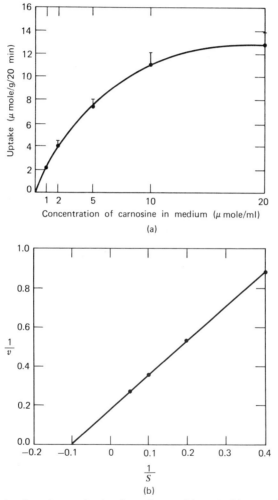

**Figure 2.20** Uptake of total carnosine by rings of everted hamster jejunum. (*a*) Uptake at 20 min over a range of concentrations. (*b*) Uptake at 2 min as Lineweaver-Burk plot. $S=$ concentration of carnosine in medium ($\mu$mole/ml). Note that $v$, in $\mu$mole/g/incubation time, represents a 20-min uptake in (a) and a 2-min uptake in (*b*). Reproduced with permission from Matthews et al., 1974, Figure 2 (adapted) and Figure 3.

(b) Are the estimates from the two graphs the same? Did you expect them to be? Why might they not be?

(c) Which type of graph should give the more reliable pair of estimates? Why?

3 The metabolic transformation of tryptophan to serotonin (5-HT) by tryptophan hydroxylase requires a cofactor, 2-amino-4-hydroxy-6,7-dimethyl-5,6,7,8-tetrahydropterin (DMPH$_4$). Ethanol inhibits this trans-

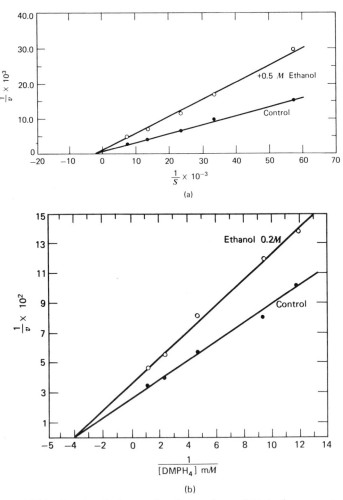

**Figure 2.21** Inhibition by ethanol of tryptophan hydroxylase activity in the supernatant fraction of rat midbrain homogenates. (*a*) With tryptophan concentration variable, 10–100 $\mu M$. DMPH$_4$ concentration, 1 m$M$. Units of $v$ are picomoles of 5-HT formed per 0.2 ml of enzyme preparation per 45 min incubation. (*b*) With DMPH$_4$ concentration variable, 50 $\mu M$–1 m$M$. Tryptophan concentration, 10 $\mu M$. Units of $v$ as in (*a*). Reproduced with permission from Rogawski et al., 1974, Figure 3 and Figure 4.

formation *in vitro* by homogenates of rat brain. From the Lineweaver-Burk plots shown in Figure 2.21, determine whether ethanol interferes with the binding of either tryptophan or $DMPH_4$ to the enzyme.

**4** Alvarado (1966) proposed that sugars and neutral amino acids, both of which are transported by sodium ion dependent mechanisms in the small intestine, might share a common carrier. Using D-galactose as the model sugar and cycloleucine as the model neutral amino acid, he obtained the data shown in Figure 2.22. $K_m$ for uninhibited D-galactose transport is 2.2 mmole/liter, and $K_I$ for the inhibition by galactose of cycloleucine transport is 2.5 mmole/liter. Do these results support Alvarado's hypothesis? Why or why not?

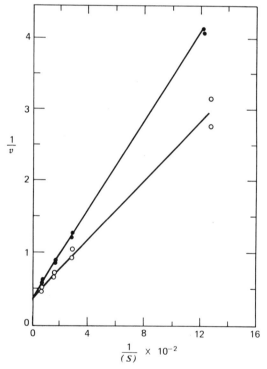

**Figure 2.22** Inhibition by D-galactose of cycloleucine uptake by rings of everted hamster intestine. O, uninhibited line; ●, with 15 m$M$ galactose added; $S$=cycloleucine concentration (moles/l); $v$=uptake velocity ($\mu$mole/ml/min). Reproduced with permission from Alvarado, 1966, Figure 1, © 1966 by the American Association for the Advancement of Science.

**5** Ochratoxin A is a mycotoxin. Suzuki et al. (1975) studied the effect of ochratoxin A on several parameters of renal function including accumulation of para-aminohippuric acid (PAH) by rat renal cortical slices *in vitro*. PAH is taken up by a saturable renal transport system.

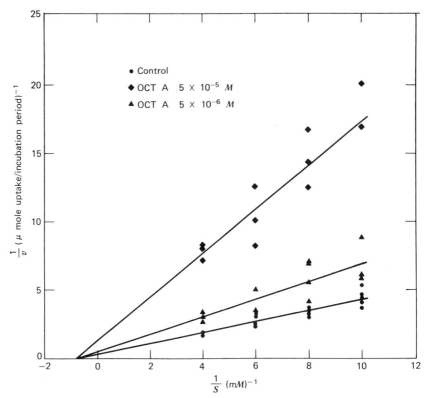

**Figure 2.23** Inhibition by ochratoxin A (OCT A) of PAH uptake by rat renal cortical slices during a 75-min incubation. $S$ = PAH concentration, $0.10 \times 10^{-3} - 0.25 \times 10^{-3} M$; $v$ = uptake velocity. Reproduced with permission from Suzuki et al., 1975, Figure 2.

From their data (Figure 2.23), would you conclude that ochratoxin A competes with PAH for its transport system or that it damages renal tissue?

6  Watabe and Akamatsu (1974) studied the biotransformation of *cis*-stilbene by a microsomal reaction system and its inhibition by the compound *trans*-stilbenimine. Microsomal oxidation of *cis*-stilbene (I) gives the epoxide intermediate *cis*-stilbene oxide (II), whose conversion to *threo*-stilbene glycol(III) is catalyzed by the microsomal enzyme epoxide hydrolase.

In one series of studies they found the amounts shown in Table 2.4 of metabolites of (I) without and with the addition of *trans*-stilbenimine. In a separate kinetic study of the inhibition by *trans*-stilbenimine of the conversion of (II) to (III) they observed the behavior shown in Figure 2.24.

(a) Are the results of the two studies consistent? Why or why not?

(b) What would you propose as the mechanism of inhibition by *trans*-stilbenimine of microsomal *cis*-stilbene metabolism?

**Table 2.4** Accumulation of *cis*-stilbene oxide(II) in the hepatic microsomal metabolism of *cis*-stilbene(I) to *threo*-stilbene glycol(III) in the presence and in the absence of *trans*-stilbenimine

| Incubation Time (min) | Control | | *trans*-Stilbenimine Added | |
|---|---|---|---|---|
| | II Formed ($\mu M$) | III Formed ($\mu M$) | II Formed ($\mu M$) | III Formed ($\mu M$) |
| 15 | 6.1 | 84.4 | 28.9 | 19.2 |
| 30 | 2.2 | 116.7 | 18.2 | 35.6 |
| 60 | 0.0 | 136.5 | 2.6 | 42.7 |

Reproduced from Watabe and Akamatsu, 1974, Table 2.

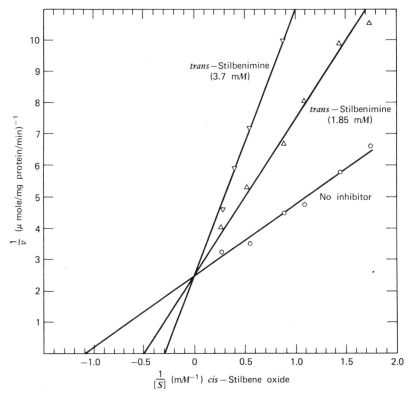

**Figure 2.24** Inhibition by *trans*-stilbenimine of rabbit liver microsomal epoxide hydrolase activity: $S$ = concentration of *cis*-stilbene oxide (m$M$), $v$ = rate of *threo*-stilbene oxide formation ($\mu$mole/mg protein/min). Reproduced with permission from Watabe and Akamatsu, 1974, Figure 1.

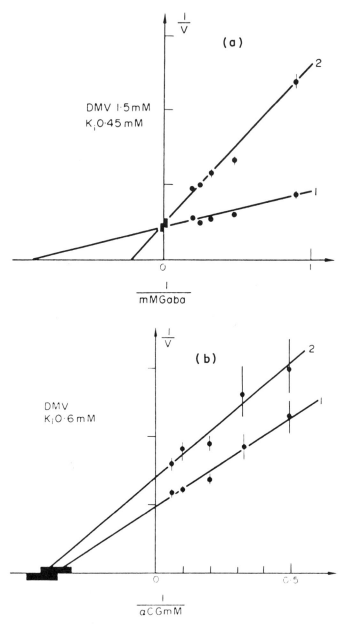

**Figure 2.25** Inhibition by DMV of the activity of GABA transaminase purified from mouse brain. 1, uninhibited lines; 2, with 1.5 mM DMV added. (a) With GABA as variable substrate; concentration in mM. (b) With α-ketoglutarate as variable substrate; concentration in mM. v=rate of transamination in arbitrary fluorometric units. Reproduced with permission from Maitre et al., 1974, Figure 3 and Figure 4.

7 Certain $\alpha$-substituted fatty acids, such as 2,2-dimethyl valeric acid (DMV), have been shown to inhibit the production of audiogenic seizures in mice. This anticonvulsant action is associated with an elevated level of $\gamma$-aminobutyric acid (GABA) in the brain. GABA is deaminated in the brain by GABA transaminase in accordance with the following reaction:

GABA + $\alpha$-ketoglutarate $\rightleftharpoons$ succinic semialdehyde + glutamate.

Maitre et al. (1974) investigated the kinetic behavior of GABA trans-aminase *in vitro* in the presence and absence of DMV. Their results are shown in Figure 2.25.

(a) What do these data suggest to you as a plausible mechanism of DMV action?

(b) What do they suggest about the order of addition of the two substrates, GABA and $\alpha$-ketoglutarate, to GABA transaminase?

8 6-Methyl tetrahydropterin is a cofactor in the hydroxylation of tryptophan to 5-hydroxytryptophan by tryptophan hydroxylase (Figure 2.26). What is the relationship of calcium ion to tryptophan hydroxylase?

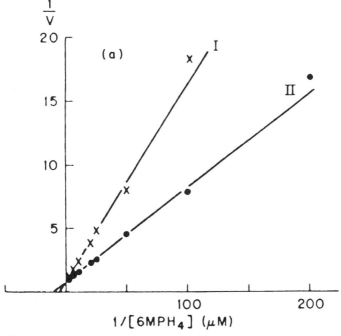

**Figure 2.26** Effect of calcium ion on activity of trytophan hydroxylase isolated from rat hind brain. I, control incubations; II, with 10 m$M$ CaCl$_2$ added. ($a$) With 6-methyl tetrahydropterin concentration variable; tryptophan concentration, 500 $\mu M$. ($b$) With tryptophan concentration variable; 6-methyl tetrahydropterin concentration, 1 m$M$; $v$ = rate of 5-HT formation (ng/mg protein/15 min incubation). Reproduced with permission from Boadle-Biber, 1975, Figure 1 and Figure 2.

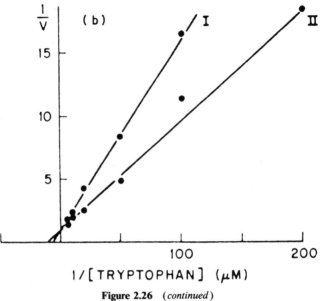

Figure 2.26 (*continued*)

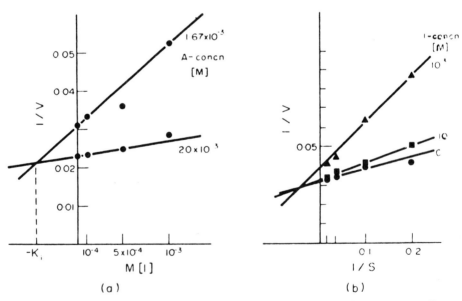

(a)

(b)

**Figure 2.27** Inhibition by ibuprofen of aminopyrine *N*-demethylation by 15,000 g of liver supernatant. (*a*) Dixon plot. I = ibuprofen concentration (*M*). (*b*) Lineweaver-Burk plot. *S* = aminopyrine concentration (m*M*); *v* = rate of *N*-demethylation. Where aminopyrine (A) and ibuprofen (I) are not variable, their concentrations are given on the appropriate graphs; *C* = control. Reproduced with permission from Reinicke and Klinger, 1975, Figure 1.

**9** Show that a graph of the form in Figure 2.14 can be used to distinguish between competitive and pure noncompetitive inhibition. How would you estimate $K_I$ from a graph of $1/v$ against I if inhibition were noncompetitive ($K_A$ unchanged)?

**10** Ibuprofen, a nonsteroid antiinflammatory agent, was studied by Reinicke and Klinger (1975) for its effect on microsomal aminopyrine $N$-demethylation. The results are reproduced in Figure 2.27. Are the two graphs consistent with each other? What kind of inhibitory action do you think ibuprofen has in this system? What is the (approximate) value of $K_I$?

**11** Can you show that in the case of uncompetitive inhibition, where the inhibitor can bind *only* to the active complex, the intercept of a Lineweaver-Burk plot is altered but the slope is not?

**Hint:** Start with the complete equation for inhibition, Equation 2.9, and eliminate terms by analogy with the treatment in Sections 2.6.1 and 2.6.2.

## REFERENCES

Alvarado, F. "Transport of sugars and amino acids in the intestine: Evidence for a common carrier." *Science*, **151**, 1010–1013 (1966).

Alvarado, F. and R. K. Crane. "Studies on the mechanism of intestinal absorption of sugars. VII. Phenylglycoside transport and its possible relationship to phlorizin inhibition of the active transport of sugars by the small intestine." *Biochim. Biophys. Acta*, **93**, 116–135 (1964).

Boadle-Biber, M. C. "Effect of calcium on tryptophan hydroxylase from rat hind brain." *Biochem. Pharmacol.*, **24**, 1455–1460 (1975).

Briggs, H. E. and J. B. S. Haldane. "A note on the kinetics of enzyme action." *Biochem. J.*, **19**, 338–339 (1925).

Brown, A. H. "Enzyme action." *Trans. Chem. Soc. (London)*, **81**, 373–389 (1902).

Calissano, P., D. Bonsignore, and C. Cartasegna. "Control of haem synthesis by feedback inhibition on human erythrocyte δ-aminolaevulate dehydratase." *Biochem. J.*, **101**, 550–552 (1966).

Chirgwin, J. M. and E. A. Noltmann. "The enediolate analogue 5-phosphoarabinonate as a mechanistic probe for phosphoglucose isomerase." *J. Biol. Chem.*, **250**, 7272–7276 (1975).

Christensen, H. N. "Reactive sites and biological transport." *Adv. Protein Chem.*, **15**, 239–314 (1960).

Cleland, W. W. "The kinetics of enzyme-catalyzed reactions with two or more substrates or products. I. Nomenclature and rate equations." *Biochim. Biophys. Acta*, **67**, 104–137 (1963).

Cohen, M. L., S. L. Chan, H. N. Bhargava, and A. J. Trevor. "Inhibition of mammalian brain acetylcholinesterase by ketamine." *Biochem. Pharmacol.*, **23**, 1647–1652 (1974).

Cuatrecasas, P. "Membrane receptors." *Annu. Rev. Biochem.*, **43**, 169–214 (1974).

Dixon, M. "The determination of enzyme inhibitor constants." *Biochem. J.*, **55**, 170–171 (1953).

Eadie, G. S. "The inhibition of cholinesterase by physostigmine and prostigmine." *J. Biol. Chem.*, **146**, 85–93 (1942).

Ege, R. "Die Verteilung der Glucose zwischen Plasma und roten Blutkörperchen. Zur Physiologie des Blutzuckers. IV." *Biochem. Z.*, **111**, 189–218 (1920).

Ege, R. "Wie ist die Verteilung der Glucose zwischen den roten Blutköperchen und der äusseren Flüssigkeit zu Erklären? Zur Physiologie des Blutzuckers. V." *Biochem. Z.*, **114**, 88–110 (1921).

Ege, R., E. Gottlieb, and N. W. Rakestraw, "The distribution of glucose between human blood plasma and red corpuscles and the rapidity of its penetration." *Am. J. Physiol.*, **72**, 76–83 (1925).

Fox, C. F. "The structure of cell membranes." *Sci. Am.*, 31–38 (February 1972).

Garrettson, L. K., J. A. Procknal, and G. Levy. "Fetal acquisition and neonatal elimination of a large amount of salicylate: Study of a neonate whose mother regularly took therapeutic doses of aspirin during pregnancy." *Clin. Pharmacol. Ther.*, **17**, 98–103 (1975).

Gershon, M. D., and R. F. Altman, "An analysis of the uptake of 5-hydroxytryptamine by the myenteric plexus of the small intestine of the guinea pig." *J. Pharmacol. Exp. Ther.*, **179**, 29–41 (1971).

Gershon, M. D., R. G. Robinson, and L. L. Ross. "Serotonin accumulation in the guinea pig myenteric plexus: Ion dependence, structure-activity relationship and the effect of drugs." *J. Pharmacol. Exp. Ther.*, **198**, 548–561 (1976).

Guidotti, G. "The structure of membrane transport systems." *Trends Biochem. Sci.*, **1**, 11–13 (1976).

Gunn, R. B., M. Dalmark, D. C. Tosteson, and J. O. Wieth. "Characteristics of chloride transport in human red blood cells." *J. Gen. Physiol.*, **61**, 185–206 (1973).

Hanes, C. S. "CLXVII. Studies on plant amylases. I. The effect of starch concentration upon the velocity of hydrolysis by the amylase of germinated barley." *Biochem. J.*, **26**, 1406–1421 (1932).

Henri, V. "Recherches physico-chimiques sur les diastases," *Arch. Fisiol.*, **1**, 299–324 (1904).

Hofstee, B. H. J. "On the evaluation of the constants $V_m$ and $K_m$ in enzyme reactions." *Science*, **116**, 329–331 (1952).

Iversen, L. L. and M. J. Neal. "The uptake of ($^3$H)GABA by slices of rat cerebral cortex." *J. Neurochem.*, **15**, 1141–1149 (1968).

Keilin, D. and T. Mann. "On the haematin compound of peroxidase." *Proc. R. Soc. London*, **122**, 119–133 (1937).

Klinghoffer, K. A. "Permeability of the red cell membrane to glucose." *Am. J. Physiol.*, **111**, 231–242 (1935).

Kyte, J. "Structural studies of sodium and potassium ion-activated adenosine triphosphatase. The relationship between molecular structure and the mechanism of active transport." *J. Biol. Chem.*, **250**, 7443–7449 (1975).

LeFevre, P. G. "Evidence of active transfer of certain nonelectrolytes across the human red cell membrane." *J. Gen. Physiol.*, **31**, 505–527 (1948).

LeFevre, P. G. "The evidence for active transport of monosaccharides across the red cell membrane." *Symp. Soc. Exp. Biol.*, **8**, 118–135 (1954).

LeFevre, P. G. "Rate and affinity in human red blood cell sugar transport." *Am. J. Physiol.*, **203**, 286–290 (1962).

LeFevre, P. G. "Sugar transport in the red blood cell: Structure-activity relationships in substrates and antagonists." *Pharmacol. Rev.*, **13**, 39–70 (1961).

Levine, B. S. and S. D. Murphy. "Effect of piperonyl butoxide on the metabolism of dimethyl and diethyl phosphorothionate insecticides." *Toxicol. Appl. Pharmacol.*, **40**, 393–406 (1977).

Lin, S. K., A. A. Moss, and S. Riegelman. "Iodipamide kinetics: Capacity-limited biliary excretion with simultaneous pseudo-first-order renal excretion." *J. Pharm. Sci.*, **66**, 1670–1674 (1977).

Lineweaver, H. and D. Burk. "The determination of enzyme dissociation constants." *J. Am. Chem. Soc.*, **56**, 658–666 (1934).

Maitre, M., L. Ciesielski, and P. Mandel. "Effect of 2-methyl-2-ethyl caproic acid and 2-2-dimethyl valeric acid on audiogenic seizures and brain gamma aminobutyric acid." *Biochem. Pharmacol.*, **23**, 2363–2368 (1974).

Masing, E. "Sind die roten Blutkörper Durchgängig für Traubenzucker?" *Arch. Ges. Physiol.*, **149**, 227–249 (1912).

Matthews, D. M., J. M. Addison, and D. Burston. "Evidence for active transport of the dipeptide carnosine (β-alanyl-L-histidine) by hamster jejunum *in vitro*." *Clin. Sci. Mol. Med.*, **46**, 693–705 (1974).

Mayer, R. T. and R. A. Prough. "Characterization of a metabolite–cytochrome P-450 complex derived from the aerobic metabolism of an insect juvenile hormone analog by rat microsomal fractions." *Toxicol. Appl. Pharmacol.*, **38**, 439–454 (1976).

Michaelis, L. and M. Menten. "Die Kinetik der Invertinwirkung." *Biochem. Z.*, **49**, 333–369 (1913).

Miller, D. M. "The kinetics of selective biological transport. I. Determination of transport constants for sugar movements in human erythrocytes." *Biophys. J.*, **5**, 407–415 (1965).

Nelson, J. A. "Effects of dichlorodiphenyltrichloroethane (DDT) analogs and polychlorinated biphenyl (PCB) mixtures on 17β-($^3$H)-estradiol binding to rat uterine receptor." *Biochem. Pharmacol.*, **23**, 447–451 (1974).

Neufeld, J. A. "The enzymology of inherited mucopolysaccharide storage disorders." *Trends Biochem. Sci.*, **2**, 25–26 (1977).

Reinicke, C. and W. Klinger. "Influence of ibuprofen on drug-metabolizing enzymes in rat liver *in vivo* and *in vitro*. *Biochem. Pharmacol.*, **24**, 145–147 (1975).

Reiser, S. and P. A. Christiansen. "Intestinal transport of amino acids as affected by sugars." *Am. J. Physiol.*, **216**, 915–924 (1969).

Rogawski, M. A., S. Knapp, and A. J. Mandell. "Effects of ethanol on tryptophan hydroxylase activity from striate synaptosomes." *Biochem. Pharmacol.*, **23**, 1955–1962 (1974).

Skou, J. C. "Enzymatic aspects of active linked transport of Na$^+$ and K$^+$ through the cell membrane." *Prog. Biophys. Mol. Biol.*, **14**, 133–166 (1964).

Suzuki, S., Y. Kozuka, T. Satoh, and M. Yamazaki. "Studies on the nephrotoxicity of ochratoxin A in rats." *Toxicol. Appl. Pharmacol.*, **34**, 479–490 (1975).

von Figura, K. and H. Kresse. "Quantitative aspects of pinocytosis and intracellular fate of N-acetyl-α-D-glucosaminidase in Sanfilippo B fibroblasts." *J. Clin. Invest.*, **53**, 85–90 (1974).

Watabe, T. and K. Akamatsu, "Accumulation of an epoxy intermediate during the hepatic microsomal metabolism of *cis*-stilbene to *threo*-stilbene glycol due to the inhibition of epoxide hydrolase by *trans*-stilbenimine." *Biochem. Pharmacol.*, **23**, 1845–1850 (1974).

Widdas, W. F. "Inability of diffusion to account for placental glucose transfer in the sheep and consideration of the kinetics of a possible carrier transfer." *J. Physiol.*, **118**, 23–39 (1952).

Widdas, W. F. "Kinetics of glucose transfer across the human erythrocyte membrane." *J. Physiol.*, **120**, 23P–24P (1953).

Wilbrandt, W. "The relation between rate and affinity in carrier transports." *J. Cell. Comp. Physiol.*, **47**, 137–145 (1956).

Wilbrandt, W. "Minireview. Recent trends in membrane transport research." *Life Sci.*, **16**, 201–212 (1975).

Wilbrandt, W. and T. Rosenberg. "Die Kinetik des enzymatischen Transports." *Helv. Physiol. Acta*, **9**, C86–C87 (1951).

Wilbrandt, W., S. Frei, and T. Rosenberg. "The kinetics of glucose transport through the human red cell membrane." *Exp. Cell. Res.*, **11**, 59–66 (1956).

Wilbrandt, W. and T. Rosenberg. "The concept of carrier transport and its corollaries in pharmacology." *Pharmacol. Rev.*, **13**, 109–183 (1961).

Winter, C. G. and H. N. Christensen. "Migration of amino acids across the membrane of the human erythrocyte." *J. Biol. Chem.*, **239**, 872–878 (1964).

# 3

---

# Acute Exposure with
# First-Order Disposition

**3.1**  First-order processes

**3.2**  Diffusion across biological membranes

    3.2.1  First-order nature of diffusion

    3.2.2  Physical factors that determine the rate of diffusion

**3.3**  The one-compartment body model

**3.4**  Half-life and volume of distribution in the one-compartment body model

**3.5**  How to estimate kinetic parameters using the one-compartment body model

    3.5.1  From plasma data

    3.5.2  From cumulative excretion data

    3.5.3  From excretory rate data

**3.6**  The one-compartment body model with parallel elimination processes

**3.7**  The two-compartment body model

**3.8**  Half-life and volume of distribution in the two-compartment body model

**3.9**  How to estimate kinetic parameters using the two-compartment body model

**3.10**  The peripheral compartment: First-order absorption and first-order elimination in a one-compartment model

    3.10.1  $k_a > k_e$

    3.10.2  $k_a \leqslant k_e$

    3.10.3  $k_a \ll k_e$

**3.11**  First-order absorption and first-order elimination in a two-compartment model

**3.12**  The area under the curve

**3.13**  The concept of clearance

**3.14**  More complex models

**3.15**  Computer fitting of multiple exponential kinetic data

**Appendix 3.1**  Derivation of the Bateman function for first-order absorption from a depot and first-order elimination from a single compartment

**Appendix 3.2**  Derivation of the expression for $t_{\max}$ from the Bateman function

## 3.1 FIRST-ORDER PROCESSES

The preceding chapter pointed out that at low substrate concentrations the rate of a saturable process is dependent on substrate concentration. In other words, as long as a saturable system is not near saturation, it will behave as if it were not saturable. Intuitively this is reasonable. Does the rate equation applicable to a saturable system predict this behavior?

For the expression

$$v = \frac{V_m A}{K_m + A},$$

when the substrate concentration is low relative to $K_m$, or $A \ll K_m$, then

$$v \approx \left(\frac{V_m}{K_m}\right)(A). \tag{3.1}$$

Equation 3.1 is descriptive of a first-order process as defined in Chapter 1, for which $k$, the first-order rate constant, is equal to $(V_m/K_m)$.

Since all multireactant processes are in principle saturable, this kind of first-order process has sometimes been called "pseudo first-order," with the implication that it appears to be first order with respect to A only because B is far from saturated within the concentration range of A under consideration. For example, whereas passive diffusion is a classical first-order process, it is possible to imagine a membrane the entire surface of which is covered with molecules about to diffuse. That the integrity of a biological system so overcrowded with any one kind of molecule would be in serious jeopardy is not relevant here. The point is that saturation of even passive diffusion is theoretically possible. Nonetheless we will consider that mechanisms such as passive diffusion are first order, and ignore the participation of the membrane in the process—except, of course, to the extent that it controls the magnitude of the first-order rate constant $k$.

There is another useful way to approach the kinetics of diffusion. Fick's first law states that the rate of diffusion of a solute down a concentration gradient is proportional to the magnitude of the gradient itself:

$$\frac{dM}{dt} = -DA\frac{dC}{dx}, \tag{3.2}$$

where $M$ is the mass and $C$ the concentration of the solute; $D$ is the diffusion constant, which has the dimensions distance$^2$/time; $A$ is the cross-sectional area of the diffusion volume; and $dC/dx$ is the concentration gradient over an infinitesimally small distance $dx$. When Fick's first law is restated for diffusion across a membrane barrier of thickness $dx$, the concentration

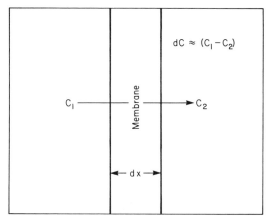

**Figure 3.1** Application of Fick's law to diffusion resulting from a concentration difference across a membrane.

gradient $dC$ is approximated by the concentration difference across the membrane, illustrated in Figure 3.1. Therefore, assuming that $C_1 > C_2$,

$$\frac{dM_1}{dt} = -\frac{DA}{dx}(C_1 - C_2). \tag{3.3}$$

Since $dx$, the thickness of the membrane, is a constant, $AD/dx$ is the first-order rate constant for diffusion across the membrane.

Equation 3.3 describes a net transfer or an approach-to-equilibrium process across the membrane. Net transfer from $C_1$ to $C_2$ continues only as long as $C_1$ is greater than $C_2$. When $C_1$ is equal to $C_2$ at equilibrium, the net transfer rate $dM_1/dt$ is zero. Since there is no change in either the quantity or the identity of solute molecules in the whole system, which includes the volume within which the solute concentration is $C_1$, the volume within which it is $C_2$, and the membrane volume, the system is a *closed* system and the stable state eventually reached is a true equilibrium. Assuming that the membrane volume $A\,dx$ is negligible relative to the other two volumes, the system is a *closed two-compartment system*. It is represented schematically in Figure 3.2, where $\alpha$ is the rate constant for net transfer from compartment 1 to compartment 2.

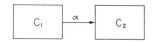

**Figure 3.2** The closed two-compartment model.

## 3.2  DIFFUSION ACROSS BIOLOGICAL MEMBRANES

### 3.2.1  First-Order Nature of Diffusion

Fick's law states that transfer of freely diffusible molecules across a biological membrane should be first order. Chapter 2 stated that lipid-soluble molecules are able to diffuse relatively freely through the nonpolar interior of biological membranes. There is a body of experimental evidence that demonstrates that transfer of many simple lipid-soluble compounds obeys Fick's law. Since electrolytes are in general not lipid-soluble in their ionized forms, this group of compounds is restricted to nonelectrolytes and to the uncharged electrolyte forms.

Figure 3.3 illustrates the first-order nature of transfer into cerebrospinal fluid for 14 different drugs. The ordinate values represent the difference between the plasma concentration of drug and its concentration in the cerebrospinal fluid, or $C_1 - C_2$ in terms of Fick's law, Equation 3.3. These differences are normalized by division by the plasma concentration of drug,

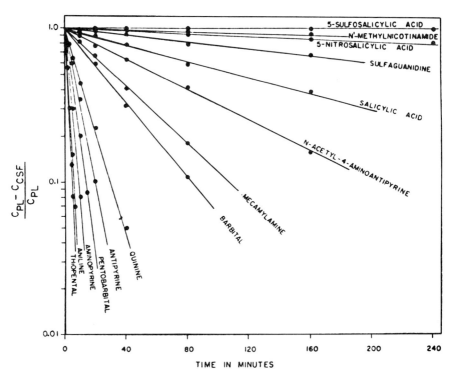

**Figure 3.3**  Relative rates of entry of drugs into cerebrospinal fluid (CSF): $C_{CSF}$, concentration of drug in CSF; $C_{PL}$, concentration of free drug in plasma. Each point represents the mean of values from three to five dogs. Reproduced with permission from Brodie et al., 1960, Figure 1, © 1960 by The Williams & Wilkins Co., Baltimore.

maintained at a constant level by a continuous infusion. The rates of entry of all 14 drugs are directly proportional to the differences between the drug concentrations on the two sides of the membrane. All the drugs obey Fick's law.

Similar data have been obtained for transport in both directions across the stomach wall (Shore et al., 1957; Schanker et al., 1957; Hogben et al., 1957); for absorption from the intestinal tract (Hogben et al., 1959; Schanker et al., 1958; Schanker, 1959), from the lung (Enna and Schanker, 1972; Burton and Schanker, 1974) and through the skin (Trehearne, 1956); for uptake by the erythrocyte (Sha'afi et al., 1971); for passage into the brain (Mayer et al., 1959); and for absorption from subcutaneous and intramuscular injection sites (Ballard et al., 1968; Schou, 1961). Some of these studies have been reviewed (Schanker, 1962, 1964; Hogben, 1960).

Drug and toxicant transfer processes cannot always be characterized by first-order kinetics. In particular, excretion from liver or kidney may not be first order. The kidney and the liver are organs whose function is to excrete foreign compounds and toxic metabolic products, while at the same time conserving and regulating the body's supply of essential nutrients. Accordingly specialized transfer systems have evolved for this purpose. Many drugs and toxicants are actively secreted into the urine or the bile and may be actively reabsorbed in the kidney as well (see Section 4.5). The carrier mechanisms by which foreign compounds are transported in the kidney and liver are also used by endogenous compounds, so that competition can occur. Such competition for carrier sites is potentially significant physiologically, particularly for reabsorption in the kidney, an active transport process that is designed to capture and conserve essential amino acids and monosaccharides.

Wherever in the body specialized carrier transport systems for essential nutrients are found, there is always the possibility that structurally similar drugs or toxicants may be actively transported by the same mechanisms. Such transport systems are located in the gastrointestinal tract and in the placenta as well as in the kidney and liver. Penetration of drugs into the fetus is generally thought to be by simple diffusion except for the occasional drug that may bear a structural resemblance to an actively transported essential nutrient (Ginsburg, 1971). A few drugs or toxicants structurally related to essential nutrients are known to be actively absorbed from the gastrointestinal tract (Schanker and Jeffrey, 1961). However, insufficient experimental information is available in either of these areas to provide material for discussion or to permit general conclusions to be drawn.

The presence of an active transport mechanism does not, of course, preclude the operation of a parallel first-order process. Net diffusion must be presumed to occur wherever a concentration gradient exists, provided physical factors are reasonably favorable to diffusional transfer. One example is the parallel absorption by diffusion and by carrier transport of phenol red in the rat lung, a rare instance of lung absorption of a foreign compound by an active process (Enna and Schanker, 1973).

In general it is reasonable to assume as a working hypothesis that absorption and distribution of exogenous compounds are first order. In this chapter we consider the kinetics of compounds whose elimination mechanisms are also first order. Chapter 4 deals with the behavior of compounds whose kinetics, particularly elimination kinetics, are not first order.

### 3.2.2 Physical Factors that Determine the Rate of Diffusion

The physical factors that control the rate of diffusion of a nonelectrolyte or of the uncharged form of an electrolyte include its solubility, its size, and its degree of ionization in the fluid medium on both sides of the membrane. These factors are considered individually.

#### *Lipid Solubility*

The degree of lipid solubility of a compound is expressed by its partition coefficient. Originally the partition coefficient was expressed in terms of an oil-water partitioning. The organic solvent-water partition coefficient is in common use today. The organic phase is often chloroform, hexane or heptane, or ether. The partition coefficient is determined by shaking an appropriate quantity of the drug together with water and the chosen organic solvent and allowing the drug to reach an equilibrium between the two phases. The concentration of the drug is measured in each of the two phases, and the partition coefficient is calculated by means of the formula

$$\text{partition coefficient} = \frac{\text{concentration in organic phase}}{\text{concentration in aqueous phase}}.$$

Absolute values of partition coefficients are not very meaningful, but the rank order within a homologous series of compounds is generally about the same from one organic solvent to another and can be used effectively in correlations.

Late in the nineteenth century Overton suggested that the rates of penetration of nonelectrolytes into plant cells paralleled their oil-water partition coefficients. Gryns (1896) and Hedin (1897) reached the same conclusion from their studies of penetration into erythrocytes. Extensive experimental work supporting this suggestion was carried out by Collander and Bärlund (1933) and later by Collander (1954) using the large plant (algal) cell *Chara ceratophylla* and the plant cell *Nitella*. These studies demonstrated that molecular size as well as partition coefficient was a factor in determining the rapidity of entry into the cell. In general smaller molecules such as methanol, ethanol, and water were found to penetrate more rapidly then would have been expected based on their partition coefficients alone, while the passage of very large molecules was hindered.

Following these classic studies on plant cell models, a series of publications by Brodie, Schanker, Hogben, and their co-workers established that the rate constants for transport of a number of drugs across the intestinal wall were roughly correlated with the partition coefficients of the drugs (Hogben et al., 1959; Schanker et al., 1958; Shore et al., 1957). Subsequently, detailed studies by this group demonstrated that the same correlation existed for transfer from plasma into brain (Mayer et al., 1959) and into cerebrospinal fluid (Brodie et al., 1960). Table 3.1 demonstrates the rough proportionality between the first-order rate constant for transfer into cerebrospinal fluid and the heptane-water partition coefficients of the uncharged forms of some of the drugs shown in Figure 3.3.

Still more recent work has established that a large number of drugs including antipyrine, pentobarbital, phenobarbital, salicylic acid, procaine amide, and several antibiotics are absorbed from the rat lung at rates that correlate with their chloroform-water partition coefficients (Enna and Schanker, 1972; Burton and Schanker, 1974). Similarly, the uptake rates of a series of lipophilic amides by human and canine erythrocytes were found to be proportional in magnitude to the amides' ether-water partition coefficients (Figure 3.4) (Sha'afi et al., 1971).

Figure 3.4 illustrates two additional points that are important in connection with diffusion across membranes. First, there are marked differences in the ease with which the same substance can penetrate corresponding membranes of different species. Thickness and lipid composition of membranes, which affect the permeability of the membrane itself, are highly variable with species. Clearly the erythrocyte membrane of the dog is much more permeable to diffusion by this series of amides than is that of man. Species-related differences in diffusion rate constants are common (Jacobs and Glassman, 1937). Where they exist, they are reflected in species-related differences in overall pharmacokinetic behavior.

The second point to note in connection with Figure 3.4 is that valeramide and butyramide behave differently from their branched chain analogues

**Table 3.1** Partition coefficients and transfer rate constants for selected drugs

| Drug | Heptane-Water Partition Coefficient of Un-Ionized Form of Drug | Transfer Rate Constant $(min^{-1})$ |
|---|---|---|
| Thiopental | 3.3 | 0.50 |
| Aniline | 1.1 | 0.40 |
| Aminopyrine | 0.21 | 0.25 |
| Pentobarbital | 0.05 | 0.17 |
| Antipyrine | 0.005 | 0.12 |
| Barbital | 0.002 | 0.026 |
| N-Acetyl-4-aminoantipyrine | 0.001 | 0.012 |
| Sulfaguanidine | $<0.001$ | 0.003 |

From Brodie et al., 1960, Table 2.

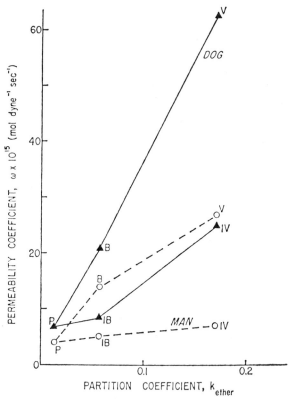

**Figure 3.4** Relationship between permeability coefficient and partition coefficient for lipophilic amides in red cell membranes of man and dog: P, propionamide; B, butyramide; V, valeramide; IB, isobutyramide; IV, isovaleramide. Reproduced from Sha'afi et al., 1971, Figure 4, by copyright permission of the Rockefeller University Press.

isovaleramide and isobutyramide in both species; propionamide falls on both lines. This observation is considered further in the next subsection.

### Molecular Size

It has already been pointed out that very small molecules diffuse more rapidly, and very large molecules more slowly, than consideration of their partition coefficients alone would suggest. Within a homologous series of organic compounds of reasonable size, the diffusion rate constant may well increase with molecular weight as the lengthening carbon chain confers increasing lipophilicity on the molecule. However, the effect of lipophilicity on transfer rate is less pronounced for large than for small molecules. The effect of molecular size can be demonstrated by relating the quotient

$$\frac{\text{transfer rate constant}}{\text{partition coefficient}}$$

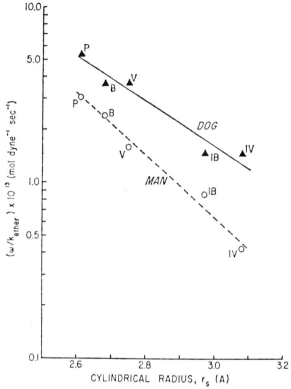

**Figure 3.5** Permeability of red cells of man and dog to lipophilic amides as a function of the cylindrical radius of the solute. Symbols as in Figure 3.4. Reproduced from Sha'afi et al., 1971, Figure 5, by copyright permission of the Rockefeller University Press.

to molecular radius. When this is done for the homologous series of lipophilic amides in Figure 3.4, the dependence of diffusion rate on molecular size is clearly apparent (Figure 3.5). Larger molecules are retarded in their passage through membranes by frictional resistance and, in the case of branched chain compounds such as isobutyrate and isovalerate, by steric hindrance as well.

Very small molecules are likely to be more polar (less lipophilic) than their larger congeners. Small molecules with a significant degree of hydrophilicity may move through membrane pores. Pores, or channels, exist in all membranes. Water, essential inorganic ions such as sodium and potassium, and small organic molecules such as methanol, ethanol, and urea are able to pass freely through these aqueous membrane channels. Water-soluble molecules whose diameters exceed about $4 \times 10^{-4}$ $\mu$m, however, are in general excluded from the cell interior unless, like the essential sugars and amino acids, they are transported by specialized mechanisms.

Blood capillary walls are composed of endothelial cells whose junctions allow the passage of water-soluble molecules larger than $4 \times 10^{-4}$ $\mu$m in diameter. Permeability of the capillary wall to larger water-soluble molecules suggests that its pores are of the order of $30 \times 10^{-4}$ $\mu$m in diameter. Water-soluble molecules having radii greater than about $30 \times 10^{-4}$ $\mu$m (or having molecular weights greater than about 60,000) are generally excluded from transcapillary passage. For molecules whose radii are less than $30 \times 10^{-4}$ $\mu$m, the rate of transcapillary movement is inversely proportional to the spherical radius of the molecule, as originally shown by Pappenheimer and his co-workers (1951, 1953). Table 3.2 gives the molecular weight, the radius of a sphere equivalent in its physical behavior to the molecule in question, the diffusion coefficient (for free diffusion; $D$ in the statement of Fick's law), and the capillary permeability of a series of water-soluble molecules of increasing size. Clearly permeability of the capillary wall to molecules in this series is not directly proportional to the free diffusion coefficients of these molecules. The decrease in permeability with increasing molecular size and weight is much greater than would be expected on the basis of the diffusion coefficients alone, suggesting that mechanical hindrance is an important factor influencing the rates of transfer of hydrophilic as well as of lipophilic compounds.

To illustrate this point Pappenheimer developed the concept of restricted pore area, the capillary surface area that would be required to allow observed transfer rates if transfer were not restricted by molecular size. Restricted pore area is dependent on the substance being transferred. The dependence of restricted pore area on molecular radius (of an equivalent sphere) is shown in

**Table 3.2**  Molecular weight and size, free diffusion coefficient, and capillary permeability for selected water-soluble compounds

| Molecule | Radius of Equivalent Sphere (Å) | Molecular Weight | $D \times 10^5$ (cm$^2$/sec) | Capillary Permeability (cm$^3$/sec/100 g, Perfused Hind Leg of Cat) |
|---|---|---|---|---|
| (Water) | (1) | 18 | 3.20 | 3.7 |
| NaCl | 1.4 | 58 | 1.53 | 2.2 |
| Urea | 1.6 | 60 | 1.95 | 1.83 |
| Glucose | 3.6 | 180 | 0.91 | 0.64 |
| Sucrose | 4.4 | 342 | 0.74 | 0.35 |
| Raffinose | 5.6 | 594 | 0.56 | 0.24 |
| Inulin | 15.2 | 5,500 | 0.21 | 0.036 |
| Myoglobin | 19.0 | 17,000 | 0.15 | 0.005 |
| Hemoglobin | 31.0 | 68,000 | 0.094 | 0.001 |
| Serum albumin | | 69,000 | 0.085 | 0.000 |

From Pappenheimer, 1953, Table 2; Pappenheimer et al., 1951, Table 5; and Renkin, 1964, Table 1.

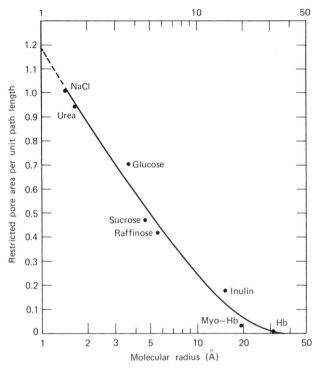

**Figure 3.6** Restricted diffusion as a function of molecular size in the capillary circulation of the perfused hind leg of the cat. The molecule is considered to be a sphere of equivalent diffusion coefficient. Restricted pore area is given per unit path length in capillaries of 100 g of muscle. Reproduced with permission from Pappenheimer, 1953, Figure 4.

Figure 3.6. Note that capillary pore size prevents the passage of albumin and hemoglobin as well as of all larger proteins out of the blood (see Table 3.2).

There is variability in capillary permeability with tissue. Glomerular capillaries and the capillaries in the liver are especially permeable to large molecules. Brain capillaries, in contrast, are surrounded by a sheath of closely juxtaposed glial cells. Water-soluble molecules leaving the systemic circulation and entering the brain exhibit transfer rates consistent with the premise that transfer across the glial cell membranes, not through capillary pores, is the rate-determining step.

### Degree of Ionization

The ionized forms of most exogenous materials fall into the class of compounds that cannot cross cell membrane walls either by diffusion or through aqueous channels, although they may be able to pass through the pores of the capillary wall. As a result of his studies of artificial model membranes, Osterhout (1925, 1933) was the first to propose that electrolytes diffuse through membranes only in their un-ionized forms. This principle is now firmly established. Ionized drug forms are hydrophilic rather than lipophilic. They tend to be highly solvated (surrounded by "cages" of water molecules), and their partition coefficients are very low. Diffusion of a partially ionized drug can be considered in terms of diffusion of the un-ionized form alone. Therefore the rate of diffusion of a partially ionized drug and its total concentrations at steady state across a membrane are dependent on the pH's of the fluids on both sides of the membrane. The effect of pH is on the concentration gradient of the diffusing or un-ionized species, not on the rate constant for its diffusion.

The degree of ionization of an acidic or basic drug is related to the pH of the medium in which it is dissolved by the Henderson-Hasselbalch equation:

$$\mathrm{pH} = \mathrm{p}K_a + \log \frac{\text{base form}}{\text{acid form}}, \tag{3.4}$$

where $\mathrm{p}K_a$ is the negative logarithm of the acid dissociation constant:

$$K_a = \frac{(\mathrm{H}^+)(\mathrm{A}^-)}{(\mathrm{HA})} \qquad \text{for an acid}$$

$$K_a = \frac{(\mathrm{H}^+)(\mathrm{B})}{(\mathrm{HB}^+)} \qquad \text{for a base.}$$

At a pH equal to its $\mathrm{p}K_a$ the drug will be 50% ionized. At pH's above the $\mathrm{p}K_a$ more drug will exist in the base form ($\mathrm{A}^-$ or B) than in the acid form; at pH's below the $\mathrm{p}K_a$ more drug will be in the acid form (HA or $\mathrm{HB}^+$) than in the base form. Acidic drugs therefore will diffuse more rapidly at low than at high pH, and basic drugs more rapidly at high than at low pH, since correspondingly more of the drugs will be in the un-ionized forms capable of diffusion.

Marked pH differences are maintained between the systemic blood and the contents of the gastrointestinal tract, from which exogenous compounds are absorbed into the blood and into which they may be excreted. The pH of the blood is about 7.4. The pH of the gastrointestinal tract increases from the range 1–3 in the stomach (variable with the amount and quality of food ingested) to 5–7 in the upper small intestine, to as much as 8 in the lower small intestine and colon.

Schanker et al. (1958) found that weakly acidic ($\mathrm{p}K_a > 3$) and weakly basic ($\mathrm{p}K_a < 7.8$) drugs were readily absorbed from the rat small intestine, where the pH of the absorbing surface was estimated to be about 5.3 (Hogben et al., 1959). These data are graphed in Figure 3.7. When the pH of the intestinal contents was raised through the range 4–8 by perfusing the small intestine *in situ* with strongly buffered solutions of the drugs, the absorption of acidic drugs was decreased and that of basic drugs was increased (Table 3.3).

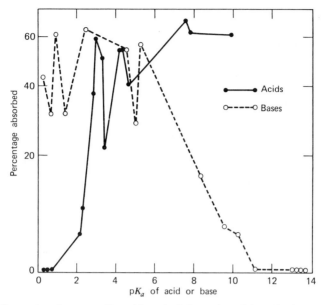

**Figure 3.7** Comparison between $pK_a$ and intestinal absorption of drugs in the rat. Reproduced with permission from Schanker et al., 1964, Figure 4, © 1964 by Academic Press Inc. (London) Ltd.

**Table 3.3** Intestinal absorption of drugs from solutions of various pH values

| | | Percentage Absorbed[a] | | | |
|---|---|---|---|---|---|
| | | pH of the Intestinal Solution | | | |
| Drug | $pKa$ | 3.6–4.3 | 4.7–5.0 | 7.2–7.1 | 8.0–7.8 |
| **Bases** | | | | | |
| Aniline | 4.6 | 40±7 (9) | 48±5 (5) | 58±5 (4) | 61±8 (10) |
| Aminopyrine | 5.0 | 21±1 (2) | 35±1 (2) | 48±2 (2) | 52±2 (2) |
| p-Toluidine | 5.3 | 30±3 (3) | 12±3 (2) | 65±4 (3) | 64±4 (2) |
| Quinine | 8.4 | 9±3 (3) | 11±2 (2) | 41±1 (2) | 54±5 (4) |
| **Acids** | | | | | |
| 5-Nitrosalicyclic | 2.3 | 40±0 (2) | 27±2 (2) | <2 (2) | <2 (2) |
| Salicylic | 3.0 | 64±4 (4) | 35±4 (2) | 30±4 (2) | 10±3 (6) |
| Acetylsalicylic | 3.5 | 41±3 (2) | 27±1 (2) | — | — |
| Benzoic | 4.2 | 62±4 (2) | 36±3 (4) | 35±4 (3) | 5±1 (2) |
| p-Hydroxypropiophenone | 7.8 | 61±5 (3) | 52±2 (2) | 67±6 (5) | 60±5 (2) |

From Hogben et al., 1959, Table 1, © 1959 by the Williams & Wilkins Co., Baltimore.

[a] Expressed as the mean ± the range; figures in parentheses indicate number of animals.

Excretion of drugs into the gastric juice from the plasma is similarly dependent on their dissociation constants. Strong acids are poorly excreted, weak acids and bases fairly rapidly excreted, and strong bases very rapidly excreted (Shore et al., 1957). Conversely, strong acids and very weak bases are well absorbed from the stomach, whereas strong bases are not (Hogben et al., 1957).

Partitioning of drugs across the gastric mucosa is frequently used as an illustration of the effect of pH gradients on the transmembrane diffusion of ionizable compounds. It is a particularly vivid example because the pH difference across the gastric mucosa is so great. Consider the partitioning across the blood-gastric interface of salicylic acid, an acid with a $pK_a$ of 3.0, and of quinine, a base with a $pK_a$ of about 8. (Since the capillary wall is porous, it is presumably the membranes of the epithelial cells lining the stomach that determine the rates of absorption and secretion.) The physical situation is diagrammed in Figure 3.8.

In the plasma there will be 10,000 molecules of salicylate for every molecule of salicylic acid:

$$7 - 3 = \log \frac{\text{salicylate}}{\text{salicylic acid}} = 4,$$

whereas in the gastric contents there will be 100 molecules of salicyclic acid for every molecule of salicylate:

$$1 - 3 = -2 = \log \frac{\text{salicylate}}{\text{salicylic acid}}.$$

At steady state across the membrane barrier the concentrations of the diffusing species, un-ionized salicylic acid, will be equal but the total drug concentrations will not (Figure 3.9). Of a total of 1,000,201 molecules of drug, 1,000,100 or 99.99%, will be present in the plasma. It is clear that salicylic acid will be readily absorbed from the stomach but poorly excreted into the stomach.

For the basic drug quinine the situation is reversed. In the plasma there will be 10 molecules of the acid or ionized form of the drug for every

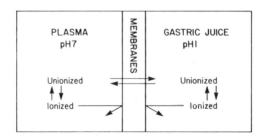

**Figure 3.8**  Model for partitioning across the gastric mucosa.

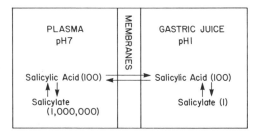

**Figure 3.9** Partitioning of salicylic acid across the gastric mucosa.

molecule of uncharged quinine:

$$7-8=-1=\log\frac{\text{quinine}}{\text{quinine H}^+},$$

whereas in the gastric juice there will be 10,000,000 molecules of the ionized form for every molecule of quinine:

$$1-8=-7=\log\frac{\text{quinine}}{\text{quinine H}^+}.$$

Again, the concentrations of quinine across the membrane interface will be equal at steady state but the total drug concentrations will not, as shown in Figure 3.10. Of a total of 10,000,012 molecules of quinine, 10,000,001 will be present in the gastric contents at steady state.

Passive renal reabsorption from forming urine (see Section 4.5) is strongly dependent on urinary pH. Urine pH can be manipulated within the limited range of 5–8 to alter drug excretion. Administration of bicarbonate promotes the excretion of acidic drugs both by causing a very slight shift from tissues to blood (blood is highly buffered and its pH changes only a fraction of a unit) and by decreasing reabsorption from the more alkaline urine. At the same time reabsorption of basic drugs is increased. For example, the renal clearance of tocainide (see Section 3.13), a primary amine, in adult males is 50 ml/min. When bicarbonate is given to maintain urine pH at $\geqslant 7.4$, renal

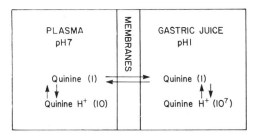

**Figure 3.10** Partitioning of quinine across the gastric mucosa.

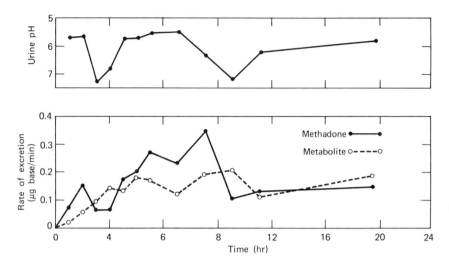

**Figure 3.11** Influence of urine pH on rate of excretion of methadone and of its metabolite after oral administration of 5 mg of methadone to a human subject. Adapted with permission from Baselt and Casarett, 1972, Figure 3.

reabsorption is greatly enhanced and renal clearance of tocainide drops to 13 ml/min (Lalka et al., 1976). On the other hand, acidification of the urine with ammonium chloride impairs the reabsorption of bases and therefore increases their rate of excretion. An example of this behavior is shown in Figure 3.11. Methadone, used as a heroin substitute in the treatment of heroin addiction, is a weak base with a $pK_a$ of 8.6. As Figure 3.11 shows, normal variations in urine pH have a marked influence on the rate of methadone excretion. Increases in urine pH are associated with decreases in methadone excretion rate. On the other hand, the rate of excretion of the measured methadone metabolite is affected little if at all by urine pH.

The metabolite, an *N*-demethylated compound, has sufficiently greater polarity than its parent that it is a very weak acid with a $pK_a$ of 10.4. At pH 7 it would be 99.96% in the un-ionized form:

$$7 = 10.4 + \log\frac{\text{metabolite-}}{\text{metabolite}} \quad \text{and} \quad \frac{\text{metabolite}}{\text{metabolite-}} = 2500;$$

and at pH 6 it would be more than 99.99% in the un-ionized form:

$$6 = 10.4 + \log\frac{\text{metabolite-}}{\text{metabolite}} \quad \text{and} \quad \frac{\text{metabolite}}{\text{metabolite-}} = 25,000.$$

The metabolite is such a weak acid that at these pH's virtually all of it is present in the undissociated or diffusible form, so that a pH change within the urinary pH range has little effect on it.

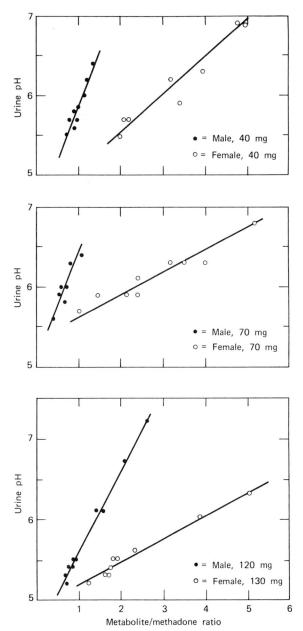

**Figure 3.12** Urinary concentration ratio of metabolite to methadone as a function of urine pH in three male and three female subjects taking 40, 70, or 120 or 130 mg of methadone daily. Reproduced with permission from Baselt and Casarett, 1972, Figure 5.

If metabolite reabsorption is independent of pH while reabsorption of parent methadone is favored at higher urine pH's, it is to be expected that the ratio of metabolite to methadone in excreted urine will be directly dependent on urine pH. Figure 3.12 shows that this expectation is correct. Note the clear-cut difference between males and females.

Of course, ionizable compounds will not actually be in a steady state across body membrane interfaces. Both the pH difference across the membrane and the flow rates of the body fluids in which an ionizable drug or toxicant is dissolved and carried past the membrane will affect the concentration gradient of the diffusible or un-ionized molecular species. Therefore net transfer will be dependent on flow rates as well as on pH and $pK_a$. If flow rates are not rapid, or if approximately constant total concentrations can be maintained artificially in a rapidly flowing body fluid such as blood, a steady state may be approached and the amount actually transferred will be a good index of the steady state behavior of the compound. On the other hand, if rapid flow should effectively clear all transferred material immediately from the area of the transfer site, the amount transferred will be controlled only by the amount of diffusible material available to be transferred and by the physical factors that determine the transfer rate constant. In the next section we consider the body as a single compartment and examine the kinetic behavior of a compound that is transferred out of that compartment by a first-order process and immediately cleared from the transfer site area.

## 3.3   THE ONE-COMPARTMENT BODY MODEL

In the human body true equilibrium conditions do not exist. Indeed, true equilibrium conditions would not be compatible with survival. Nutrients are continually being absorbed and utilized either for energy production or storage or for structural needs. The child grows, the adult gains or loses weight (or both, sequentially), and compartment volumes fluctuate accordingly. Drugs and toxicants are absorbed, transformed, and eliminated. A dynamic steady state, in which there is no change in the quantity but there is a change in the identity of the solute molecules of a particular type present in the system, may or may not be reached at any time during the passage of a foreign compound through the body.

In the two-compartment microsystem described in Section 3.1, suppose that $C_2$ is and remains effectively zero during the transfer process. Physiologically this is not as unreasonable as it may sound at first: it describes such common processes as rapid transport away from an absorption site, excretion in exhaled air, or irreversible loss into the urine. Let us consider the situation in which a drug is eliminated through the kidney by filtration without reabsorption. The model is schematically simple (Figure 3.13). It is a linear one-compartment open model: linear because all the rate processes characterizing it are first order; open because there is loss from the system; and

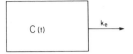

Figure 3.13 The linear one-compartment open model.

obviously it includes only one compartment. $k_e$ is the overall rate constant for elimination. Since excretion is an essentially irreversible process, $C_2$ is in fact zero in this model. The form of the symbol for concentration within the compartment indicates that concentration is a function of time.

Note that there is no arrow for input into the system. For the time being we will consider that the input process is infinitely rapid; therefore, it has been completed before we take any measurements. Another way of stating this assumption is that mixing of drug within the single compartment is instantaneous and homogeneous. We will relax this limitation in Section 3.10; however, absorption is frequently very much faster than elimination and, of course, materials administered intravenously are very rapidly, although not instantaneously, admixed with the blood.

Note also that it is implicit in this discussion of diffusion that the substance diffusing is present in true solution in body fluids. Section 3.4 discusses briefly some of the effects of binding to plasma proteins, but detailed consideration of the consequences of binding to plasma or tissue proteins or sequestration in intracellular fat is deferred until Chapter 4.

When $C_2$ is zero the statement of Fick's first law (Equation 3.3) becomes

$$\frac{dC(t)}{dt} = -k_e C(t) \tag{3.5}$$

or

$$\frac{dC}{C} = -k_e \, dt. \tag{3.6}$$

Integrating, and applying the boundary condition that $C = C_0$ at $t_0$, we find that

$$C = C_o e^{-k_e t} \tag{3.7}$$

or

$$\ln C = \ln C_0 - k_e t. \tag{3.8}$$

Equation 3.7 states that when the concentration $C$ of drug in the blood is measured at convenient time intervals and graphed against time $t$, it will be found to decay exponentially. The amount of drug remaining in the body will decline smoothly with time as shown in Figure 3.14.

How rapidly will the amount of drug remaining in the body decline? It is obvious that the disappearance of drug is faster when $k_e$ is larger. After all, $k_e$

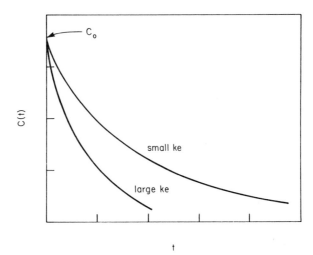

**Figure 3.14**   Concentration, time plots for the linear one-compartment open model with large and small $k_e$.

represents the only way out of the compartment, and the bigger the door, the more rapid the escape of drug. Therefore we would like to be able to estimate $k_e$. The only way to estimate $k_e$ from data graphed as in Figure 3.14 is to approximate the tangent to the curve at some concentration (any concentration) $C$, since Equation 3.6 states that $k_e = -(dC/dt)/C$.

Now how is $C_0$ to be estimated? At time zero, $e^{-k_e t} = 1$ and $C = C_0$. But since a measurement cannot be made at time zero, the only way to estimate $C_0$ is to extrapolate the dieaway curve to the ordinate. Both the extrapolation of a curve and the estimation of a tangent to that curve are uncertain operations strongly subject to bias. Therefore the form of Equation 3.7 is not very useful.

Equation 3.8, however, states that if the same concentration data are graphed semilogarithmically against time, the graph will be a straight line with ordinate intercept $\ln C_0$ and slope $-k_e$ as shown in Figure 3.15a. Since slopes and intercepts of straight lines are readily calculable by utilizing standard statistical methods, Equation 3.8 is to be preferred to Equation 3.7.

The elimination of a reasonable number of foreign compounds does seem to conform to the predictions of a simple one compartment open model. One example is shown in Figure 3.15b, from a study by Bradley and Bond (1975). The toxicity to mice of lipopolysaccharide (LPS) isolated from the bacterium *E. coli* was investigated with and without coadministration of pactamycin, an antibiotic that enhances LPS toxicity. It had been proposed among other possible mechanisms for this synergism that pactamycin might delay the disappearance of LPS from the blood. The data in Figure 3.15b clearly rule out this possibility.

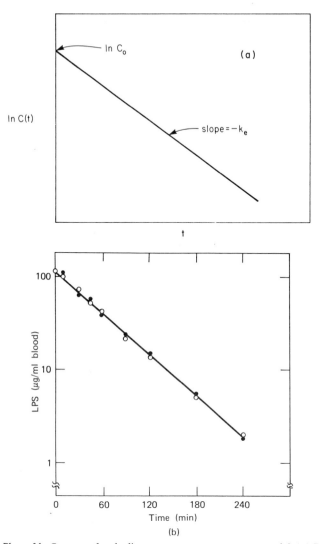

**Figure 3.15** Plots of $\ln C$ versus $t$ for the linear one-compartment open model. (*a*) Predicted. (*b*) Observed clearance of *E. coli* lipopolysaccharide (LPS) from blood of mice injected intravenously with 1 mg LPS/kg alone (○) or together with 2 mg of pactamycin/kg (●). (*b*) Reproduced with permission from Bradley and Bond, 1975, Figure 2.

### 3.4  HALF-LIFE AND VOLUME OF DISTRIBUTION IN THE ONE-COMPARTMENT BODY MODEL

Only two parameters are required to define a straight line. In Figure 3.15*b* the ordinate intercept is $\ln C_0$, from which $C_0$ is seen to be somewhat greater than 100 μg LPS per milliliter of blood; and the slope is $-k_e$, from which $k_e$ can be estimated to be about 0.014 min$^{-1}$. $k_e$ is called a microscopic rate constant, or microconstant, because it is associated with a single specific process. Later on we shall see that not all kinetically determined rate constants are microconstants.

Two additional (but not independent) pieces of information can also be extracted from Figure 3.15$b$. When $C = C_0/2$, by substituting in Equation 3.8 we can calculate that

$$\ln C_0 - \ln 2 = \ln C_0 - k_e t_{1/2}$$

where the subscript designates $t_{1/2}$ as the half-life, the time required for the concentration to drop to half its initial value $C_0$.

$$t_{1/2} = \frac{\ln 2}{k_e} = \frac{0.693}{k_e}. \tag{3.9}$$

The half-life, like $k_e$, is independent of the dose and of the time period of measurement. It can easily be read directly from a semilogarithmic plot. For example, by inspection of Figure 3.15$b$ it is apparent that the blood concentration of LPS falls to half its initial value in 50 min. Irrespective of where on the straight line the estimate is made, the half-life will be 50 min. $k_e$ can usually be determined more easily from the half-life than by calculating the slope of the line. In this case

$$k_e = \frac{0.693}{t_{1/2}} = \frac{0.693}{50 \text{ min}} = 0.014 \text{ min}^{-1}.$$

The half-life is an important parameter. It is used more often than $k_e$ to characterize the kinetics of elimination, although the two parameters give identical information. The special utility of the half-life lies in its more obvious physical significance. It is immediately meaningful to be told that the half-life of LPS is 50 min. We can (almost) instantaneously estimate that 75% of the LPS will be gone in 100 min, $87\frac{1}{2}\%$ in 150 min, and so on. To be told that $k_e$ for LPS is 0.014 min$^{-1}$ is less immediately illuminating.

The second additional useful piece of information is the magnitude of the volume of distribution. The ordinate intercept of a semilogarithmic concentration, time graph can be used to estimate the volume of distribution $V_d$ whenever the total dose $D$ is known, since

$$\frac{D}{V_d} = C_0. \tag{3.10}$$

Of course $D$ must represent the quantity of material actually present in solution in the compartment, which is not necessarily equivalent to the total dose administered. Compounds inhaled or given orally are almost never completely absorbed; if fully absorbed, they may be metabolized and/or excreted before they even reach the systemic circulation. Compounds injected intravenously enter the systemic circulation directly, but they may not be in solution in plasma water. When the volume of distribution is estimated, it is assumed that the compound is uniformly in solution throughout that volume, which is not necessarily the case for materials carried by the plasma. Highly lipophilic compounds may travel with the lipid subfraction of the plasma, which is only about 0.4% of total plasma weight. Polar exogenous compounds such as drugs are transported bound to plasma proteins, particularly to albumin. In the initial steps of many assays for materials present in the plasma proteins are precipitated, releasing bound materials. The contribution of this bound fraction causes the measured concentration of the compound in plasma fluid to be higher than the *in vivo* concentration. This, of course, in turn causes the apparent volume of distribution to be smaller than the real volume. It is not at all uncommon for as much as 80% of a drug to be bound to plasma proteins. Binding of this magnitude has a very large effect on the apparent volume of distribution. If a drug is 80% bound, its apparent volume of distribution—assuming that both bound and free drug were measured experimentally—would be only one-fifth the actual volume. If binding to plasma proteins is suspected, its magnitude can be estimated in a separate *in vitro* experiment and the measured plasma concentrations corrected accordingly.

Provided $D$ is known with certainty and the concentration of the compound in plasma water has been determined, $V_d = D/C_0$, and $V_D$ is a real volume. This relationship has been used to advantage in classical physiology. Model compounds, selected for their solubility and diffusional attributes, have been used for the estimation of body water volumes. Evans blue, a large molecular weight dye that does not traverse capillary or red cell membranes, is used to determine plasma water volume. Sodium and chloride ions, which are largely excluded from the cell interior, have been used to determine extracellular fluid volume. Highly lipophilic materials diffuse readily across most membranes and can be used to estimate total body water.

For example, Soberman et al. (1949) compared total body water volume estimates in human subjects given both the drug antipyrine and deuterium oxide intravenously. Distribution of deuterium oxide, or heavy water, into total body water is complete within about an hour, after which its behavior presumably cannot be distinguished from that of the water with which it is admixed. Plasma deuterium oxide concentrations were measured at 2, 3, and 5 hr after intravenous administration of 50 g of deuterium oxide, and the three estimates were averaged. Body water volume was calculated as 50 g/average $D_2O$ concentration in plasma. Antipyrine also penetrates all body water subcompartments rapidly, equilibrating in total body water within an hour and a half and undergoing only negligible excretion. However, the plasma concentration of antipyrine must be corrected for its slow metabolism. Accordingly plasma antipyrine concentrations were measured at 2, 3, and

**Table 3.4**  Total body water in normal subjects determined by antipyrine and by deuterium oxide ($D_2O$) dilution

| Subject Number | Sex | Weight (kg) | Total Body Water-Antipyrine (liters) | Total Body Water-$D_2O$ (liters) |
|:---:|:---:|:---:|:---:|:---:|
| 1 | F | 45.0 | 22.2 | 22.6 |
| 2 | F | 73.4 | 28.8 | 30.8 |
| 3 | M | 66.5 | 34.2 | 35.8 |
| 4 | M | 69.5 | 35.0 | 33.4 |
| 5 | M | 70.0 | 39.9 | 39.8 |
| 6 | M | 52.2 | 28.7 | 28.8 |
| 7 | M | 55.5 | 30.5 | 33.6 |
| 8 | M | 49.1 | 28.4 | 29.2 |

Adapted from Soberman et al., 1949, Table V.

5 hr after administration of 1 g of antipyrine and back-extrapolated to time zero (assuming first-order metabolism) to obtain $C_0$. Body water volume was calculated as $1 \text{ g}/C_0$. Table 3.4 shows that in eight normal subjects the agreement between total body water estimates obtained by the two methods was excellent.

In the study represented in Figure 3.15b the average dose of LPS injected intravenously was 24 $\mu$g. Since the initial concentration was about 105 $\mu$g of LPS per milliliter of blood, the volume of distribution is estimated to be $24\mu$g of LPS/$105 \ \mu$g/ml $= 0.23$ ml. This volume is unrealistically small even for a 24-g mouse, which should have a blood volume of about 1.7 ml and a plasma water volume of about 1.0 ml. LPS is a complex molecule containing both lipid and polysaccharide components and possessing antigenic properties. It is entirely reasonable that it should travel in association with plasma proteins, as the low apparent volume of distribution suggests that it does.

## 3.5  HOW TO ESTIMATE KINETIC PARAMETERS USING THE ONE-COMPARTMENT BODY MODEL

### 3.5.1  From Plasma Data

It is apparent from the development in Section 3.4 that the plasma concentration of a compound may be determined periodically and graphed semilogarithmically against time to estimate the two independent parameters $k_e$ and $C_0$, which define the kinetic expression describing a one-compartment open system. Although the blood is certainly more accessible than other tissues, it is not always as useful as might be wished. Small laboratory animals may not have enough blood to support the repetitive closely spaced monitoring required for a good kinetic study, even if the assay used is so sensitive that only a small volume of blood need be taken. On the other hand, if the assay used is not especially sensitive it may not be possible to detect the compound in the plasma after a short time, even in the larger laboratory animals and in humans, from whom relatively large volumes of blood can be taken repeatedly. In addition, the prospect of repeated blood sampling is not particularly appealing to human subjects. Therefore it is fortunate that there are other less intrusive methods of estimating kinetic parameters.

### 3.5.2    From Cumulative Excretion Data

Whenever for one reason or another it is not convenient to sample plasma, cumulative excretion may be measurable. Let us suppose that the compound is excreted exclusively in the urine and let us call the total amount excreted after an infinite amount of time $U_\infty$. $U_\infty$ is, of course, equal to the dose $D$. Then $U_\infty - U$ is the amount yet to be excreted at time $t$. It is equal to $B$, the amount in the body at time $t$, where $B = CV_D$. Therefore,

$$(U_\infty - U) = B = V_D C_0 e^{-k_e t} \tag{3.11}$$

and

$$\ln(U_\infty - U) = \ln(V_D C_0) - k_e t, \tag{3.12}$$

and a graph of $\ln(U_\infty - U)$ against time will be a straight line with intercept $\ln(V_D C_0)$ and slope $-k_e$ as shown in Figure 3.16a.

This technique allows $k_e$, but not $V_D$, to be estimated. It is straightforward and precise, and is commonly used in investigations both with humans and with laboratory animals. It may be applied to data from any measurable route of excretion. An example of its application is shown in Figure 3.16b, from a study by Nelson and O'Reilly (1960).

Sulfisoxazole, a sulfonamide, is excreted solely into the urine. A single oral dose of 850 mg of sulfisoxazole was administered to human volunteers and total urine output was collected for the following 72 hr, by which time little or no detectable sulfisoxazole was present. The total amount $U_\infty$ of sulfioxazole excreted and the amount $U$ excreted by time $t$ were calculated by multiplying the measured concentration of sulfisoxazole in each urine sample by the sample volume and summing the results. A semilogarithmic graph of $(U_\infty - U)$ against time is shown in Figure 3.16b for one of the subjects. The data demonstrate excellent fit to a straight line that intersects the ordinate at a point corresponding to 850 mg, the total dose. It is apparent that the total dose was absorbed. The negative slope of the line is 0.082 hr$^{-1}$, indicating that the half-life of sulfisoxazole in this subject is 8.5 hr.

Although this technique has the advantages of simplicity and precision, its proper application requires that $U_\infty$ be known with assurance. If a urine sample is missed or lost, or if sampling is not carried far enough in time, it

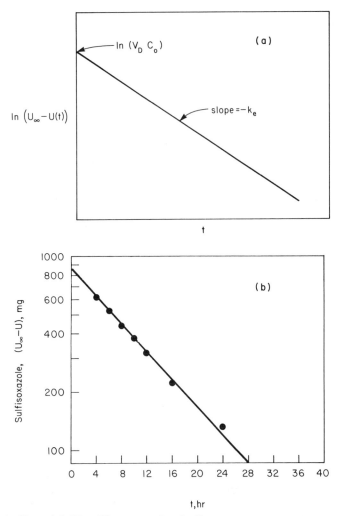

**Figure 3.16** Plots of $\ln(U_\infty - U)$ versus $t$ for the linear one-compartment open model. (*a*) Predicted. (*b*) Observed ln (amount of unexcreted sulfisoxazole) against time following oral administration of 850 mg of sulfisoxazole to a human subject. Data from Nelson and O'Reilly, 1960, Table 1.

cannot be used. The next technique does not have this drawback, but it is less precise.

### 3.5.3  From Excretory Rate Data

If $U_\infty$ is not known, the *rate* of urinary excretion may be approximated by measuring the amounts of the compound contained in sequential timed urine fractions. From Equation 3.11,

$$U = U_\infty - V_D C_0 e^{-k_e t} = V_D C_0 (1 - e^{-k_e t}). \qquad (3.13)$$

Differentiating to obtain the rate of excretion into the urine at time $t$,

$$\frac{dU}{dt} = k_e V_D C_0 e^{-k_e t},$$     (3.14)

or

$$\ln\left(\frac{dU}{dt}\right) = \ln(k_e V_D C_0) - k_e t.$$     (3.15)

Although $dU/dt$ is not measurable experimentally, it may be approximated by $\Delta U/\Delta t$, the amount $\Delta U$ excreted during a small time interval $\Delta t$. The graph of $\ln(\Delta U/\Delta t)$ against time should approximate a straight line whose intercept is $\ln(k_e V_D C_0)$ and whose slope is $-k_e$. In practice the concentration of the compound is measured in aliquots of timed urine samples and multiplied by the sample volume to estimate $\Delta U$. $\Delta U/\Delta t$ is calculated and plotted semilogarithmically against time, where $t$ is taken as the *midpoint* of $\Delta t$.

This technique can also be used to estimate kinetic parameters using data from any measurable route of excretion. An example is given in Figure 3.17. Rat livers were perfused with D-tubocurarine, a neuromuscular blocking agent, in an artificial rat blood perfusate, and total bile was collected at 15-min intervals. Figure 3.17 shows the rate of excretion of D-tubocurarine

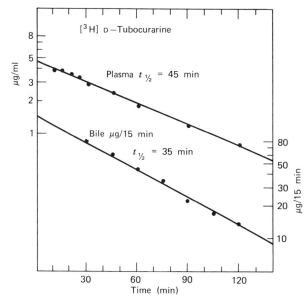

**Figure 3.17** Relationship of plasma D-tubocurarine (TC) and rate of TC excretion in bile to time during perfusion of rat livers with artificial rat blood containing TC. Points represent the means of data from four experiments. Reproduced from Meijer et al., 1976, Figure 3, © 1976 by the Williams & Wilkins Co., Baltimore.

into the bile, expressed as micrograms per 15-min period and plotted semi-logarithmically against time, as well as the concentrations of $D$-tubocurarine in the perfusate during the same time period. The ordinate intercept of the excretion rate line, $k_e V_D C_0$ or $k_e D$, is about 135 $\mu$g per 15 min. Since the total amount of $D$-tubocurarine dissolved in the perfusate was 600 $\mu$g,

$$k_e = \frac{135 \ \mu g / 15 \ \text{min}}{600 \ \mu g}$$

$$= 0.015 \ \text{min}^{-1},$$

from which

$$t_{1/2} = \frac{0.693}{0.015} \ \text{min} = 46 \ \text{min}.$$

This estimate of $t_{1/2}$ is actually in better agreement with the $t_{1/2}$ determined from plasma (perfusate) dieaway data, 45 min, than with the $t_{1/2}$ determined directly from the slope of the excretion rate line in Figure 3.17, 35 min.

Because of the degree of control possible in an *in vitro* experiment and the consequent steady rate of bile flow, the data in Figure 3.17 do not demonstrate the lack of precision usually characteristic of a semilogarithmic graph of excretion rate against time.

In this study the plasma data do not permit an accurate estimate of $V_D$. The ordinate intercept of the plasma line in Figure 3.17 suggests that $C_0$ is about 4.6 $\mu$g/ml, from which

$$V_D = \frac{600 \ \mu g}{4.6 \ \mu g / ml} = 130 \ \text{ml}.$$

But the plasma volume, an independent experimental variable, was actually 70 ml. The explanation of this discrepancy is that adsorption of $D$-tubocurarine onto the walls of the perfusion apparatus has effectively removed it from accessibility for plasma analysis. There is a rapidly established equilibrium between adsorbed and dissolved $D$-tubocurarine so that all the $D$-tubocurarine is available for biliary excretion; this is demonstrated by noting that use of the total dose to calculate $t_{1/2}$ from the excretion data gives a reasonable $t_{1/2}$ estimate.

Note that the effect on $V_D$ of adsorption onto the perfusion apparatus is in a direction opposite to the effect of binding to plasma proteins exemplified by the lipopolysaccharide study discussed in Section 3.4. To anticipate the effect of sequestration on $V_D$, the key question to ask is: What effect does this kind of sequestration have on measured concentrations? In the perfusion study with $D$-tubocurarine, measured concentrations were lower than they would have been in the absence of adsorption, although the total dose was available for excretion. Consequently the estimated $V_D$ is too large. In the lipopolysaccharide study, measured concentrations were higher than they would have been had protein-bound LPS not been freed during the analytical procedure; consequently the estimated $V_D$ is too small.

Even when $V_D$ does not represent a real volume of distribution it is still a useful proportionality constant relating concentration to dose. As such it can be used in subsequent calculations despite its lack of physiological significance. For example, in the $D$-tubocurarine study hepatic clearance would be estimated as $k_e V_D$, or

$$= (0.015 \text{ min}^{-1})(130 \text{ ml})$$

$$= 2.0 \text{ ml/min}.$$

This value is identical to the experimental value for hepatic clearance of $D$-tubocurarine calculated by multiplying the experimentally fixed flow of plasma through the liver (16.5 ml/min) by the experimentally determined extraction efficiency (12%). Clearance is discussed further in Section 3.13.

### 3.6 THE ONE-COMPARTMENT BODY MODEL WITH PARALLEL ELIMINATION PROCESSES

It is extremely unusual for a foreign material, particularly if it is an organic compound, to be eliminated by only one pathway. Materials relatively unaltered by metabolism may be excreted largely or occasionally even entirely by a single route. For example, cadmium is probably normally excreted almost exclusively through the bile, although kidney damage may permit its release into the urine. More commonly, and especially in the case of organic compounds, metabolic processes produce one or more metabolites whose polarity and stability differ from those of the parent compound and of the other metabolites. The various compounds may be excreted by any one or more of the possible excretory routes: into the urine, bile (feces), or expired air, or into the usually quantitatively less important excretions such as sweat, milk, skin, hair, or nails.

Let us suppose that a material is partly metabolized and partly excreted unchanged into the urine and the bile. The microconstants for these three distinct processes are $k_m$ (metabolism), $k_u$ (urine), and $k_b$ (bile). Schematically the model can be represented as in Figure 3.18. It is still a one-compartment open model with first-order elimination, but now the overall elimination constant $k_e$ is equal to the sum of the microconstants for the three parallel elimination processes, $k_u$, $k_m$, and $k_b$:

$$\frac{dC}{dt} = -k_e C = -(k_m + k_u + k_b)C. \tag{3.16}$$

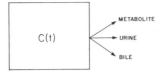

**Figure 3.18**  The linear one-compartment open model with parallel routes of elimination.

When only plasma concentration data for parent compound are available, then only $k_e$ and $V_D$ can be estimated, since as before

$$\ln C = \ln C_0 - k_e t. \tag{3.8}$$

But when the product of one of the parallel processes—urine concentration, for example—is measured, it must be remembered that the rate constant governing the transfer from plasma to urine is $k_u$ and *not* $k_e$:

$$\frac{dU}{dt} = k_u C V_D = k_u V_D C_0 e^{-k_e t}, \tag{3.17}$$

$$\ln\left(\frac{\Delta U}{\Delta t}\right) = \ln(k_u V_D C_0) - k_e t. \tag{3.18}$$

Integrating Equation 3.17, applying the boundary condition that $U=0$ at $t=0$, and substituting $U_\infty$ for its equivalent $k_u V_D C_0 / k_e$, we find that

$$U_\infty - U = \left(\frac{k_u V_D C_0}{k_e}\right) e^{-k_e t}, \tag{3.19}$$

$$\ln(U_\infty - U) = \ln\left(\frac{k_u V_D C_0}{k_e}\right) - k_e t. \tag{3.20}$$

Therefore graphs of either $\ln(U_\infty - U)$ or $\ln(\Delta U/\Delta t)$ against time are straight lines with slope $-k_e$. However, a graph of $\ln(\Delta U/\Delta t)$ against time intersects the ordinate at the point $\ln(k_u V_D C_0)$, whereas the corresponding intercept of a graph of $\ln(U_\infty - U)$ against time is $\ln(k_u V_D C_0 / k_e)$. Either graph can be used for the estimation of $k_e$ and, if $D$ is known, of $k_u$. Neither, of course, can be used to estimate $V_D$ unless $C_0$ is also known. Biliary excretion may be treated the same way to obtain $k_b$. The rate of appearance of metabolite within the model compartment may be used to obtain an estimate of $k_m$ only when excretion of metabolite is slow relative to its formation. Otherwise the methodology of Section 3.10 is more appropriate.

Another point is important in connection with the measurement of metabolite concentration within the model compartment. It cannot be assumed that the volume of distribution of the parent compound is necessarily the volume of distribution of the metabolite. As is suggested by Figure 3.18, transformation of parent compound into metabolite is equivalent to its exit from the single compartment. The metabolite enters its own volume of distribution, which probably is not congruent with the volume of distribution of its parent. Therefore metabolite plasma concentration measurements cannot be converted into amounts of metabolite unless the volume of distribution of the metabolite is known from independent measurements.

If metabolite is assayed in the urine, the situation is entirely different. It is then not known whether the constant estimated from the slope is actually $k_e$ or is $k_\mu^M$, the microconstant for excretion of metabolite into the urine. The slowest of any sequence of steps will control the overall rate; in this case, the rate of appearance of metabolite in the urine. If the rate constant for formation of metabolite is much larger than the rate constant for its excretion, the slopes of $\ln(\Delta U/\Delta t)$, $t$ and $\ln(U_\infty - U)$, $t$ graphs for metabolite will be $-k_u^M$ and the ordinate intercepts will also be related to $k_u^M$. If the rate constant for excretion of metabolite is much larger than the rate constant for its formation, the slopes of such graphs will be $-k_e$, and very little metabolite will accumulate within the system. In this case, the ordinate intercepts of the urinary excretion graphs will be related to $k_m$. If the relationship between the two rate constants $k_m$ and $k_u^M$ is intermediate between these two extremes, $\ln(U_\infty - U)$, $t$ and $\ln(\Delta U/\Delta t)$, $t$ graphs will not be linear unless formation of metabolite is rapid relative to the time the first measurement is taken.

It is not obvious intuitively why the slopes of graphs representing different processes should be identical. It is perhaps helpful to bear in mind that the rates of all the competing parallel processes are controlled by the quantity of material available for transfer and metabolism. This quantity, in turn, declines at a rate that is the sum of all the simultaneous rates of loss: at a rate determined by $k_e$.

Figure 3.19$a$ is a graph of $\ln(U_\infty - U)$ against time in two human subjects given medazepam, a commercially available antianxiety agent. Figure 3.19$b$ presents the cumulative urinary excretion data from which the amounts yet to be excreted were calculated. Both figures are from a study by Schwartz and Carbone (1970) using $^{14}$C-labeled medazepam, and all amounts are amounts of $^{14}$C rather than of medazepam. Note that the urine of subject H-15 was not monitored long enough to permit an estimate of $U_\infty$. To get around this insufficiency, the investigators adopted an arbitrary value for total excretion that linearized the relationship between $\ln(U_\infty - U)$ and time. For subject H-16, $U_\infty$ was estimated directly from the experimental data in Figure 3.19$b$ as 63%$D$, a figure indicating that medazepam is not excreted solely in the urine but by some other route or routes as well. From the transformation in Figure 3.19$a$ the authors estimated that the half-lives of $^{14}$C in subjects H-16 and H-15 were 2.5 and 12 days, respectively. These half-lives corresponded well with plasma $^{14}$C half-lives, which were 15 days in subject H-15 and 2.5 days in subject H-16. Of course the half-lives estimated from plasma and from urine data in the same subject will be identical if the one-compartment open model accurately describes the system, since the slope of the appropriate plot is in each case $-k_e$. Nonetheless it would be better in principle to use

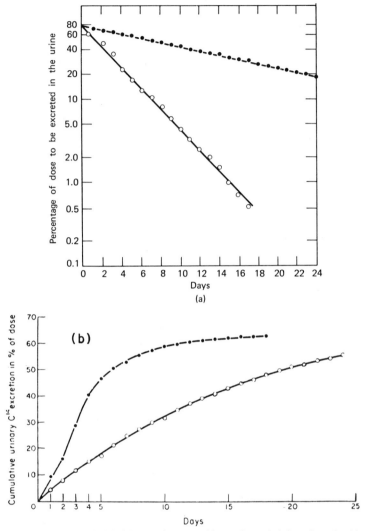

**Figure 3.19** Excretion of radiolabel by two human subjects after administration of a 30-mg oral dose of [14C] medazepam hydrochloride. (a) Ln ($U_\infty - U$), $t$ for subjects H-15 (●) and H-16 (O). (b) $U, t$ for subjects H-15 (O) and H-16 (●). Reproduced with permission from Schwartz and Carbone, 1970, Figures 6 and 7.

the alternate data analysis technique rather than to fix an arbitrary value of $U_\infty$, which forces the data to conform to the assumed kinetic model.

This is an appropriate point at which to introduce an important warning. Radiolabeled compounds are used frequently in pharmacokinetic studies. Assays for radiolabel are rapid and sensitive and require only small sample volumes so that repeated closely spaced assays in the same animal are feasible. However, these assays are not specific. What is being measured is the amount of a particular radionuclide, not the amount of a particular kind of molecule. Radiolabeled inorganic compounds usually present a less serious potential problem in this regard than do radiolabeled organic compounds, which can undergo extensive metabolism. When a toxicant or drug is metabolized, the labeled atom may be lost from the parent molecule, may be retained in the parent or in one or more metabolites structurally related to the parent, or may even be incorporated into a structurally unrelated but important metabolite such as acetate, which enters active body pools. Whatever pathways it may take, as long as radiolabel is incorporated into more than one kind of molecule, measurement of total radioactivity is nearly always useless kinetically, representing as it does a mixture of compounds uncharacterized either quantitatively or qualitatively. The $^{14}C$ half-lives determined by Schwartz and Carbone from plasma and urine data in the medazepam example do not represent the half-lives either of medazepam or of any of its radiolabeled metabolites. That plasma and urine data could be represented by straight lines on semilogarithmic plots suggests, however, that all radiolabeled compounds were in a dieaway phase during the period of measurement.

As a general rule, unless it has been established that the radionuclide is associated with only one kind of molecule, the use of total radioactivity in kinetic calculations is not productive and may be misleading. Radioactivity measurement may, of course, be used to quantitate individual compounds following qualitative separation by one of the many available methods such as paper or column chromatography.

In the medazepam study the authors stated that they chose to use a $\ln(U_\infty - U)$ plot because a graph of $\ln(\Delta U/\Delta t)$ against time was very erratic. Partly because urination is sporadic rather than continuous, graphs of $\ln(\Delta U/\Delta t)$ are often difficult to interpret. Houston and Levy (1976) circumvented this difficulty in a study of salicylamide metabolism in rats by stimulating urination at preselected intervals. Salicylamide (SAM) itself is not detected in the urine after intravenous administration, although it is rapidly cleared from the plasma. Houston and Levy found that the mean plasma half-life of SAM in a group of five rates was 13.2 min, or $k_e = 0.0525$ min$^{-1}$. Figure 3.20 is a graph of $\ln(\Delta U/\Delta t)$ against time for the two metabolites of SAM measured in the urine, salicylamide glucuronide (SAMG) and salicylamide sulfate (SAMS). The slopes of the two lines are similar, suggesting a half-life of about 1.7 or 1.8 hr for excretion of each metabolite, but they are much less steep than the slope of the line for loss of parent compound from the plasma. This observation suggests that the overall excretion rate constant is probably smaller than the formation rate constant for both metabolites. Let us see whether that suggestion is correct.

The negative slopes of the $\ln(\Delta U/\Delta t)$, $t$ graphs represent the overall elimination rate constants $k_e^M$ for the compartments from which the urinary

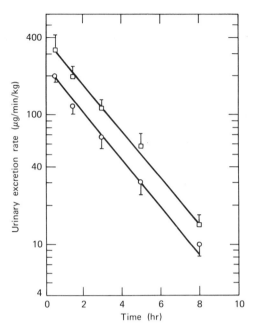

**Figure 3.20**  Average urinary excretion rates of SAMG (O) and SAMS (□) by a group of five rats after intravenous injection of salicylamide, 100 mg/kg. Reproduced with permission from Houston and Levy, 1976, Figure 3, © 1976 by the Williams & Wilkins Co., Baltimore.

metabolites were transferred. Therefore

$$k_e^{SAMG} \cong k_e^{SAMS} = \frac{0.693}{1.7 \text{ hr}} = 0.41 \text{ hr}^{-1} \quad \text{or} \quad 0.0068 \text{ min}^{-1}.$$

To estimate the values of the formation rate constants, we note that 52.8% of the total intravenous dose of 100 mg of SAM per kilogram was excreted in the urine as SAMS and 33.5% was excreted as SAMG. Therefore

$$k_f^{SAMG} = (0.0525 \text{ min}^{-1})(0.335) = 0.0176 \text{ min}^{-1}$$

and

$$k_f^{SAMS} = (0.0525 \text{ min}^{-1})(0.528) = 0.0277 \text{ min}^{-1},$$

where $k_f^M$ is the rate constant for formation of metabolite that will appear in the urine.

Notice the restriction placed on $k_f^M$. This restriction is necessary because $k_f^M$ was calculated from the total amount of metabolite excreted in the urine, which is not necessarily the total amount formed. If metabolite is excreted only in the urine, then $k_f^M$ is the rate constant for total metabolite formation. In this case $k_e^M = k_u^M$ and $(k_f^{SAMS} + k_f^{SAMG}) = k_m^{SAM}$.

This equivalence can be tested by comparing $k_e^M$ with $k_u^M$ calculated from the ordinate intercepts of the $\ln(\Delta U/\Delta t)$, $t$ graphs. Since the estimate of "dose" of SAMS or SAMG used in the calculation of $k_u^M$ is the cumulative amount excreted in the urine, and since this figure appears in the denominator of the calculation

$$k_u^M = \frac{\text{antilog of ordinate intercept}}{\text{dose}},$$

if the cumulative amount excreted in the urine is less than the total amount of metabolite formed the apparent $k_u^M$ calculated in this way will be found to be greater than $k_e^M$.

For SAMG the ordinate intercept is about 220 $\mu$g/min/kg and the "dose" is $(0.335)(100 \text{ mg/kg}) = 33.5 \text{ mg/kg}$. Therefore

$$k_u^{\text{SAMG}} = \frac{0.220 \text{ mg/min/kg}}{33.5 \text{ mg/kg}} = 0.0066 \text{ min}^{-1}.$$

For SAMS the ordinate intercept is about 400 $\mu$g/min/kg and the "dose" is $(0.528)(100 \text{ mg/kg}) = 52.8 \text{ mg/kg}$. Therefore

$$k_u^{\text{SAMS}} = \frac{0.400 \text{ mg/min/kg}}{52.8 \text{ mg/kg}} = 0.0076 \text{ min}^{-1}.$$

Within the accuracy of estimating from the graph, it may be concluded that both metabolites are excreted entirely in the urine and that the excretion rate constants $k_e^M$ for the two metabolites are very similar to each other and about one-third the corresponding formation rate constants $k_f^M$, where $(k_f^{\text{SAMS}} + k_f^{\text{SAMG}}) = k_m^{\text{SAM}}$. The appropriate model is given in full in Figure 3.21 with values assigned to the rate constants.

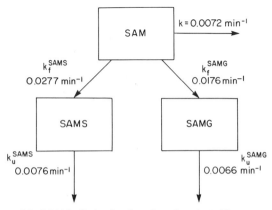

**Figure 3.21**  Model of SAM elimination based on data from Houston and Levy, 1976.

## 3.7   THE TWO–COMPARTMENT BODY MODEL

Instantaneous and homogeneous mixing is a contradiction in practical terms. Even a foreign compound injected intravenously and physically restricted to the plasma will not distribute itself instantaneously throughout the plasma volume. The very process of mixing takes time. Furthermore, the body is not a single compartment and seldom acts as if it were. If the compound enters any tissues other than the plasma it must cross membrane barriers that delay still more its distribution throughout its final volume. In fact, the materials whose behavior seems to conform reasonably well to the predictions of a one-compartment open model are those whose distribution is rapid and is therefore essentially complete before the first sample is taken for analysis.

What is the result of adding a single distributive or peripheral compartment to our basic model? Schematically the linear two-compartment open model shown in Figure 3.22 appears to be only slightly more complex than the linear one-compartment open model, although now there are three microconstants instead of one. Note that excretion from compartment 2, the peripheral compartment, is assumed to be zero or at least negligible. In fact it is not always negligible, and loss from peripheral compartments (e.g., through the skin) can be taken into account, as we discuss in Section 3.14. For the moment we restrict ourselves to the simplest form of the linear two-compartment open model, in which the compound is assumed to be distributed homogeneously throughout compartment 1 at time zero and eliminated only from compartment 1.

It is evident at the outset that $k_{12}$ must be either roughly the same order of magnitude as $k_e$ or greater than $k_e$. Otherwise excretion from compartment 1 would be so rapid relative to distribution that the existence of the peripheral compartment would not be kinetically demonstrable. Whenever distribution into the peripheral compartment is significant, however, it will alter the time course of observable concentration change in the central compartment. During the distributional phase there is net transfer out of compartment 1. Depending on the relative magnitudes of $k_{12}$ and $k_e$, a larger or smaller part of the material lost from compartment 1 accumulates in compartment 2. At the instant in time at which the concentration in compartment 2 has become equal to the concentration in compartment 1, compartment 2 is poised in a dynamic steady state. Then the direction of net transfer reverses. The distributional phase is complete and, provided $k_{21} \geqslant k_e$, the whole system behaves

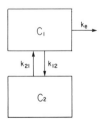

**Figure 3.22**  The linear two-compartment open model.

subsequently like a single compartment with a rate constant for excretion that we will call $\beta$, which is the rate constant for whole body loss. It is not a microconstant but it is related to the microconstant $k_e$, since

$$(\beta)(\text{total body burden}) = (k_e)(\text{amount in compartment 1}), \quad (3.21)$$

from which it also follows that

$$\frac{\beta}{k_e} = \text{fraction of body burden contained in compartment 1}.$$

The requirement that $k_{21}$, like $k_{12}$, is of the same order of magnitude as or is larger than $k_e$ is important. If $k_{21}$ is smaller than $k_e$, the system will not degenerate into one apparent compartment following the distributional phase. Instead compartment 1 will empty more rapidly than compartment 2, and the terminal dieaway phase will represent loss from compartment 2 at a rate determined by $k_{21}$. In this case compartment 2 is an example of a deep compartment. Discussion of deep compartments is deferred until later in this chapter. For the time being we assume that $k_e < k_{12}$ and $k_e < k_{21}$.

How does the two-compartment open model behave mathematically?

The degree of complexity introduced into the equations for $C_1$ and $C_2$ simply by adding one peripheral compartment to the simplest open model is staggering at first.

$$C_1 = \frac{D}{V_1(\alpha - \beta)} \left[ (k_{21} - \beta)e^{-\beta t} - (k_{21} - \alpha)e^{-\alpha t} \right] \quad (3.22)$$

and

$$C_2 = \frac{k_{12}D}{V_2(\alpha - \beta)} \left[ e^{-\beta t} - e^{-\alpha t} \right] \quad (3.23)$$

where

$$\alpha = \tfrac{1}{2}\left[ (k_{12} + k_e + k_{21}) + \sqrt{(k_{12} + k_e + k_{21})^2 - 4k_{21}k_e} \right] \quad (3.24)$$

and

$$\beta = \tfrac{1}{2}\left[ (k_{12} + k_e + k_{21}) - \sqrt{(k_{12} + k_e + k_{21})^2 - 4k_{21}k_e} \right]. \quad (3.25)$$

Let us examine some of the implications of these relationships. To begin with, note that if $k_e = 0$, $\beta = 0$, and $\alpha = (k_{12} + k_{21})$. This observation suggests that terms in $\beta$ should have something to do with excretion from the system and terms in $\alpha$ should have something to do with distribution into the peripheral compartment. In fact, $\alpha$ is the rate constant for net transfer out of compartment 1 during the distributional phase, taking into account both distributive and excretory processes; and $\beta$ is the rate constant, now defined, for whole body loss. In the closed two-compartment system with which we began this chapter, $k_e = 0$ and $\alpha = (k_{12} + k_{21})$. In the open two-compartment system $\alpha$ is a function of $k_e$ as well as of $k_{12}$ and $k_{21}$; if both $k_{12}$ and $k_{21}$ are zero, $\alpha = k_e$.

It is apparent that $\alpha$, which is the sum of two positive terms, is always larger than $\beta$, which is the difference between the same two terms. Mathematically speaking, the larger the absolute magnitude of the exponent of a negative exponential, the faster that exponential decays. Therefore the term in $e^{-\alpha t}$ in the expression for $C_1$ (Equation 3.22) will always decay faster than the term in $e^{-\beta t}$. (Although $\alpha$ and $\beta$ appear both in the exponents and in the linear multiplicative constants of the two terms in Equation 3.22, the exponentials dominate.) As another example recall that the larger $k_e$ is, the more rapidly material is lost from the one-compartment open system.

If the term in $e^{-\alpha t}$ approaches zero faster than the term in $e^{-\beta t}$, at some time the term in $e^{-\alpha t}$ will have become negligible relative to the term in $e^{-\beta t}$. Thereafter the term in $e^{-\beta t}$ will dominate the expression for $C_1$, while at earlier times $C_1$ will reflect both terms. In other words, once the term in $e^{-\alpha t}$ has become negligible relative to the term in $e^{-\beta t}$ a constant dynamic relationship has been established between $C_1$ and $C_2$ and the system has degenerated into one apparent compartment whose rate constant for excretion is $\beta$. When the term in $e^{-\alpha t}$ is dropped from the equation for $C_1$,

$$C_1 \approx \left( \frac{D(k_{21} - \beta)}{V_1(\alpha - \beta)} \right) e^{-\beta t}, \qquad (3.26)$$

or

$$\ln C_1 \approx \ln \left( \frac{D(k_{21} - \beta)}{V_1(\alpha - \beta)} \right) - \beta t, \qquad (3.27)$$

so that a graph of the terminal segment of the $C_1$ dieaway curve is a straight line whose slope is $-\beta$ and whose ordinate intercept is $\ln[D(k_{21} - \beta)/V_1(\alpha - \beta)]$. The resemblance of Equation 3.27 to the rate equation for a one-compartment model is obvious.

What is happening to $C_2$ during all this time? We know, of course, that it increases initially, peaks, then declines. We also know that it must reach its maximum at that time point at which distributional steady state has been achieved—that is, when $e^{-\alpha t}$ is effectively zero. To predict the behavior of $C_2$ after this point, we can drop the term in $e^{-\alpha t}$ from Equation 3.23 for $C_2$, so that

$$C_2 \approx \left( \frac{k_{12} D}{V_2(\alpha - \beta)} \right) e^{-\beta t}, \qquad (3.28)$$

or

$$\ln C_2 \approx \ln\left(\frac{k_{12}D}{V_2(\alpha - \beta)}\right) - \beta t. \tag{3.29}$$

Clearly, after distributional steady state has been achieved the concentration of material in compartment 2 declines in parallel with the concentration in compartment 1. This is the only intuitively satisfactory conclusion, of course, since we have already determined that after distributional steady state has been reached the system behaves as if it were one compartment. But there is another important point in connection with Equation 3.29.

The alert reader will have been disturbed by the distinction made between $k_{12}$ and $k_{21}$. After all, all transfers in this model are considered to be by passive diffusion. How, then, can the rate constant for transfer in one direction across a membrane be different from the rate constant for transfer in the opposite direction for the same compound across the same membrane?

Properly, transfers are expressed in terms of amounts. At either equilibrium or steady state, the *amounts* transferred in both directions are equal. But since analytical assays are made in terms of concentrations, and since we often do not have the information that would enable us to convert concentrations to amounts, kinetically determined transfer constants contain a "hidden" volume term. An example may illustrate this point more clearly. Consider the closed two-compartment model for which $k_{12}$ is the microconstant for forward transfer and $k_{21}$ is the microconstant for transfer in the reverse direction, as in Figure 3.23. At equilibrium the concentrations $C_1$ and $C_2$ are equal and the amounts of solute diffusing in both directions per unit of time are also equal:

$$C_1 = C_2 \quad \text{and} \quad \frac{dM_1}{dt} = -k_{12}M_1 = \frac{dM_2}{dt} = -k_{21}M_2$$

$$= -k_{12}V_1C_1 = -k_{21}V_2C_2.$$

Therefore, since $C_1 = C_2$,

$$k_{12}V_1 = k_{21}V_2 = k_t, \tag{3.30}$$

where $k_t$ is the true transfer microconstant. For this reason kinetically determined microconstants vary with the volume out of which the solute is diffusing.

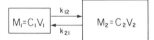

**Figure 3.23** The linear closed two-compartment model. The schematic diagram is drawn to make it clear that the volumes $V_1$ and $V_2$ of the two compartments are not equal.

Now we can return to Equation 3.29 and substitute $k_{21}/V_1$ for its equivalent $k_{12}/V_2$:

$$\ln C_2 \approx \ln\left(\frac{k_{21}D}{V_1(\alpha-\beta)}\right) - \beta t. \tag{3.31}$$

When Equation 3.31 is compared with Equation 3.27,

$$\ln C_1 \approx \ln\left(\frac{(k_{21}-\beta)D}{V_1(\alpha-\beta)}\right) - \beta t, \tag{3.27}$$

it is apparent that although $C_1$ dieaway parallels $C_2$ dieaway after distribution steady state has been reached, $C_2$ is not equal to $C_1$. In fact, $C_2$ is always larger than $C_1$, although it approaches $C_1$ when $k_{21} \gg \beta$:

$$\frac{C_2}{C_1} = \frac{k_{21}}{k_{21}-\beta}.$$

Why should this be so?

There is always at least a slight lag as solute is transferred from compartment 2 to compartment 1 to compensate for excreted solute. The magnitude of the lag is a function of the readiness with which the readjustment takes place. When $k_{21}$ is large, transfer from compartment 2 to compartment 1 is rapid and $C_2$ is only slightly larger than $C_1$. When $k_{21}$ is small, however, transfer is slow and $C_2$ may be much larger than $C_1$.

We now have all the information we need to sketch the expected behavior of the concentrations of solute in both compartments of a two-compartment open model. In a linear coordinate system the dependence of $C_1$ on $t$ (Figure 3.24$a$) is not readily distinguishable from the behavior predicted by a one-compartment open model. But since Equation 3.22 expresses $C_1$ as the sum of two exponential terms, a graph of $\ln C_1$ against time is not linear either. Instead it is the resultant of the superposition of two log linear segments: the first represents net transfer out of compartment 1, and the second represents net loss from the whole system. When $\ln C_1$ is graphed against time the earlier points show positive deviations from the straight line approximated by the later points, as shown in Figure 3.24$b$. Figure 3.24$b$ also shows that $C_2$ peaks at about the time distribution is complete (about the time the graph of $\ln C_1$ against time achieves linearity) and that thereafter $\ln C_2$ declines in parallel with, but above, $\ln C_1$.

A good example of concentration changes in kinetically differentiable tissues relative to concentration changes in the plasma is provided by the classic study by Brodie et al. (1952) of thiopental distribution in the dog. Figure 3.25 shows that the liver, representative of the viscera or of well-perfused tissues in general, has already reached a steady state relationship

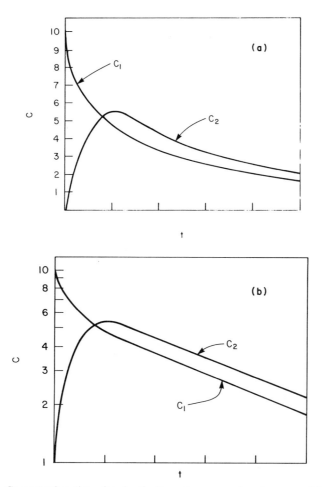

**Figure 3.24** Concentration, time plots for the linear two-compartment open model. (*a*) $C, t$ for the central $(C_1)$ and peripheral $(C_2)$ compartments. (*b*) $\ln C, t$ for the central $(C_1)$ and peripheral $(C_2)$ compartments.

with the plasma by the first sampling time. Total thiopental concentrations are shown; liver total concentrations are higher than plasma total concentrations because the degree of sequestration by tissue binding differs in the two compartments (Bischoff and Dedrick, 1968).

Thiopental concentration in muscle, representative of lean, moderately to poorly perfused tissue, peaks later, between 15 and 30 min after administration, and thereafter declines in parallel with the plasma concentration. But thiopental concentration in adipose tissue, representative of a deep compartment, continues to increase for 6 hr after thiopental administration. This behavior is characteristic of deep compartments, for which $k_{21}$ is $< k_e$.

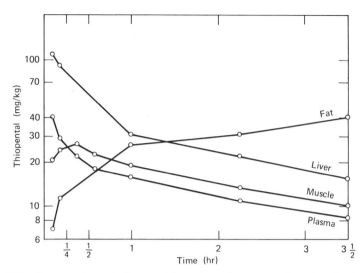

**Figure 3.25** Concentrations of thiopental in various tissues of a dog after the intravenous administration of 25 mg/kg. Reproduced with permission from Brodie et al., 1952, Figure 1, © 1952 by the Williams & Wilkins Co., Baltimore.

Whenever the rate constant for return of a solute from a peripheral compartment to the central compartment is very small, the time lag for this transfer will be particularly large. There may be a large difference between concentration in the peripheral compartment and concentration in the central compartment even after a single exposure. The difference is magnified by repetitive exposures; as we shall see in Chapter 5, the steady state level of a compound in a peripheral tissue is inversely proportional to the magnitude of $k_{21}$, and if $k_{21}$ is very small the steady state concentration may be very large indeed. Fat and bone are nearly always deep compartments, and skeletal muscle may be also.

The fetus has been shown to be a deep compartment in the few such kinetic studies that have been carried out. This observation has profound implications with respect to extrapolation from small laboratory animals with their brief gestation periods of around 20 days to humans chronically exposed over a gestation period of 9 months. Figure 3.26 is taken from a recent study by Olson and Massaro (1977). Following a single subcutaneous injection of methylmercury into pregnant mice, maternal blood mercury concentrations declined steadily during the 7-day measurement period (Figure 3.26*a*). However, the amount of mercury present in each fetus continued to increase during the same period (Figure 3.26*b*); in other words, there is a 7-day or greater time lag between administration of methylmercury to the mother and establishment of a maternal-fetal steady state relationship. The potential for methylmercury accumulation in the fetus with continuing maternal exposure to methylmercury is very high.

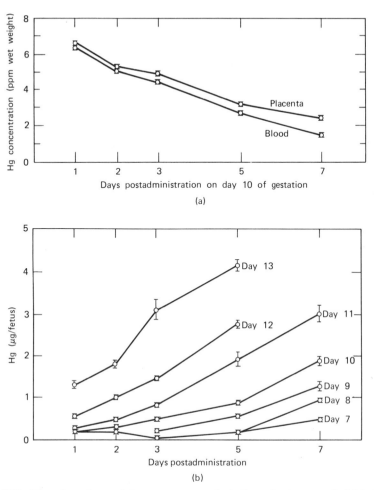

**Figure 3.26**   Time dependence of tissue mercury content after subcutaneous administration of radiolabeled methylmercuric chloride, 5 mg/kg, to pregnant mice. (*a*) In placenta and maternal blood after administration on day 10 of gestation. (*b*) In whole fetus after administration on days 7–13 of gestation. Reproduced with permission from Olson and Massaro, 1977, Figure 1 (adapted) and Figure 2.

## 3.8   HALF-LIFE AND VOLUME OF DISTRIBUTION IN THE TWO-COMPARTMENT BODY MODEL

The expression for $C_1$ is of the general form

$$C_1 = A_0 e^{-\alpha t} + B_0 e^{-\beta t},$$

where

$$A_0 = \frac{D(\alpha - k_{21})}{V_1(\alpha - \beta)}$$

and

$$B_0 = \frac{D(k_{21}-\beta)}{V_1(\alpha-\beta)}.$$

When the distributional phase is complete, the expression for $C_1$ reduces to

$$C_1 \approx B_0 e^{-\beta t} \qquad \text{or} \qquad \ln C_1 = \ln B_0 - \beta t.$$

When the concentration of solute is assayed in the central compartment as a function of time and graphed against time in a semilogarithmic coordinate system, the constant $\beta$ is readily estimated. It is the negative slope of the terminal linear segment of the curve. Like $k_e$, $\beta$ may be used to calculate a half-life:

$$t_{1/2} = \frac{\ln 2}{\beta} = \frac{0.693}{\beta}.$$

The half-life calculated using the rate constant $\beta$ is called the biological half-life, whereas the half-life calculated using the microconstant $k_e$ is the half-life of residence in the central compartment. The biological half-life is always calculated using the slope of the terminal linear portion of the dieaway curve. In the one-compartment body model, of course, the biological half-life is identical to the half-life of loss from the plasma, $\ln 2/k_e$.

An apparent volume of distribution can also be estimated, by back-extrapolation of the $\beta$ segment to the ordinate. This process is shown in Figure 3.27.

$$V_{\text{extrap}} = \frac{D}{B_0} = \frac{V_1(\alpha-\beta)}{k_{21}-\beta}.$$

Since $\alpha$ and $\beta$ are functions of all the rate constants of the system, it should be obvious that in a multicompartment system $V_{\text{extrap}}$ and $\beta$ need not have any physiological significance. Recall that unless protein or other binding intervenes, the volume of distribution calculated for a one-compartment system is a real volume of distribution. The volume of distribution estimated by back-extrapolation of the $\beta$ segment to the ordinate is only an approximation to the total volume, $V_1 + V_2$, of the two-compartment system. If the compound had been distributed homogeneously throughout both compartments at time zero, $V_{\text{extrap}}$ would be equal to $V_1 + V_2$, since the $\beta$ phase in fact represents degeneration of the two-compartment system to a one-compartment system of volume $V_1 + V_2$. But the compound was not distributed homogeneously throughout both compartments at time zero; it was all in compartment 1. And since it was all in compartment 1, more

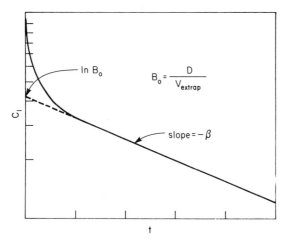

**Figure 3.27** Estimation of $\beta$ and $V_{\text{extrap}}$ from a plot of $\ln C_1$ versus $t$.

material was excreted during the distributional phase than would have been excreted under the assumptions made in back-extrapolating the $\beta$ segment of the curve. Quite apart from any considerations of protein binding or other forms of sequestration, $V_{\text{extrap}}$ will always overestimate the actual volume $V_1 + V_2$ in an open system. The longer the distributional phase, the more serious the overestimation will be. On the other hand, if the length of the distributional phase were to become vanishingly small (which is the same as specifying that the system were to be forced toward one compartment of volume $V_1 + V_2$), then $V_{\text{extrap}}$ would be an accurate estimate of $V_1 + V_2$.

A better, but not necessarily good, approximation of the volume $V_1 + V_2$ is provided by another volume of distribution defined for the two-compartment model during the $\beta$ phase of dieaway. This volume is $V_\beta$. It relates total body burden to plasma concentration during the $\beta$ phase:

$$V_\beta = \frac{\text{total body burden}}{\text{plasma concentration, } \beta \text{ phase}}, \tag{3.32}$$

and is therefore a particularly useful volume parameter irrespective of its accuracy as an approximation of $V_1 + V_2$. From Equation 3.21 it follows that $V_\beta = k_e V_1 / \beta$, from which also $\beta V_\beta = k_e V_1$. Both these volume parameters, $V_\beta$ and $V_{\text{extrap}}$, are considered in greater detail in Section 5.4.

We will find that there are other ways to estimate volumes of distribution, nearly all of which consistently either over- or underestimate the physiological volumes they are supposed to approximate. Since for so many reasons kinetically determined volumes of distribution usually do not correspond to real physiological volumes, it has often been suggested that kinetic volumes of distribution should be regarded, and used, simply as proportionality constants having the dimensions of volumes. The suggestion has merit in that it is easy to be misled into equating kinetically determined volumes of distribution with actual volumes. On the other hand, as we have already seen, sometimes useful inferences about the behavior of a compound can be made by comparing the kinetically determined volume of distribution with reasonable estimates, obtained independently, of its actual volume of distribution. On balance it is probably more worthwhile to retain an awareness of the conceptual origin of the kinetic volume of distribution than to view it only as a proportionality constant.

### 3.9  HOW TO ESTIMATE KINETIC PARAMETERS USING THE TWO-COMPARTMENT BODY MODEL

The presence in the expression for $C_1$ of two decaying exponentials suggests that the dieaway curve can be resolved into two straight line segments. This process is variously called feathering, curve stripping, or the method of residuals. It is carried out as follows:

$$C_1 = A_0 e^{-\alpha t} + B_0 e^{-\beta t}$$

1  Graph $\ln C_1$ against time as in Figure 3.28a.

2  Extrapolate the terminal straight line portion of the curve back to the ordinate. The negative slope of this segment is $\beta$ and its intercept is $\ln B_0$, where $V_{\text{extrap}} = D/B_0$.

3  At times $t_1$, $t_2$, $t_3$, etc., corresponding to the points on the early part of the experimental curve that show a positive deviation from the $\beta$ segment, read from the $\beta$ segment the $C_1$ values that would have been measured if distribution had been instantaneous and homogeneous throughout both compartments. Call these values $C_1'$.

4  Calculate $C_1 - C_1'$ for times $t_1$, $t_2$, $t_3$, etc.

5  Plot $C_1 - C_1'$ against time. This graph should be a straight line with intercept $\ln A_0$ and slope $-\alpha$.

6  The microscopic rate constants $k_e$, $k_{12}$, and $k_{21}$ may now be obtained directly from the values of $\alpha$, $\beta$, $A_0$ and $B_0$:

$$k_e = \frac{\alpha\beta}{k_{21}}, \tag{3.33}$$

$$k_{21} = \frac{A_0\beta + B_0\alpha}{A_0 + B_0}, \tag{3.34}$$

$$k_{12} = \alpha + \beta - k_e - k_{21}. \tag{3.35}$$

Figure 3.28b is an example of feathering taken from a study by Borchard et al. (1975) of polychlorinated biphenyl (PCB) pharmacokinetics in sheep.

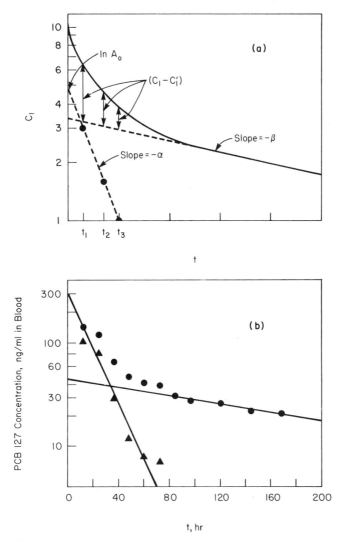

**Figure 3.28** Estimation of $\alpha$, $\beta$, $A_0$, and $B_0$ from a plot of $\ln C_1$ versus $t$: feathering. (*a*) Technique applied to idealized curve. (*b*) Technique applied to data from elimination phase of PCB component 127 in sheep: $\bullet$, experimentally determined concentrations in blood; $\blacktriangle$, feathered points determining $\alpha$ line. (*b*) Data from Borchard et al., 1975, Table II.

The data shown are for a particular component, 127, of a commercial mix of PCB isomers; $B_0$ is 45 ng/ml, and the authors calculated that $\beta$ is 0.0043 $hr^{-1}$, so that the biological half-life is about 161 hr or nearly a week. When the points on the extrapolated portion of the $\beta$ line are subtracted from the corresponding experimental values and the differences graphed, they define the $\alpha$ line, whose ordinate intercept is 300 ng/ml and whose slope is $-0.065$

$hr^{-1}$. Therefore the half-life of distribution is about 11 hr.

$$k_{21} = \frac{[(300)(0.0043)+(45)(0.065)]\ (ng/ml)\ (hr^{-1})}{(300+45)\ ng/ml}$$

$$= 0.012\ hr^{-1},$$

$$k_e = \frac{(0.0043)(0.065)\ (hr^{-1})}{(0.012)}$$

$$= 0.023\ hr^{-1},$$

and

$$k_{12} = (0.0043+0.065-0.012-0.023)\ (hr^{-1})$$

$$= 0.034\ hr^{-1}.$$

Since $\beta/k_e$ is $0.0043/0.023$ or 0.19, only 19% of the total body burden is in the central compartment during the terminal dieaway phase when the body is presumably in a steady state.

Note that the points that determine the $\alpha$ line mirror the irregularities in the experimental points. The "best" $\alpha$ line can be defined by linear regression techniques; but since it is determined by small differences between large numbers, its slope is very sensitive even to small variations in the experimental points. Practically speaking, observations during the distributional phase should be made as close together as possible if the $\alpha$ line is to be defined with any reasonable degree of certainty. Problem 10 at the end of Chapter 4 is a good illustration of the uncertainty in an $\alpha$ line based on only 4 or 5 points.

### 3.10  THE PERIPHERAL COMPARTMENT: FIRST-ORDER ABSORPTION AND FIRST-ORDER ELIMINATION IN A ONE-COMPARTMENT MODEL

Up to this point the process of entry into a compartment has been neglected. It has been assumed that absorption and homogeneous mixing occur instantaneously. Clearly this is not the case for the peripheral compartment of a two-compartment system, which can be represented schematically as in Figure 3.29 and for which we already know that

$$C_2 = \frac{k_{12}D}{V_2(\alpha-\beta)}\left[e^{-\beta t}-e^{-\alpha t}\right]. \qquad (3.23)$$

This expression takes into account simultaneous loss from the central compartment during the absorption (distribution) phase as well as the continuing contribution to $D$ of material leaving the peripheral compartment.

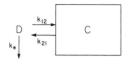

**Figure 3.29** First-order absorption and first-order elimination in the peripheral compartment of a two-compartment open model with simultaneous loss from the central compartment.

There are other common situations in which the appearance of a compound obeys first-order kinetics. One is first-order formation of metabolite. In this case the compartment volume $V$ is the volume of distribution of the metabolite. The model is shown schematically in Figure 3.30, where $k_e$ for the parent compound is $(k_u + k_b + k_m)$ and $k_e^M$ is the rate constant of elimination of the metabolite. The differential equations for this system are

$$\frac{dC}{dt} = k_m A - k_e^M C V \tag{3.36}$$

and

$$\frac{dA}{dt} = -(k_m + k_u + k_b)A = -k_e A, \tag{3.37}$$

where $A$ is the amount of parent compound remaining at time $t$.

Integrating Equation 3.37 and substituting the resulting expression for $A$ into Equation 3.36,

$$\frac{dC}{dt} = k_m D e^{-k_e t} - k_e^M C V. \tag{3.38}$$

Integrating (this integration requires the use of an integrating factor; see Appendix 3.1) and applying the boundary condition that $C_0 = 0$,

$$C = \frac{k_m D}{(k_e - k_e^M)V} \left( e^{-k_e^M t} - e^{-k_e t} \right). \tag{3.39}$$

The simplest form of this type of expression, for first-order absorption from a depot and first-order elimination from the single compartment, corresponds to the schematic diagram in Figure 3.31, where

$$\frac{dC}{dt} = k_a A - k_e C V \tag{3.40}$$

and

$$\frac{dA}{dt} = -k_a A, \tag{3.41}$$

where $A$ is the amount remaining at the depot site at time $t$.

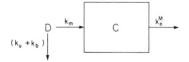

**Figure 3.30** First-order metabolism and first-order elimination of metabolite with simultaneous parallel routes of parent compound elimination.

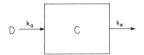

Figure 3.31  First-order absorption from a depot and first-order elimination.

Substituting the integrated form of Equation 3.41 into Equation 3.40 and integrating as before (see Appendix 3.1),

$$C = \frac{k_a D}{V(k_a - k_e)} (e^{-k_e t} - e^{-k_a t}). \qquad (3.42)$$

This function describes the one-compartment body model with first-order (e.g., oral) absorption and excretion by a first-order process.

The analogies in the structures of Equations 3.23, 3.39, and 3.42 are apparent. All three equations represent biphasic behavior of the general form shown in Figure 1.6d. Let us examine Equation 3.42 further. Its behavior depends on the relative magnitudes of $k_a$ and $k_e$, and the discussion that follows is divided accordingly into three sections.

### 3.10.1  $k_a > k_e$

When $k_a > k_e$ the negative exponential $e^{-k_a t}$ will decay rapidly compared to the negative exponential $e^{-k_e t}$. There is a sharp initial rise in concentration during the short absorption phase, after which the expression for $C$ reduces to

$$C \cong \left( \frac{D}{V} \right) \left( \frac{k_a}{k_a - k_e} \right) e^{-k_e t} \qquad (3.43)$$

or

$$\ln C \cong \ln \left( \frac{D}{V} \right) \left( \frac{k_a}{k_a - k_e} \right) - k_e t. \qquad (3.44)$$

Therefore when $k_a > k_e$ the terminal portion of a graph of $\ln C$ against time is a straight line: its slope is $-k_e$, and it can be back-extrapolated to the ordinate to give an estimate of the quantity $(k_a/(k_a - k_e))(D/V)$ as shown in Figure 3.32a.

The value of the ordinate intercept together with the value of $D$ (provided it is known; remember that $D$ represents the amount absorbed unchanged) may be used to estimate the volume of distribution. As is the case whenever other processes operate in parallel with elimination, the volume of distribution estimated by back-extrapolating the dieaway segment is not equal to the actual volume of distribution. Since the ordinate intercept is actually larger than $D/V$ by the factor $k_a/(k_a - k_e)$, the quantity $D/V$ will always be

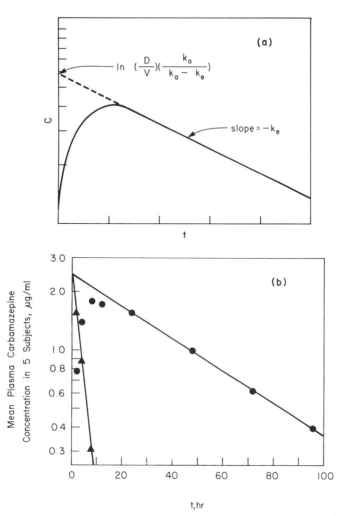

**Figure 3.32** Plots of $\ln C$ versus $t$ for the linear one-compartment open model with first-order absorption; $k_a \gg k_e$. (*a*) Predicted, showing extrapolation of terminal portion to ordinate. (*b*) Observed plasma concentration of carbamazepine as a function of time after oral administration of a single 200-mg dose; means of data from five human subjects (●). The feathered line is also shown (▲). (*b*) Data from Gérardin et al., 1976, Table II.

overestimated in this back-extrapolation process, and consequently the quantity $V$ will be underestimated. The error becomes smaller as $k_e$ becomes smaller relative to $k_a$.

The reason for the overestimation of $D/V$ is not difficult to understand. Absorption continuing throughout the early part of the time course of concentration change tends to shift the excretory phase to later times, causing the intercept of the back-extrapolated terminal slope to be larger than it would have been had absorption been instantaneous. Note that as $k_a$ becomes very large, this model is forced toward the one-compartment open model with instantaneous and homogeneous mixing, and the ordinate intercept approaches the true $D/V$ value.

An experimental example of this model with $k_a \gg k_e$ is shown in Figure 3.32*b*. The data are taken from a study by Gérardin et al. (1976) of the pharmacokinetics of carbamazepine, an anticonvulsant used in the treatment of epilepsy. Five adult male volunteers took tablets containing 200 mg of carbamazepine, and the plasma concentration of the drug was monitored at intervals for the following 168 hr. Figure 3.32*b* gives the mean plasma concentration data up to 96 hr, corrected for body weight differences and graphed in a semilogarithmic coordinate system. Since the terminal portion of the curve is effectively linearized by the transformation, the authors applied to the data a computer program appropriate to a one-compartment open model. The terminal half-life was found to be 37.7 hr; $k_e$ is therefore 0.018 hr$^{-1}$. Back-extrapolation from the terminal phase of the graph gives an intercept of 2.4 $\mu$g/ml. The authors calculated independently that $D/V$ was about 2.1 $\mu$g/ml, so that in this case the ordinate intercept is not a gross overestimate of the true $D/V$, suggesting that $k_a$ is substantially greater than $k_e$.

To confirm this supposition $k_a$ may be estimated by feathering. The feathering process is exactly analogous to that which was used to obtain $\alpha$ for the two-compartment open system. Early points on the experimental curve that deviate from the back-extrapolated segment of its terminal linear portion are subtracted from the corresponding points of the back-extrapolated segment and the differences are graphed semilogarithmically against time. The result should be a straight line with slope $-k_a$. When this procedure is followed for the data of Figure 3.32*b*, $k_a$ is estimated to be 0.316 hr$^{-1}$, or $17 \times k_e$.

An interesting and useful feature of this function is that the time $t_{\max}$ at which it peaks is independent of the dose:

$$t_{\max} = \frac{\ln k_a - \ln k_e}{k_a - k_e}. \tag{3.45}$$

(See Appendix 3.2 for this derivation.) Therefore it may occasionally be possible to obtain an estimate of $k_a$ even if only the concentrations around the maximum can be measured, provided an estimate of $k_e$ is available from an independent experiment. This option can be useful when the assays available are not particularly sensitive, so that the entire curve cannot be characterized; or when absorption is so rapid that a sufficient number of points cannot be obtained on the rising portion of the curve for feathering.

For example, the experimental curve of Figure 3.32*b* peaks at some time between 9 and 10 hr. Using the authors' value of 9.6 hr and substituting in

Equation 3.45,

$$9.6 \text{ hr} = \frac{\ln k_a - \ln 0.018}{(k_a - 0.018) \text{ hr}^{-1}}.$$

The value of $k_a$ that satisfies this equation is $0.316 \text{ hr}^{-1}$. Of course, $k_e$ could have been calculated if $k_a$ were known.

For most compounds and routes of administration $k_a$ is larger than $k_e$. Wagner has exploited the relationship between partition coefficient and membrane transfer rate constant to develop a means of predicting gastric absorption rate constants $k_a$ from partition rate constants within a homologous series of compounds (1975b).

### 3.10.2  $k_a \leqslant k_e$

When $k_a \leqslant k_e$, absorption continues throughout the entire elimination process and the terminal phase of the graph is not linear. An example of this type of behavior is shown in Figure 3.33.

Tylosin is an antibiotic used in veterinary medicine. A single dose of tylosin was given intramuscularly, the recommended route of administration, to a normal dog. Absorption from an intramuscular depot is often slow; in this case it continues throughout the entire elimination phase. For comparison the $\beta$ phase of the plasma dieaway curve for the same dose of tylosin

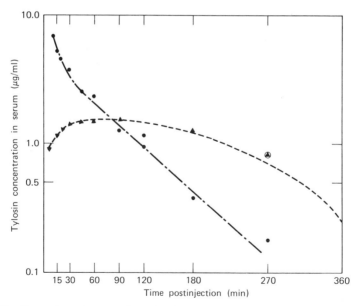

**Figure 3.33** Comparison of mean plasma levels of tylosin activity in six beagles given single intravenous (●) and intramuscular (▲) injections, both 10 mg/kg. Reproduced with permission from Weisel et al., 1977, Figure 1.

given intravenously is also shown. Since absorption and elimination take place simultaneously following the intramuscular injection, the peak serum concentration when tylosin is given by this route is not as high as that observed after the intravenous injection, which "peaks" at time zero; but elevated concentrations persist over an extended time period.

### 3.10.2  $k_a \ll k_e$

In rare instances $k_a \ll k_e$. In this case a phenomenon aptly named "flip-flop" occurs. Inspection of Equation 3.42 will show that since the exponential with the larger negative exponent decays faster, the negative terminal slope is either $k_a$ or $k_e$, whichever is smaller. If $k_a \ll k_e$, the terminal phase of the graph is linear, but its slope is $-k_a$ instead of $-k_e$. Although concentrations will not rise very high if $k_a \ll k_e$, the only way to resolve unequivocally the question whether a terminal slope represents $-k_a$ or $-k_e$ is to perform an independent experiment in which the compound is given intravenously and $k_e$ is measured.

A good example of flip-flop is the behavior of benzathine penicillin G injected intramuscularly. The half-life of soluble penicillins such as sodium penicillin G is short: about 0.5 hr, whether the penicillin is given orally or intramuscularly (Eagle et al., 1953; Nichols et al., 1955). A great deal of effort has been expended in the development of slow release dosage forms of penicillin, to extend the duration of action of a single dose of the antibiotic.

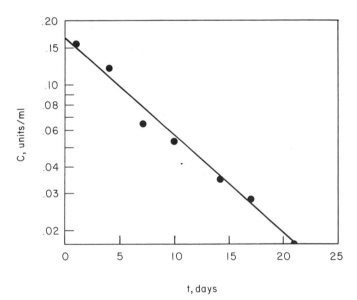

**Figure 3.34** The plasma concentration of benzathine penicillin G as a function of time after intramuscular administration of a single dose ($1.2 \times 10^6$ U) to 20 adult males. Data from Wright et al., 1959, Table I.

Benzathine penicillin G is one such slow release medication. When it was injected intramuscularly its half-life was found to be 6.5 days (Figure 3.34), which represents the half-life of appearance in the plasma rather than the half-life of elimination. Although $1.2 \times 10^6$ units of penicillin were injected, the maximum observed plasma concentration was 0.16 unit/ml, in agreement with the expectation that concentrations should be low whenever $k_a \ll k_e$.

### 3.11 FIRST–ORDER ABSORPTION AND FIRST–ORDER ELIMINATION IN A TWO–COMPARTMENT MODEL

Probably the most generally useful single model describing acute oral exposure is the two-compartment model with first-order absorption and disposition, shown schematically in Figure 3.35. There may also, of course, be more than one peripheral compartment. Multicompartment body models are discussed in Section 3.14. On the other hand, if distribution is very rapid relative to absorption [if $(k_{12} + k_{21}) \gg k_a$], this model tends to reduce to the one-compartment body model described in the preceding section.

As long as $k_a \geq (k_{12} + k_{21})$, a graph of $\ln C_1$ against time will take the general form shown in Figure 3.36a. The mathematical expression for $C_1$ is

$$C_1 = \frac{k_a D}{V_1} \left[ \left( \frac{k_{21} - \alpha}{(k_a - \alpha)(\beta - \alpha)} \right) e^{-\alpha t} \right.$$

$$+ \left( \frac{k_{21} - \beta}{(k_a - \beta)(\alpha - \beta)} \right) e^{-\beta t}$$

$$\left. - \left( \frac{k_{21} - k_a}{(\alpha - k_a)(k_a - \beta)} \right) e^{-k_a t} \right] \tag{3.46}$$

The values of $\beta$, $\alpha$, and $k_a$ may be estimated by successive feathering. Note that in this system too, flip-flop can occur, and an independent experiment may be necessary to distinguish between $\alpha$ and $k_a$.

An example of feathering in a two-compartment model with first-order absorption is given in Figure 3.36b, from Nayak et al. (1974). Methaqualone, an anticonvulsant, was given orally to eight adult male subjects and its serum level followed for 25 hr. The authors estimated graphically that $k_a = 1.40$ hr$^{-1}$, $\alpha = 0.58$ hr$^{-1}$, and $\beta = 0.032$ hr$^{-1}$. Note that $k_a$ and $\alpha$ are very similar.

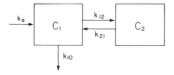

**Figure 3.35** The linear two-compartment open model with first-order absorption.

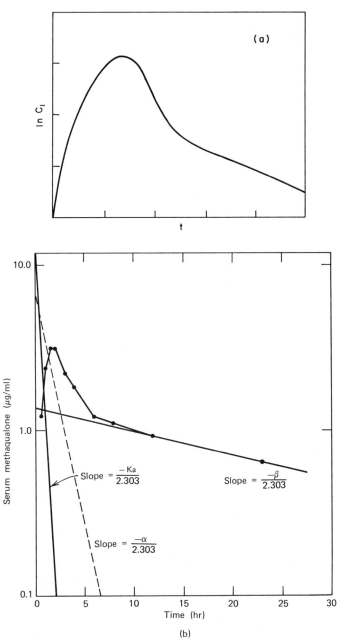

**Figure 3.36** Plots of $\ln C$ versus $t$ for the linear two-compartment open model with first-order absorption; $k_a > (k_{12} + k_{21})$. (*a*) Predicted. (*b*) Observed mean serum methaqualone levels following oral administration of a 300 mg tablet to eight human subjects. (*b*) Reproduced with permission from Nayak et al., 1974, Figure 1.

Given their standard deviations of 0.32 and 0.55 $hr^{-1}$, respectively, one is not distinguishable from the other. Also note that the $k_a$ line is determined by only two points in this example. As the authors point out, it is not possible to conclude on the basis of these data alone whether $k_a$ or $\alpha$ is larger.

## 3.12   THE AREA UNDER THE CURVE

The area under the curve of a graph of concentration versus time, from time zero to time $t$, can be represented by the definite integral of the expression for concentration as a function of time, within the stated time boundaries:

$$\text{AUC} = \int_0^t C\, dt. \tag{3.47}$$

Under certain conditions the area under the curve AUC is related to the total amount of material absorbed. If first-order kinetics adequately describe all absorption, distribution, and excretion processes and if no storage or delay compartment intervenes ahead of monitored compartments, the area under the curve can be used to estimate the total internal dose. For example, for the simplest one-compartment body model with instantaneous intravenous administration,

$$(\text{AUC})_\infty = C_0 \int_{t=0}^{t=\infty} e^{-k_e t} = \frac{C_0}{k_e} = \frac{D}{Vk_e}. \tag{3.48}$$

Since $D$ should be known when a compound is given intravenously, perhaps it would be more useful to consider the $(\text{AUC})_\infty$ for a one-compartment model with first-order absorption. Interestingly, this proves to be identical to the $(\text{AUC})_\infty$ for a one-compartment model with instantaneous injection:

$$(\text{AUC})_\infty = \frac{k_a D}{V(k_e - k_a)} \int_{t=0}^{t=\infty} (e^{-k_a t} - e^{-k_e t}) = \frac{D}{Vk_e}. \tag{3.49}$$

In this case, of course, $D$ represents the total dose absorbed, which is not necessarily equal to the total dose administered. The equation

$$(\text{AUC})_\infty = \frac{D}{Vk_e}$$

can be used to obtain an estimate of the actual internal total dose whenever first-order linear kinetics apply, irrespective of the route of administration.

The AUC may be estimated by using the trapezoidal rule: draw straight line segments between adjacent experimental points and sum the areas of all the trapezoids thus formed. It may also be estimated by using a planimeter, or by cutting out and weighing a piece of paper the shape of the unknown area and comparing it with the weight of a piece of paper of known area. Or the experimental line may be fit and the AUC estimated by application of a digital computer program (see Section 3.15).

The dose determined from the area under the curve may differ from the administered dose for two reasons. First, absorption may be incomplete. In this case the AUC allows estimation of the total dose absorbed. Second, the compound may be absorbed but may never reach the systemic circulation. If, for example, the compound is metabolized in or eliminated from the liver, the lung, or the gastrointestinal tract, the amount absorbed unchanged from an oral dose will be relatively less than the amount absorbed unchanged from another administration site. For example, Chiou (1975) showed that in man up to 38% of an oral dose of chloroform is metabolized in the liver and up to about 17% is excreted intact from the lung before the chloroform reaches the systemic circulation. This is perhaps the most common example of the *first-pass effect*. A first-pass effect can occur in any organ or tissue capable of metabolism or elimination, provided the absorbed material enters the tissue in question before reaching the systemic circulation or central compartment. Figure 3.37 expresses this statement schematically.

The AUC can be used to estimate the quantity of a drug or toxicant absorbed unchanged from time zero to time $t$. It is often used to assess the availability of drug from a commercial formulation, and much has been written on its exploitation for this purpose. An excellent article on the subject is one from a series published during 1968–1969 by J. G. Wagner (1968). The techniques used are discussed only briefly here.

Wagner and Nelson (1963) showed that the amount $A$ of drug absorbed unchanged to time $t$ is

$$A = CV + Vk_e \int_0^t C\, dt = CV + Vk_e(\text{AUC}). \qquad (3.50)$$

Since $(\text{AUC})_\infty$ is $D/k_e V$ (Equations 3.48 and 3.49), the fraction of the

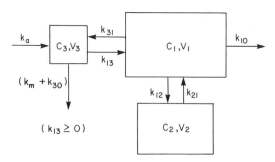

**Figure 3.37**   A linear open model with first-order absorption and first-pass elimination.

projected total internal dose that will have been absorbed by time $t$ is

$$\frac{A}{D} = \frac{C + k_e(\text{AUC})}{k_e(\text{AUC})_\infty}. \tag{3.51}$$

Remember that $D$ represents the internal dose or the amount absorbed unchanged. In practice the areas are usually calculated from a computer fit or by means of the trapezoidal rule, and $k_e$ is estimated from the slope of terminal dieaway data. The Wagner-Nelson method assumes first-order elimination in a one-compartment model but is independent of any assumption concerning the mechanism or kinetic order of drug absorption. It may be adapted to the two-compartment open model, provided absorption is first order and, in this case, it may be used to estimate all the microconstants of the two-compartment system (Wagner, 1974).

Loo and Riegelman developed an analogous expression for the amount of drug absorbed to time $t$ in a two-compartment open system without regard to the kinetic order of the absorption process (1968). The Loo-Riegelman expression contains an extra term representing amount of drug in the peripheral compartment at time $t$, and its application requires that $k_{12}$, $k_{21}$, and $k_e$ be known from an independent intravenous study. The uses and limitations of the two methods have been compared in detail by Wagner (1975a).

In the study of salicylamide (SAM) metabolism carried out by Houston and Levy and used as an example of the estimation of kinetic parameters in a one-compartment open model with parallel elimination processes in Section 3.6, areas under the curve were also estimated. SAM was administered either intravenously (100 mg/kg) or orally (500 mg/kg) to groups of five rats, and the AUCs from 0 to 90 min were estimated for parent SAM and for the two metabolites SAMS and SAMG. For SAM but not for SAMS and SAMG, AUC from 0 to 90 min was a good approximation to $(\text{AUC})_\infty$ since little SAM remained in the plasma after this time whether administration was oral or intravenous. The AUCs are given in Table 3.5.

**Table 3.5** Area under the plasma concentration, time curve from 0 to 90 min for SAM, SAMG, and SAMS after oral and intravenous administration; means of values from five rats

| Compound | AUC after 100 mg/kg Intravenously ($\mu$g min/ml) | AUC after 500 mg/kg Orally ($\mu$g min/ml) |
|---|---|---|
| SAM | 1320 | 1028 |
| SAMG | 1070 | 3146 |
| SAMS | 1085 | 2252 |

Data from Houston and Levy, 1976, Tables 2 and 4.

The oral availability of SAM may be estimated directly from the AUCs, since they approximate $(AUC)_\infty$, with a correction for the difference in doses:

$$\text{oral availability of SAM} = \frac{(AUC)_\infty \text{ oral}}{(AUC)_\infty \text{ i.v.}}$$

$$= \left[ \frac{(1028)\ (\mu g/ml)\ min}{(5)(1320)\ (\mu g/ml)\ min} \right] (100)$$

$$= 16\%.$$

The AUCs for SAMS and SAMG cannot be so directly interpreted, since neither is an approximation to $(AUC)_\infty$. However, two general inferences can be drawn.

First, since oral administration of SAM results in greatly increased AUCs for SAMS and SAMG at a total internal SAM dose somewhat less than that of the intravenous study (cf. 1028 with 1320), we can assume that an important component of the incomplete oral availability is first-pass metabolism of SAM, either in the gastrointestinal tract or in the liver, with distribution of the metabolites into the plasma compartment.

Second, it is to be expected that $(AUC)_\infty$ for the two metabolites after intravenous administration of SAM will be approximately equal:

$$(AUC)_{\infty\ SAMS} = \frac{52.8\ mg/kg}{(3.0\ l/kg)(0.0076\ min^{-1})} = 2300\ (\mu g/ml)\ min$$

$$(AUC)_{\infty\ SAMG} = \frac{(33.5\ mg/kg)}{(2.3\ l/kg)(0.0066\ min^{-1})} = 2200\ (\mu g/ml)\ min$$

$$= \frac{D}{Vk_e},$$

where the volumes of distribution were estimated by Houston and Levy from renal clearance data as discussed in the next section. Table 3.5 shows that by 90 min after intravenous injection of SAM the two AUCs are already about equal.

### 3.13   THE CONCEPT OF CLEARANCE

The clearance $Cl_{total}$ of an intravenously administered compound is defined as

$$Cl_{total} = \frac{D}{\int_0^\infty C\,dt} \quad \text{or} \quad \frac{D}{(AUC)_\infty}, \tag{3.52}$$

where the denominator represents the area under the plasma $C, t$ curve from time zero to infinite time. As shown in the previous section, for any one-compartment model with first-order elimination

$$\int_0^\infty C\,dt = \frac{D}{k_e V_D},\qquad (3.48),\ (3.49)$$

so that

$$Cl_{total} = k_e V_D.\qquad (3.53)$$

Since from Equation 3.17

$$\frac{dU}{dt} = k_u V_D C_0 e^{-k_e t} = k_u V_D C,\qquad (3.17)$$

$$\frac{\frac{dU}{dt}}{C} = k_u V_D = Cl_{renal}.\qquad (3.54)$$

Therefore clearance by one of several parallel processes can be thought of as *the rate of elimination of a compound by that process divided by its concentration in the plasma*. A graph of $\Delta U/\Delta t$ against $C$ should approximate a straight line with positive slope $k_u V_D$ (Figure 3.38a). Of course if renal excretion is the sole elimination process, $Cl_{renal} = Cl_{total} = k_e V_D$. Note that the relationship between $\Delta U/\Delta t$ and $C$ is linear only as long as the elimination process is exclusively first order.

Clearance can be by any excretory pathway, although renal clearance is the most familiar. An example of pulmonary clearance of chloroform in humans is shown in Figure 3.38b. The slope of this pulmonary excretion graph represents a clearance of about 900 ml/min. This value compares well with the predicted value calculated by multiplying the extraction efficiency or fraction cleared, 0.17 (Chiou, 1975), by the pulmonary blood flow rate of 5000 ml/min:

$$0.17 \times 5000 \text{ ml/min} = 850 \text{ ml/min}.$$

Since pulmonary clearance represents diffusion from pulmonary arterial blood into alveolar air, it is a first-order process, and the relationship between the rate of excretion in expired air and concentration in the blood should always be linear.

Note that clearance is directly dependent not only on the excretory rate constant but also on the volume of the compartment being cleared. It has been pointed out by Perrier and Gibaldi (1974) that clearance is entirely independent of kinetic parameters associated with any compartment other than the compartment from which material is being eliminated. In other

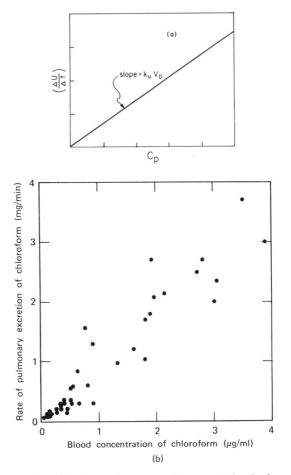

**Figure 3.38** The relationship of excretion rate to $C$, concentration in the compartment from which excretion is occurring, when excretion is first order. ($a$) Predicted, for urinary excretion. The slope of the line is $Cl_{renal}$. ($b$) Observed pulmonary excretion rate of chloroform as a function of its concentration in the blood in a group of human subjects. The slope of the line through these data is $Cl_{pulmonary}$. ($b$) Reproduced with permission from Fry et al., 1972, Figure 5.

words, clearance is always expressed in terms of microconstants instead of the hybrid kinetic rate constants characteristic of models with more than one compartment. Therefore it has been suggested that clearance may sometimes be the most meaningful measure of the elimination of a foreign compound.

Clearance has the dimensions $(vol)(time^{-1})$, and represents the volume of plasma cleared of solute per unit of time. The relationship of clearance in a tissue to the total flow rate of plasma through the tissue is a measure of the extraction efficiency of the tissue. It can often be a useful key to the sites and mechanisms of elimination of a foreign compound.

As an example, consider once again the study of SAM metabolism by Houston and Levy (1976). The clearance of parent SAM was calculated by dividing the total intravenous dose by the area under the plasma SAM concentration, time curve. $Cl_{total}^{SAM}$ was found to be 76.3 ml/min/kg. Renal clearances of the metabolites SAMS and SAMG, however, were estimated as the slopes of urinary excretion rate, plasma concentration graphs, as shown in Figures 3.39a and 3.39b. Both graphs were linear over a wide concentration range, demonstrating that elimination of both metabolites is first order. Coadministration of ascorbic acid to these rats had no effect on the renal clearance of either metabolite. The renal clearance of SAMS was about 23 ml/min/kg, from which it can be estimated by using the value of $k_u^M$ from Section 3.6 that

$$V_D^{SAMS} = \frac{Cl_{renal}^{SAMS}}{k_{u\,SAMS}^M} = \frac{23\ ml/min/kg}{0.0076\ min^{-1}} = 3.0\ l/kg.$$

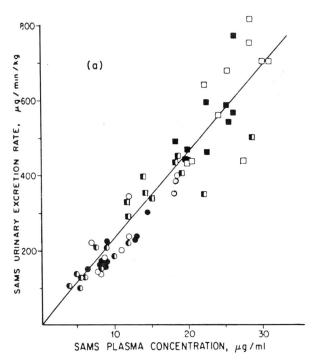

**Figure 3.39** The relationship between urinary excretion rate and plasma concentration of two metabolites of SAM in five rats administered 100 mg of SAM/kg intravenously (circles) and in five rats administered 500 mg of SAM/kg orally (squares): Open symbols, control experiments; closed symbols, with ascorbic acid, 500 mg/kg intravenously; half-open symbols, with ascorbic acid, 500 mg/kg orally. In each experiment urinary excretion rates were determined from 0 to 1 and from 1 to 2 hr and plasma concentrations were determined at 30 and 90 min. The regression line was forced through the origin. (a) Clearance of SAMS. (b) Clearance of SAMG. Reproduced with permission from Houston and Levy, 1976, Figures 7 and 8, © 1976 by the Williams & Wilkins Co., Baltimore.

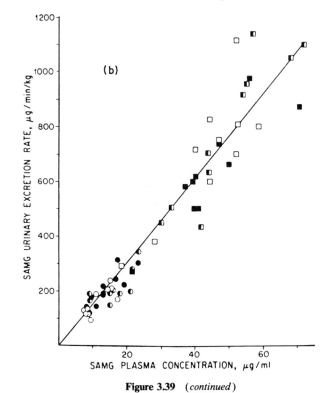

**Figure 3.39** (*continued*)

The renal clearance of SAMG was about 15 ml/min/kg, so that

$$V_D^{\text{SAMG}} = \frac{\text{Cl}_{\text{renal}}^{\text{SAMG}}}{k_{u\,\text{SAMG}}^{\text{M}}} = \frac{15\ \text{ml/min/kg}}{0.0066\ \text{min}^{-1}} = 2.3\ \text{l/kg}.$$

Similarly,

$$V_D^{\text{SAM}} = \frac{\text{Cl}_{\text{total}}}{k_e} = \frac{76.3\ \text{ml/min/kg}}{0.0525\ \text{min}^{-1}} = 1.4\ \text{l/kg}.$$

All three volumes of distribution are unreasonably large physiologically, suggesting that all three compounds are not as accessible to the analytical technique used as they are to renal extraction and excretion.

Since SAM is not excreted unchanged into the urine, clearance of parent SAM represents metabolism, which is usually considered to take place in the liver until experimental evidence suggests otherwise. In this case the mean $\text{Cl}_{\text{total}}^{\text{SAM}}$, 76.3 ml/min/kg, is slightly higher than hepatic blood flow in rats, suggesting that some SAM may be metabolized extrahepatically. Since $\text{Cl}_{\text{renal}}^{\text{SAMS}}$ and $\text{Cl}_{\text{renal}}^{\text{SAMG}}$ were calculated from urinary excretion data alone, they give no information on possible additional routes of excretion of the two metabolites.

The estimates of $V_D$ are based on the implicit assumption that there are no additional routes of excretion.

A final example has been chosen to illustrate the combined use of several of the kinetic measurements discussed in this chapter. Hinderling and Garrett (1976) administered the antiarrhythmic drug disopyramide (DP) to healthy male adult human volunteers and monitored the time course of plasma concentration change and urinary excretion of DP and of its major mono-dealkylated metabolite MP. DP was administered both orally and intravenously on separate occasions.

The fraction of an oral DP dose that reached the systemic circulation unchanged was estimated from the cumulative amounts $U_\infty$ of DP excreted into the urine after comparable oral and intravenous doses. It could equally well have been calculated from the appropriate $(AUC)_\infty$ values. This fraction was found to be 0.84. However, the apparent absorption efficiency calculated on the basis of total cumulative renal excretion of DP *plus* MP after comparable oral and intravenous doses indicated that the entire oral DP dose was absorbed. Therefore the data suggested that about 16% of the orally administered DP was metabolized either in the liver or in the intestinal wall in a first-pass metabolism.

The total clearance of DP, $Cl_{total}^{DP}$, was estimated to be $245 \pm 10$ ml/min from the $(AUC)_\infty$ value for DP given intravenously. The renal clearance of DP, $Cl_{renal}^{DP}$, was estimated to be $125 \pm 14$ ml/min from the slope of a graph of $\Delta U / \Delta t$ against $C$. The metabolic or hepatic clearance $Cl_{hepatic}^{DP}$ was taken to be the difference,

$$Cl_{hepatic}^{DP} = Cl_{total}^{DP} - Cl_{renal}^{DP},$$

on the assumption that there were no other routes of elimination of DP. $Cl_{hepatic}^{DP}$ was therefore $120 \pm 7$ ml/min. Since mean hepatic plasma flow in these subjects was 825 ml/min, the extraction efficiency (or metabolic efficiency) of the liver was $(120/825)(100) = 14\%$. This predicted value is remarkably close to the observed value of 16% metabolism on the first pass during absorption of an oral dose and identifies the liver, not the gut wall, as the site of the first-pass effect.

## 3.14  MORE COMPLEX MODELS

The addition of more peripheral compartments to the two-compartment model introduces another exponential term into the equation for $C_1$ as a function of time for each compartment added. Equation 3.55 describes a three-compartment model with elimination solely from the central compartment as shown in Figure 3.40.

$$C_1 = A_0 e^{-\alpha t} + B_0 e^{-\beta t} + C_0 e^{-\gamma t} \qquad (3.55)$$

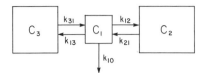

**Figure 3.40**   The linear three-compartment open model.

Resolution of the plasma dieaway curve into its component straight line segments is analogous to the procedure for the two-compartment model except that for each additional compartment another feathering step is added. Successive featherings are always made on the basis of deviations from the last line drawn. The differences between the $\gamma$ line and the experimental data define the $\beta$ line; the differences between the $\beta$ line and the early points that deviate from it define the $\alpha$ line. The third or $\alpha$ line for a three-compartment model should be linear throughout.

The kinetics of sulfate disposition in the rabbit are consistent with a three-compartment model, as shown in Figure 3.41. Resolution of the plasma sulfate dieaway curve into its three component segments gives values of $\alpha$, $\beta$, and $\gamma$ of about 14, 3.5, and 0.19 hr$^{-1}$, respectively. The biological half-life of sulfate is $0.693/\gamma$, or about 3.6 hr. It should be kept in mind that extension of

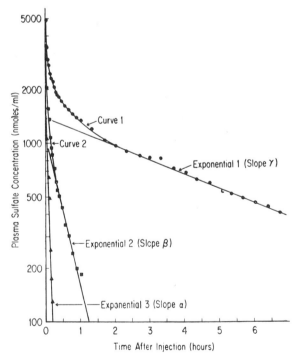

**Figure 3.41** Concentration of plasma sulfate in a rabbit following the rapid intravenous injection of 0.60 m mole of sulfate/kg. The two feathered lines derived from the ln plasma concentration, time curve are also shown. Reproduced with permission from Gunnison and Palmes, 1976, Figure 3.

the monitoring period to later times might reveal an additional, even slower dieaway segment, perhaps representing loss from a deep compartment. Therefore it is always advisable to monitor for at least 5 to 6 times what appears to be the biological half-life, to be certain that it is indeed the biological half-life.

All the models considered to this point have been mammillary models. A mammillary model consists always of a central compartment whose contents interchange with the contents of at least one peripheral compartment. Excretion from a mammillary model may be from any one or more of the compartments. Benet (1972) has pointed out that the maximum number of rate constants for which values may be estimated by sampling only from the central compartment of a mammillary model is $[2(n-1)+1]$, where $n$ is the number of compartments having rate constants directed outward, and that only one of these rate constants is unambiguously an elimination microconstant. Since the model in Figure 3.40 has three compartments and five microconstants, it may be solved for all five. However, note that two more possible microconstants were set equal to zero: $k_{20}$ and $k_{30}$. The assumption that elimination takes place from only one compartment, in this case the central compartment, allows calculation of all the microconstants. There is no way to distinguish kinetically, however, between a mammillary model with all elimination from the central compartment and a mammillary model that includes elimination from one or more peripheral compartments by sampling from the central compartment alone.

Irrespective of the number of compartments from which elimination can take place, a mammillary model with $n$ compartments will contain $n$ terms in the expression for concentration in the central compartment. Assuming that the graph of concentration as a function of time can be feathered to yield $n$ slopes, then $[2(n-1)+1]$ rate constants can be calculated. But the definition of these rate constants is ambiguous. For compartment $n$ one of the calculated rate constants is $(k_{n1}+k_{n0})$ and, unless $k_{n0}$ is known to be zero, the magnitude of $k_{n1}$ cannot be determined. Therefore there is no explicit general solution that will permit the calculation of the individual microconstants in mammillary models with loss from more than one compartment, using data obtained by sampling only the central compartment. Although it is usually ignored, this limitation also applies to the two-compartment model, as discussed by Rowland et al. (1970). Strictly speaking, all the microconstants can be calculated only if there is independent justification for selecting a model with loss from only one compartment.

Elimination either by metabolism in or by excretion from a peripheral compartment is not unusual in biological systems. Coumermycin A, a bishydroxycoumarin antibiotic whose pharmacokinetics have been studied by Kaplan (1970), and bishydroxycoumarin itself (Nagashima et al., 1968) appear to be metabolized entirely in a peripheral compartment. On the other hand, aspirin is metabolized both in the central and in a peripheral compartment (Rowland et al., 1970). Volatile materials are generally exhaled; if they have been inhaled initially, there is usually a strong first-pass effect. Many minerals are excreted in the hair. Excretion in nails, sweat, or milk may occasionally be important. It is important to remember that excretion by extrarenal and extrahepatic pathways is not necessarily excretion from a peripheral compartment in the kinetic sense of the word. Often the lung, for example, is part of the central kinetically determined compartment.

Peripheral elimination could also occur from a catenary system, which has no central compartment but consists instead of a chain of compartments through which solute travels away from its entry point. Catenary models are not ordinarily important in distribution and excretion studies except where experimental conditions place artificial constraints on the disposition of the material under study. They are, however, essential in the analysis of sequential enzyme-mediated transformations such as occur in intermediary metabolism.

It is beyond the scope of this book to develop in any detail the mathematics of multicompartment systems. The reader who is interested is referred directly to original publications on this subject. Wagner (1975) has discussed the factors important in selecting the most appropriate model, which may not necessarily be either the most accurate or the most complete model. The generalized two-compartment model appears in a publication by Rowland et al. (1970). Benet (1972) developed a generalized treatment of multicompartment mammillary models that greatly facilitates derivation of the associated kinetic equations. Benet's technique considers input only into the central compartment; Vaughan and Trainor (1975) have expanded it to include input into any or all compartments simultaneously. Equations for the three-compartment catenary model were derived by Skinner et al. (1959) for use in studies of intermediary metabolism with radiolabeled substrates; in these studies compartment volumes are replaced by the pool sizes of the key metabolic intermediates.

When disposition of one or more metabolites must be taken into account in addition to the pharmacokinetics of the parent, models become still more complex. Such systems can be treated as hybrids of more than one mammillary model with interchanges at one or more points. Generally rate constants can be estimated only by sampling multiple compartments as well as excreta.

As an example, consider the detailed kinetic study of cephapirin, an antibiotic, reported by Cabana et al. (1975). Initially, feathering of cephapirin dieaway curves after intravenous injection suggested a two-compartment model with equilibration into one tissue compartment; elimination was presumed to be from the central (plasma) compartment, and $k_{12}$, $k_{21}$, and $k_{10}$ were estimated. Cumulative urinary outputs of cephapirin and its metabolite deacetylcephapirin were measured and the data used to estimate the three microconstants for elimination by these two routes and by the total of all other, undefined routes. Since little deacetylcephapirin was found in the blood after intravenous administration of cephapirin, it was assumed that the microconstant estimated from deacetylcephapirin urinary excretion data was $k_m$. Intravenous injection of deacetylcephapirin itself permitted the estimation of $k_u^M$, which was in fact more than 9 times $k_m$. It also suggested that like its parent, deacetylcephapirin distributed between plasma and a tissue compartment and allowed estimation of the distribution microconstants.

Kinetic calculations up to this point had been based on the assumption that cephapirin was metabolized extrarenally. When the renal clearance of deacetylcephapirin was calculated by dividing the amount excreted in the urine by the area under the plasma deacetylcephapirin concentration, time curve after intravenous injection of cephapirin, it was found that renal clearance greatly exceeded a physiologically reasonable rate; therefore cephapirin must be metabolized within the kidney. The complete model is shown in Figure 3.42, where the microconstant $k_{15}$ represents simultaneous renal formation and urinary excretion of deacetylcephapirin. The microconstants $k_{15}$, $k_{16}$, and $k_{65}$ were assigned initial estimated values, then entered into a digital computer program together with fixed values of the other microconstants; in this way the values of $k_{15}$, $k_{16}$, and $k_{65}$ that gave a least squares best fit to the experimental data points for both cephapirin and deacetylcephapirin were calculated.

Two points are particularly important in connection with this study. First, note that the kinetics of cephapirin disposition are adequately described by a two-compartment open model. Second, note that if these investigators had not been specifically interested in whether cephapirin is metabolized by the kidney, there would have been no justification for the development of such a detailed kinetic model.

The degree to which a kinetic model should be refined must be dictated by the purpose of the study. Sampling from a variety of tissues, for example, will almost always reveal a multitude of peripheral compartments whose

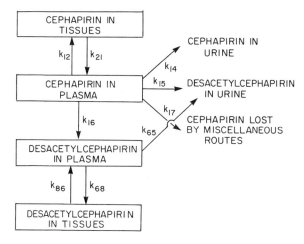

**Figure 3.42** Model of cephapirin kinetics in man. Redrawn with permission from Cabana et al., 1975, Model IV.

existence is not kinetically demonstrable by sampling from the plasma alone. In many instances differentiation of these compartments one from another will not be relevant to the study. If, however, one of the compartments contains the site of action (the biophase) of a drug or a toxicant, or is capable of sequestering large amounts of the drug or toxicant, it may be important to characterize that compartment more fully not only kinetically but physiologically and, ultimately, biochemically as well. Well-designed kinetic studies, as will become clear in later chapters, can assist in identifying the biophase of a drug or toxicant and in predicting the magnitude of potential accumulation within the sensitive tissue.

### 3.15 COMPUTER FITTING OF MULTIPLE EXPONENTIAL KINETIC DATA

Manual data plotting, curve inspection and stripping, and transformation to forms expected to be linear are always essential. These manual techniques allow the researcher to determine which of the available kinetic models is probably the most appropriate and to make decisions with regard to the proper weighting of experimental points, including the identification of outlying points.

Nonetheless, even with the aid of a calculator, manual analysis of curves representable by sequences of exponentials is tedious and prohibitively time-consuming. Digital computational fitting of kinetic data is the alternative. The digital computer will not only calculate the parameters of the assumed kinetic model much faster than is possible manually but will also provide an estimate of the overall goodness of fit, or the quality of the agreement between experimental data points and expected values calculated on the assumption that the applied kinetic model is correct. Some digital programs will also test the compatibility of the experimental data with a limited number of alternative models. Usually digital programs are fed initial estimates of the kinetic parameters obtained from manual or analog computer curve analysis, but programs can be written that will perform an initial feathering procedure to obtain these estimates.

A number of programs are available to fit multiexponential integrated curves for $C(t)$. In general, beginning with the initial estimates, these programs modify the parameters in a systematic fashion until the sum of squares of $[C(t)_{calculated} - C(t)_{experimental}]$ for all sampling times is at a minimum. There may be more than one minimum (more than one reasonable fit); to be sure of finding the "best" of all the "good" fits, the operator may feed the computer more than one set of initial parameter estimates to ensure that the same minimum is found repeatedly or, if not, that the solution giving the smallest sum of squares has been identified. Some programs incorporate a routine to ensure that the best fit has been found. If $\alpha$ and $\beta$, or $k_a$ and $k_e$, are of the same order of magnitude, the computer may find many shallow minima but no clear-cut "best" fit. This is, of course, also the case with manual data fits; note the uncertainty in the estimates of $k_a$ and $\alpha$ for the methaqualone data in Section 3.11.

The computer may modify one parameter at a time in its progress toward the minimum sum of squares. This procedure is simple but slow, and it does not always converge, or find a minimum. The Simplex procedure (Spendley et al., 1962) uses a vectorial method to spiral into the minimum, and it always converges. These are examples of direct search procedures. Gradient procedures employ partial derivatives with respect to each of the model parameters as well as values of the integrated model equation. The best known digital computer programs use gradient methods, in particular Hartley's modification of the Gauss-Newton method (Hartley, 1961). These programs include SAAM and NONLIN.

SAAM (Berman and Weiss, 1968) can accept either integrated or differential equations. It will fit more than one data set at a time so that urine and plasma data, for example, can be fit simultaneously. It can weight data points and can simulate.

NONLIN (Metzler, 1969) is slightly more versatile. It will accept either integrated or differential equations, will weight data points, fit multiple data sets simultaneously, simulate, and fit equations for saturable processes.

Specialized programs have also been written to be used in conjunction with NONLIN and SAAM. In addition, independent programs are available that will simulate data from differential equations and thus can accommodate quite complex kinetic systems.

The purpose of this book is to familiarize the reader with kinetic applications, not with computer applications. However, it is important that the student who expects to participate in active kinetics research be aware that computer curve fitting techniques will be used for all but the simplest kinetic models. The digital computer holds a central position in kinetic data analysis and interpretation.

## APPENDIX 3.1   DERIVATION OF THE EQUATION FOR FIRST-ORDER ABSORPTION FROM A DEPOT AND FIRST-ORDER ELIMINATION FROM A SINGLE COMPARTMENT

Assume that

$D$ = total dose administered into the depot at $t=0$

$A$ = amount of dose left at administration site at $t=t$

$X$ = amount absorbed at $t=t$

$k_a$ = rate constant for absorption

$k_e$ = rate constant for elimination

$$\frac{dX}{dt} = k_a A - k_e X.$$

But

$$A = De^{-k_a t},$$

so that

$$\frac{dX}{dt} = k_a D e^{-k_a t} - k_e X.$$

Multiply both sides of the equation by the integrating factor $e^{k_e t}$ and rearrange:

$$e^{k_e t}\frac{dX}{dt} + k_e X e^{k_e t} = k_a D e^{(k_e - k_a)t}.$$

The left-hand side of this equation is equal to

$$\frac{d}{dt}(X e^{k_e t}).$$

Therefore

$$X e^{k_e t} = k_a D \int e^{(k_e - k_a)t}\, dt$$

$$= \left(\frac{k_a D}{k_e - k_a}\right)(e^{(k_e - k_a)t}) + \text{constant}.$$

At $t=0$, $X=0$ and the constant of integration is therefore

$$\frac{k_a D}{k_a - k_e}.$$

Therefore

$$X e^{k_e t} = \left(\frac{k_a D}{k_e - k_a}\right)(e^{(k_e - k_a)t} - 1)$$

and

$$X = \left(\frac{k_a D}{k_e - k_a}\right)(e^{-k_a t} - e^{-k_e t}).$$

## APPENDIX 3.2 DERIVATION OF THE EXPRESSION FOR $t_{\text{max}}$

It was shown in Appendix 3.1 that

$$X = \left( \frac{k_a D}{k_e - k_a} \right)(e^{-k_a t} - e^{-k_e t}),$$

where all quantities are defined as in Appendix 3.1. Now for $X$ to be at its maximum, $dX/dt$ must be zero.

$$\frac{dX}{dt} = \left( \frac{k_a D}{k_e - k_a} \right)(k_e e^{-k_e t} - k_a e^{-k_a t}).$$

When $dX/dt = 0$,

$$k_a e^{-k_a t_{\text{max}}} = k_e e^{-k_e t_{\text{max}}};$$

$$-k_a t_{\text{max}} = \ln\left( \frac{k_e}{k_a} \right) - k_e t_{\text{max}} \quad \text{or} \quad t_{\text{max}} = \ln\left( \frac{k_e / k_a}{k_e - k_a} \right).$$

## PROBLEMS

1  Show that Equation 3.3 is dimensionally correct. What are the dimensions of $DA/dx$? Are they also the dimensions of $V_m/K_m$ in Equation 3.1? Are they consistent with the statement made by Equation 3.30?

2  Equation 3.14 is the derivative with respect to time of Equation 3.13. Equation 3.14 can also be obtained directly in differential form by consideration of the parameters that govern the rate of transfer from plasma to urine. Set up such a differential equation and show that it is equivalent to Equation 3.14.

3  Although $k_{21}$ in the two-compartment model can be smaller than $k_e$, it is never smaller than the negative terminal slope of the plasma dieaway line. Discuss why this is so.

4  Integrate Equation 3.42 and evaluate it from $t=0$ to $t=\infty$ to show that $(\text{AUC})_\infty = D/Vk_e$.

5  If $A$ is the amount of drug absorbed from an oral dose by time $t$, $A_b$ is the amount remaining in the circulation at time $t$, and $A_e$ is the amount eliminated, then

$$A = A_b + A_e.$$

Now $A_b = CV$ and, when elimination is first order,

$$\frac{d(A_e)}{dt} = k_e VC.$$

From the expressions given, and any other necessary known relationships, derive the Wagner-Nelson equation (Equation 3.50).

**6** It can be shown for Equation 3.42 that when $t = t_{max}$,

$$C_{max} = \left(\frac{D}{V}\right)\left[(m)^{1/(1-m)}\right],$$

where $m = k_a/k_e.$

Assume that $k_a = 0.004$ hr$^{-1}$ and $k_e = 0.7$ hr$^{-1}$, corresponding to absorption and elimination half-lives for benzathine penicillin G of 6.5 days and 1.0 hr, respectively. Assume further that penicillin G distributes throughout a total body water volume of 43 liters in the adult human, and calculate $C_{max}$ for the $1.2 \times 10^6$ unit dose of benzathine penicillin G used as an example in the text (Figure 3.34). How does your predicted value compare with the observed value?

**7** Show that the ordinate intercept of the feathered line from Equation 3.42 (the line with slope $-k_a$) is the same as the ordinate intercept of the back-extrapolated terminal segment (the line with slope $-k_e$).

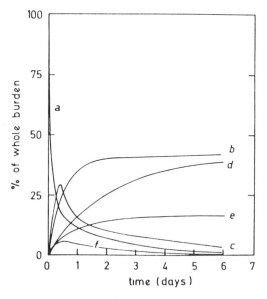

**Figure 3.43** Percentage of body burden of $^{210}$Pb in various organs and tissue of rats following a single inhalation exposure of 1 hr to [$^{210}$Pb tetraethyl. Curves; *a*, lung; *b*, cumulative digestive tract elimination (gut plus feces); *c*, blood; *d*, bone; *e*, cumulative renal elimination (kidney plus urine); *f*, liver. Reproduced with permission from Boudene et al., 1977, Figure 4.

**8** Boudène et al. (1977) administered tetraethyl lead to rats by means of an aerosol prepared from gasoline containing ($^{210}$Pb)tetraethyl, and followed for 6 days the percentage of total body burden of $^{210}$Pb found in various tissues, with the results shown in Figure 3.43. Are blood and liver part of the same kinetic compartment or do they represent different compartments? What kind of kinetic compartment is bone?

**9** Methsuximide (METH), an antiepileptic drug, is metabolized to 2-methyl-2-phenylsuccinimide (PHEN), also an antiepileptic drug, as well as to other metabolites. Dobrinska and Welling (1977) studied the pharmacokinetics of METH and PHEN in dogs after intravenous administration of 250 mg of either compound. Under these conditions METH kinetics were described by the equation

$$C = 11.7e^{-8.03t} + 6.8e^{-0.71t}$$

and PHEN kinetics by the equation

$$C = 17.1e^{-0.047t},$$

where the coefficients are expressed in $\mu g/ml$ and the numerical exponents are expressed in $hr^{-1}$. Design a model that fits the observed kinetics of METH and PHEN.

**10** Mischler et al. (1974) administered the antibiotic cephradine orally to 14 human subjects at two different dose levels, with and without supplementary treatments $A$ and $B$. The kinetic data are given, as means of 14 observations, in Table 3.6. Assume a one-compartment body model, without flip-flop.

  **(a)** Does treatment $A$ alter the absorption rate constant $k_a$? The elimination rate constant $k_e$? Give the directions of any changes.

  **(b)** Does treatment $B$ alter $k_a$? $k_e$? Give the directions of any changes.

**Table 3.6** Kinetic data for cephradine given orally to 14 adult males

| Treatment | Peak Concentration in Serum ($\mu g/ml$) | Time to Peak Serum Concentration (hr) | $t_{1/2}$ (hr) | Area under Serum Concentration Curve ($\mu g \cdot hr/ml$) | Dose (mg) |
|---|---|---|---|---|---|
| None | 44.8 | 1.1 | 0.9 | 87 | 2000 |
| $A$ | 72.2 | 1.8 | 1.5 | 254 | 2000 |
| None | 19.8 | 0.8 | 0.75 | 28 | 500 |
| $B$ | 10.9 | 2.0 | 0.83 | 25 | 500 |

Data from Mischler et al., 1974, Tables I and III.

**11** Nayak et al. (1974) (see Figure 3.36*b*) administered methaqualone to a group of eight human subjects at separate times. Since the serum concentration, time curves were not affected by the number of previous administrations of methaqualone, data for all five studies have been averaged in Table 3.7. Graph these data appropriately and feather to estimate $\beta$, $\alpha$, and $k_a$. Compare your estimates with those given in the text.

**Table 3.7** Serum methaqualone concentrations following oral administration of methaqualone to human volunteers

| $t$ (hr) | Serum Methaqualone ($\mu g/ml$) |
|---|---|
| $-0.5$ | 0.8 |
| 0.5 | 1.8 |
| 1.0 | 2.8 |
| 1.5 | 3.3 |
| 2.0 | 3.3 |
| 3.0 | 2.8 |
| 4.0 | 2.2 |
| 6.0 | 1.7 |
| 8.0 | 1.5 |
| 12.0 | 1.4 |
| 24.0 | 1.0 |

Average values based on data from Nayak et al., 1974, Table 1.

**12** About 70% of the dye phenol red is renally eliminated by the rat. 30 mg of phenol red was administered intravenously to a 275-g rat and the plasma and urine concentrations were measured as functions of time. The results are given in Table 3.8.

(a) Graph amount of phenol red yet to be excreted $(U_\infty - U)$ against time on appropriate coordinates and estimate $k_e$ and $k_u$. Is the value of the ordinate intercept consistent with the predicted value based on 70% urinary excretion?

(b) Graph $\ln(\Delta U/\Delta t)$ against time and estimate $k_e$ and $k_u$. Is the ordinate intercept consistent with the predicted value based on 70% urinary excretion?

(c) Estimate $k_e$ from the plasma concentration data and compare it with the values obtained from excretory data.

(d) Graph the rate of urinary excretion against the plasma concentration and estimate the renal clearance (as the slope). Using $V_D$

**Table 3.8** Measured plasma and urine concentrations of phenol red following intravenous administration of 30 mg to a 275-g rat; plasma samples were taken at approximate midpoints of the consecutive urine collection periods

| Time Interval of Urine Collection (min) | Urine Volume (ml) | Concentration of Phenol Red in Urine ($\mu$g/ml) | Concentration of Phenol Red in Plasma ($\mu$g/ml) |
|---|---|---|---|
| 0–5 | 1.631 | 3980 | 557.5 |
| 5–10 | 1.189 | 2720 | 352.0 |
| 10–15 | 0.675 | 3820 | 254.4 |
| 15–20 | 0.565 | 4030 | 184.0 |
| 20–25 | 0.313 | 4520 | 147.0 |
| 25–30 | 0.302 | 4160 | 103.2 |
| 30–35 | 0.103 | 3810 | 74.9 |
| 35–40 | 0.125 | 6680 | 67.7 |
| 40–50 | 0.258 | 4508 | 47.6 |
| 50–60 | 0.343 | 2740 | 32.0 |
| 60–70 | 0.268 | 1790 | 22.0 |
| 70–285 | 12.485 | 179.4 | — |

calculated from the ordinate intercept of the plasma data and $k_u$ from Problems 12a and 12b above, calculate renal clearance as $k_u V_D$. Compare your three estimates of renal clearance.

(e) In Problem 7 of Chapter 1 you calculated the rate constant for elimination of inulin from the plasma of a 275-g rat. Inulin is eliminated by glomerular filtration only. Assuming that $V_D$ for inulin in the rat is 320 ml/kg, calculate the glomerular filtration rate (the inulin clearance) for a rat of this size and compare it with the renal clearance of phenol red. Do your calculations suggest that phenol red is cleared by glomerular filtration alone in the rat kidney, or do they suggest that it is cleared by another mechanism in addition to filtration?

13  The microconstant $k_e$ is sensitive to many influences, both exogenous and endogenous, and is therefore subject to change. A change in $k_e$ will affect all the hybrid rate constants and volume terms of a two-compartment open model. Jusko and Gibaldi (1972) have simulated the behavior of $\alpha$, $\beta$, $A_0$, and $B_0$ in a two compartment open system when only $k_e$ is varied. Their results are given in Table 3.9. Parameters maintained constant were $k_{12} = 1.0$ hr$^{-1}$ and $k_{21} = 1.5$ hr$^{-1}$.

One purpose of this simulation was to show that it is not always necessary to invoke alterations in distribution microconstants or spaces to explain changes in apparent volume of distribution.

**Table 3.9**  The dependence of $\alpha$, $\beta$, $A_0$, and $B_0$ on $k_e$ for the two-compartment open model: $k_{12}$ is 1.0 hr$^{-1}$ and $k_{21}$ is 1.5 hr$^{-1}$

| Parameter | $k_e$ (hr$^{-1}$) | | | |
|---|---|---|---|---|
|  | 0.01 | 0.1 | 1.0 | 10.0 |
| $\alpha$ | 2.50 | 2.54 | 3.00 | 11.16 |
| $\beta$ | 0.006 | 0.059 | 0.50 | 1.345 |
| $A_0$ | 0.100 | 0.105 | 0.15 | 0.246 |
| $B_0$ | 0.150 | 0.145 | 0.10 | 0.004 |

Adapted from Jusko and Gibaldi, 1972, Table I, with permission of the copyright owner.

Bromsulfalein dye is used in the measurement of hepatic clearance. Clearance of bromsulfalein is altered when liver disease is present. Graph the bromsulfalein data given in Table 3.10.

(a)  Feather to estimate $\alpha$, $\beta$, $A_0$, and $B_0$ for the four subject groups with varying degrees of liver disease.

(b)  Determine the effect of liver disease on $\alpha$, $\beta$, $A_0$, and $B_0$. Is the behavior you observe qualitatively similar to the behavior predicted

**Table 3.10**  Blood levels of bromsulfalein at various intervals after intravenous administration of 5 mg/kg to four groups of individuals distinguishable on the basis of their degree of liver disease[a]

| Normal | | | Mild Liver Disease | | | Moderate Liver Disease | | | Severe Liver Disease | | |
|---|---|---|---|---|---|---|---|---|---|---|---|
| A | B | C | A | B | C | A | B | C | A | B | C |
| 7 | 6.2 | 5.42 | 12 | 6.2 | 6.66 | 9 | 6.1 | 7.16 | 9 | 6.3 | 8.01 |
| 15 | 10.3 | 2.94 | 15 | 10.4 | 4.60 | 13 | 10.8 | 6.08 | 17 | 10.7 | 7.26 |
| 15 | 15.0 | 1.67 | 16 | 15.6 | 3.33 | 10 | 15.8 | 5.32 | 17 | 15.3 | 6.69 |
| 15 | 20.1 | 0.94 | 15 | 20.3 | 2.61 | 12 | 20.4 | 4.94 | 16 | 20.7 | 6.25 |
| 15 | 25.2 | 0.61 | 16 | 25.4 | 2.04 | 11 | 25.1 | 4.40 | 18 | 25.1 | 5.90 |
| 15 | 29.8 | 0.47 | 16 | 30.2 | 1.75 | 12 | 30.2 | 4.05 | 18 | 30.0 | 5.55 |
| 12 | 35.2 | 0.35 | 16 | 34.9 | 1.55 | 11 | 35.2 | 3.62 | 16 | 34.9 | 5.25 |
| 15 | 40.0 | 0.30 | 16 | 39.2 | 1.37 | 13 | 39.9 | 3.55 | 16 | 39.6 | 4.98 |
| 15 | 44.9 | 0.25 | 16 | 44.8 | 1.18 | 12 | 45.2 | 3.32 | 18 | 45.1 | 4.76 |
| 15 | 49.9 | 0.22 | 13 | 50.0 | 1.04 | 12 | 50.2 | 3.13 | 15 | 49.8 | 4.49 |
| 14 | 55.0 | 0.22 | 13 | 54.8 | 0.88 | 12 | 55.5 | 3.00 | 18 | 55.2 | 4.37 |
| 14 | 60.1 | 0.15 | 14 | 60.3 | 0.81 | 11 | 60.1 | 2.77 | 15 | 59.9 | 4.11 |
| 12 | 65.2 | 0.15 | 14 | 64.8 | 0.68 | 12 | 64.9 | 2.71 | 17 | 65.1 | 4.04 |
| 15 | 69.7 | 0.12 | 14 | 70.1 | 0.65 | 11 | 70.2 | 2.44 | 13 | 69.3 | 3.85 |
| 14 | 75.1 | 0.10 | 15 | 74.7 | 0.63 | 12 | 75.1 | 2.41 | 18 | 75.2 | 3.72 |

From Winkler and Gram, 1961, Table 1.
[a]Column headings: A, number of measurements at each time; B, time after the injection (min); C, average concentration at each time (mg/100 ml).

by Jusko and Gibaldi? On the basis of this comparison, do you think it likely that liver disease alters the bromsulfalein distribution microconstants $k_{12}$ and $k_{21}$?

(c) In what direction does $V_{extrap}$ change as the severity of liver disease progresses? Does it become a better or a worse approximation to $V_1 + V_2$? Why? Is your conclusion intuitively reasonable?

**14** Figure 3.44 is reproduced from a paper by Mroszczak and Riegelman (1975) on the disposition of diethylstilbestrol in the rhesus monkey.

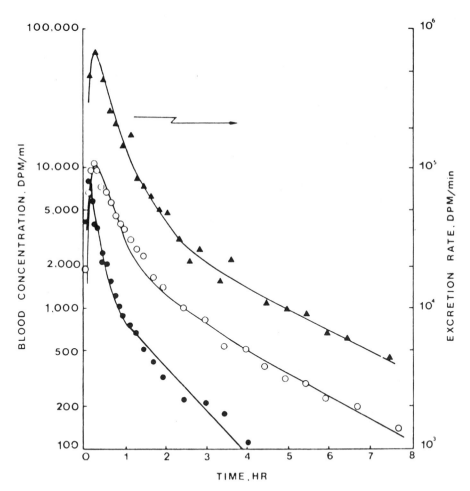

**Figure 3.44** Semilogarithmic plot of the blood levels of diethylstilbestrol (●) and diethylstilbestrol monoglucuronide (○) against time along with the biliary excretion rate of diethylstilbestrol monoglucuronide (▲) against midpoint time following intravenous administration of [$^{14}$C] diethylstilbestrol to a male rhesus monkey. Reproduced with permission from Mroszczak and Riegelman, 1975, Figure 5.

What is the rate determining step in the sequence

$$(DES)_{plasma} \xrightarrow{k_m} (DES\ monoglucuronide)_{plasma}$$

$$\xrightarrow{k_b^M} (DES\ monoglucuronide)_{bile?}$$

What relationship between the two rate constants would cause the terminal slopes of the ● and ▲ lines to be equal? The terminal slopes of the ● and ○ lines?

**15**  Cyclacillin, a semisynthetic penicillin, was found during routine safety evaluation to be nephrotoxic in male but not in female rats. The data in Table 3.11 are taken from a report of the followup investigation of this toxicity (Tucker et al., 1974). The cyclacillin was given orally. ACHC is its major metabolite, but cyclacillin is also excreted directly into the urine. Assume that in both sexes 32% of the total dose of cyclacillin was absorbed and 22% of the oral dose appeared in the urine ($U_\infty$) as cyclacillin.

**Table 3.11** Plasma concentrations of cyclacillin and of its metabolite ACHC at intervals after oral administration of cyclacillin to male and female rats; means of values from three animals per sex

| Time (hr) | Plasma Cyclacillin after 100 mg/kg Orally ($\mu$g/ml) | |
|---|---|---|
| | Males | Females |
| 1.0 | 115 | 150 |
| 1.5 | 120 | 115 |
| 2.0 | 95 | 75 |
| 3.0 | 70 | 55 |
| 4.0 | 20 | 15 |
| 6.0 | 5 | 10 |

| Time (days) | Plasma ACHC after 400 mg of Cyclacillin/kg Orally ($\mu$g/ml) | |
|---|---|---|
| | Males | Females |
| 0.25 | 22.5 | 22.5 |
| 0.5 | 22.0 | 18.5 |
| 1.0 | 24.0 | 14.0 |
| 2.0 | 21.0 | 11.5 |
| 4.0 | 18.0 | 4.5 |
| 6.0 | 17.0 | 2.5 |
| 8.0 | 14.0 | 1.0 |
| 10.0 | 14.0 | 0.5 |
| 12.0 | 11.5 | 0.2 |

From Tucker et al., 1974; data read from Figures 10 and 11.

(a) What is $k_e^C$, the overall rate constant for elimination of cyclacillin from the plasma, for male rats? For female rats?

(b) What is $k_e^A$, the overall rate constant for elimination of ACHC from the plasma, for male rats? For female rats?

(c) Estimate $k_u^C$, the microscopic rate constant for cyclacillin excretion into the urine, and $k_m^C$, the microscopic rate constant for cyclacillin transformation to ACHC, for both male and female rats. **Hint:** $k_e^C = k_u^C + k_m^C$.

(d) On the basis of these values, what do you propose as the direct cause of cyclacillin nephrotoxicity in the male rat?

16 Spironolactone protects against the toxicities of a number of compounds including indomethacin. In an effort to determine the mechanism of this protection, Klaassen (1976) studied the kinetics of indomethacin distribution and biliary excretion in control rats (CON) and in rats given spironolactone (SP). The total dose of indomethacin was 8 mg/kg. What possible mechanism for spironolactone action would you suggest based on the kinetic evidence given in Figure 3.45?

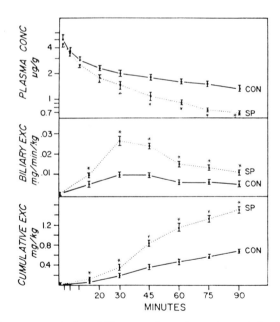

**Figure 3.45** Plasma concentration, biliary excretion rate, and cumulative biliary excretion of $^{14}C$ after administration of [$^{14}C$] indomethacin to rats. Data are expressed as microgram equivalents of indomethacin: CON, controls; SP, spironolactone pretreated. Means ± standard error for 12–14 rats. Asterisk indicates value significantly different from control value. Reproduced with permission from Klaassen, 1976, Figure 2.

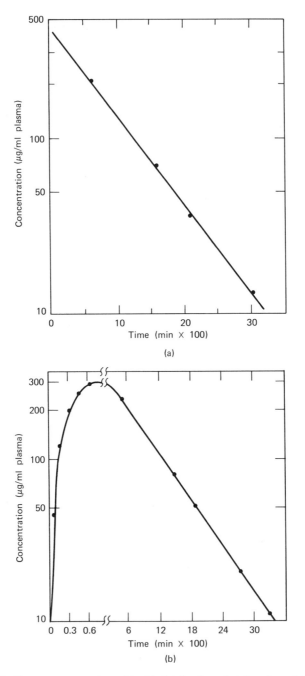

**Figure 3.46** Plasma concentration of barbital following administration of 200 mg/kg to rats either (a) intracardially or (b) orally. Reproduced with permission from Meshali and Nightingale, 1976, Figure 1 (adapted) and Figure 2.

17  Figure 3.46 represents the plasma concentration of barbital as a function of time in control rats given a single dose of 200 mg/kg either intravenously (Figure 3.46*a*) or orally (Figure 3.46*b*). Meshali and Nightingale (1976) estimated that the two rate constants characterizing curve *b* were 0.017 and 0.0011 min$^{-1}$. Which of them is $k_e$? Can you be sure? Do you think that most of the oral dose was absorbed? Why or why not?

18  Bromobenzene, a hepatotoxin, is metabolized by the liver microsomal fraction and ultimately excreted partly in the bile. Table 3.12 gives excretion data taken from a study by Sipes et al. (1974) for bromobenzene metabolites in control rats and in rats pretreated with phenobarbital, a microsomal enzyme inducer, and with SKF 525A, a microsomal enzyme inhibitor. Graph the data appropriately and answer the following questions, based on the following schematic model:

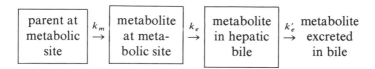

(a)  Do the data suggest that the overall rate of metabolite excretion ($k_e$ and/or $k_e'$) varies with treatment? Do they suggest that the rate of metabolite formation varies with treatment?

(b)  Does it appear that the alteration in bile flow rate caused by pretreatment has altered any of the kinetic parameters of this system? If so, which?

19  Albert et al. (1975) administered single 50-mg doses of the antihistamine diphenhydramine to a healthy adult male as an intravenous infusion and as an oral solution. From their data given in Table 3.13, determine the availability of the oral solution to the systemic circulation. (Estimate the AUC from 24 hr to infinity by dividing the plasma concentration at 24 hr by $\beta$, having estimated $\beta$ from the 12- and 24-hr plasma concentrations after intravenous administration.)

20  Levodopa, a drug used in the treatment of Parkinsonism, is less available systemically after oral than after intravenous administration. Cotler et al. (1976) administered radiolabeled levodopa to dogs by three different routes; intravenous (1), hepatoportal (2), and oral (3), identified by the corresponding numbers in the schematic diagram below:

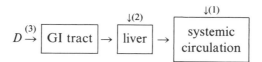

**Table 3.12** Effects of pretreatment of rats with phenobarbital (80 mg/kg i.p. for 3 days) and SKF 525-A (75 mg/kg i.p. 2 hr before) on the biliary excretion of bromobenzene metabolites and on bile flow[a]

| Time after Bromobenzene (min) | Pretreatment | | | | | |
| --- | --- | --- | --- | --- | --- | --- |
| | None | | Phenobarbital | | SKF 525-A | |
| | Bromobenzene Metabolites (μmole) | Volume of Bile (ml) | Bromobenzene metabolites (μmole) | Volume of Bile (ml) | Bromobenzene Metabolites (μmole) | Volume of Bile (ml) |
| 0–30 | 2.9 ± 0.38 | 0.59 ± 0.04 | 9.1 ± 1.1* | 1.00 ± 0.06* | 0.80 ± 0.10* | 0.39 ± 0.02** |
| 30–60 | 4.6 ± 0.51 | 0.55 ± 0.07 | 4.7 ± 0.56 | 0.80 ± 0.04*** | 3.4 ± 0.30** | 0.42 ± 0.03 |
| 60–90 | 2.9 ± 0.43 | 0.55 ± 0.06 | 2.1 ± 0.19 | 0.70 ± 0.05 | 2.8 ± 0.42 | 0.45 ± 0.04 |
| 90–120 | 2.1 ± 0.14 | 0.47 ± 0.03 | 1.4 ± 0.08* | 0.60 ± 0.04 | 2.1 ± 0.37 | 0.42 ± 0.03 |
| 120–150 | 1.3 ± 0.12 | 0.42 ± 0.04 | 0.67 ± 0.23* | 0.58 ± 0.04 | 1.6 ± 0.28 | 0.40 ± 0.04 |
| 150–180 | 0.8 ± 0.05 | 0.45 ± 0.03 | 0.76 ± 0.08 | 0.58 ± 0.06 | 1.0 ± 0.15 | 0.46 ± 0.07 |

From Sipes et al., 1974, Table 1.

[a] $^{14}$C-Bromobenzene was administered i.v. at a dose of 20 mg/kg (130 μmole/kg, sp. act. 2 μCi/μmole). Each value is the mean of data from five to six rats ±SE.

*$P < 0.01$ compared to control rats.

**$P < 0.05$ compared to control rats.

**Table 3.13** Plasma diphenhydramine concentration following oral and intravenous administration of 50 mg to an adult male subject

| Time (hr) | Plasma Diphenhydramine Concentration (ng/ml) | |
| --- | --- | --- |
| | Oral Dose | Intravenous Dose |
| 0.25 | 4.15 | 31.0 |
| 0.50 | 6.36 | 89.1 |
| 1.0 | 54.2 | 179 |
| 1.5 | — | 170 |
| 2.0 | 64.2 | 147 |
| 4.0 | 38.8 | 80.3 |
| 6.0 | 27.2 | 41.5 |
| 8.0 | 18.5 | — |
| 12.0 | 11.9 | 18.2 |
| 24.0 | 6.4 | 8.2 |

From Albert et al., 1975, Table II.

Mean $(AUC)_\infty$s for levodopa itself for four dogs were (1) 23.2, (2) 21.2, and (3) 9.7 $\mu$g hr/ml. Mean $(AUC)_\infty$ for total $^{14}$C was constant and independent of the route of administration. Assume that there are four possible mechanisms for the reduced oral availability of levodopa: incomplete absorption, metabolism in the liver, excretion from the liver to the gastrointestinal tract, and metabolism in the gastrointestinal tract.

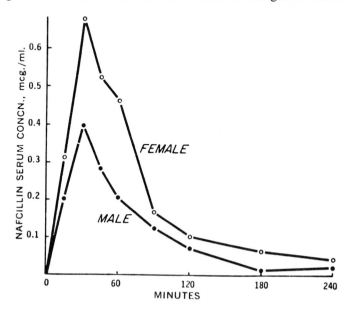

**Figure 3.47** Mean serum concentration of nafcillin in male and female beagle dogs after oral administration of 25 mg/kg. Reproduced with permission from Poole et al., 1970, Figure 3.

Which of these mechanisms is or are supported by the data given, and why?

21  When the monobasic penicillin nafcillin was administered to male and female beagle dogs at a dose level of 25 mg/kg, Poole (1970) observed a clear-cut sex-related difference in its pharmacokinetic behavior (Figure 3.47). The mean biological half-life of nafcillin, determined from plasma concentration data after a single intravenous dose, was 10 min in both sexes. Discuss possible origins of the observed difference.

**Table 3.14**  Serum levels of dimethylsulfoxide (DMSO) and dimethylsulfone (DMSO$_2$), and urinary excretion of DMSO and DMSO$_2$, after dermal administration of 1 g DMSO/kg to a human subject

| Time (hr) | DMSO in Serum ($\mu$g/ml) | DMSO$_2$ in Serum ($\mu$g/ml) | DMSO in Urine (cumulative % of dose) | DMSO$_2$ in Urine (cumulative % of dose) |
|---|---|---|---|---|
| 1 | 287 | Trace[a] | | |
| 2 | 507 | 23 | 0.2 | <0.1 |
| 4 | 488 | 33 | 1.2 | <0.1 |
| 8 | 560 | 56 | 3.0 | 0.1 |
| 16 | 479 | 119 | 6.4 | 0.3 |
| 24 | 337 | 229 | 9.7 | 0.8 |
| 36 | 156 | 340 | 12.1 | 1.7 |
| 48 | Trace[a] | 464 | 13.2 | 3.1 |
| 72 | 0 | 514 | 13.3 | 5.7 |
| 96 | | 460 | 13.3 | 7.8 |
| 120 | | 306 | 13.3 | 10.6 |
| 144 | | 245 | | 12.2 |
| 168 | | 86 | | 13.9 |
| 192 | | 130 | | 15.6 |
| 216 | | 108 | | 16.4 |
| 240 | | 114 | | 17.1 |
| 264 | | 95 | | 17.5 |
| 288 | | 59 | | 17.7 |
| 312 | | 48 | | 18.0 |
| 336 | | | | 18.2 |
| 340 | | | | 18.4 |
| 384 | | | | 18.4 |
| 408 | | | | 18.5 |
| 432 | | | | 18.6 |
| 456 | | | | 18.7 |

From Hucker et al., 1967, Table 2 and Table 3.
[a] Defined as <25 $\mu$g/ml of DMSO and <10 $\mu$g/ml of DMSO$_2$.

**22** The data in Table 3.14 are taken from a study by Hucker et al. (1967) in which dimethylsulfoxide (DMSO) was applied to the skin of a human volunteer and its absorption and disposition studied. The dose given was 1 g per kilogram of body weight. Serum and urine levels of DMSO and of its metabolite dimethylsulfone ($DMSO_2$) were monitored. You may assume that DMSO kinetics are first order throughout and that urinary excretions of DMSO and $DMSO_2$ represent the only pathways for excretion of DMSO. From the data given construct a reasonable compartmental model for DMSO kinetics. Assign approximate values to rate constants wherever possible.

**23** Regårdh et al. (1974) studied the pharmacokinetics of the $\beta$-receptor antagonist metoprolol and its metabolites in man. When the drug was given by intravenous infusion to five subjects it was found that the mean $k_e$ value was 0.450 hr$^{-1}$ and the volume of the central compartment for metoprolol was 2.2 l/kg. The mean weight of the five subjects was 66 kg. Use this information and Figure 3.48 to answer the following.

**(a)** Estimate $Cl_{total}^{metoprolol}$, $Cl_{renal}^{metoprolol}$, and $Cl_{renal}^{metabolites}$.

**(b)** What is the value of $k_m$ for total metabolism?

**(c)** Discuss the propriety of lumping all the metabolites together under the analysis for total metabolite radioactivity. Why is this procedure either justified or not justified in the calculation of clearance?

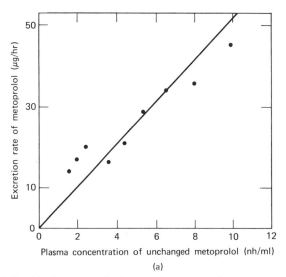

(a)

**Figure 3.48** Relationship between urinary excretion rate and plasma concentration; mean values from five human subjects. (*a*) Tritiated metoprolol. (*b*) Total tritiated metabolites. Reproduced from Regårdh et al., 1974, Figures 7 and 8.

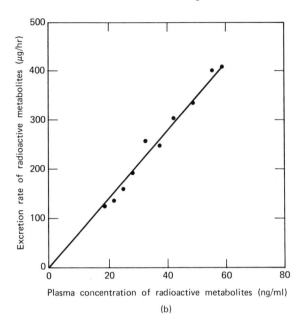

Figure 3.48 (*continued*)

## REFERENCES

Albert, K. S., M. R. Hallmark, E. Sakmar, D. J. Weidler, and J. G. Wagner. "Pharmacokinetics of diphenhydramine in man." *J. Pharmacokinet. Biopharmaceut.*, 3, 159–170 (1975).

Ballard, B. E. "Biopharmaceutical considerations in subcutaneous and intramuscular drug administration. *J. Pharm. Sci.*, 57, 357–378 (1968).

Baselt, R. C. and L. J. Casarett. "Urinary excretion of methadone in man." *Clin. Pharmacol. Ther.*, 13, 64–70 (1972).

Benet, L. Z. "General treatment of linear mammillary models with elimination from any compartment as used in pharmacokinetics." *J. Pharm. Sci.*, 61, 536–541 (1972).

Berman, M. and M. F. Weiss. *User's Manual for SAAM*, National Institutes of Health, Bethesda, Md., 1968.

Bischoff, K. B. and R. L. Dedrick. "Thiopental pharmacokinetics." *J. Pharm. Sci.*, 57, 1346–1351 (1968).

Borchard, R. E., M. E. Welborn, W. B. Weikhorst, D. W. Wilson, and L. G. Hansen. "Pharmacokinetics of polychlorinated biphenyl components in swine and sheep after a single oral dose." *J. Pharm. Sci.*, 64, 1294–1299 (1975).

Boudène, C., D. Malet, and R. Masse. "Fate of $^{210}$Pb inhaled by rats." *Toxicol. Appl. Pharmacol.*, 41, 271–276 (1977).

Bradley, S. G. and J. S. Bond. "Toxicity, clearance, and metabolic effects of pactamycin in combination with bacterial lipopolysaccharide." *Toxicol. Appl. Pharmacol.*, 31, 208–221 (1975).

Brodie, B. B., E. Bernstein, and L. C. Mark. "The role of body fat in limiting the duration of action of thiopental." *J. Pharmacol. Exp. Ther.*, **105**, 421–426 (1952).

Brodie, B. B., H. Kurz, and L. S. Schanker. "The importance of dissociation constant and lipid-solubility in influencing the passage of drugs into the cerebrospinal fluid." *J. Pharmacol. Exp. Ther.*, **130**, 20–25 (1960).

Burton, J. A. and L. S. Schanker. "Absorption of antibiotics from the rat lung." *Proc. Soc. Exp. Biol. Med.*, **145**, 752–756 (1974).

Cabana, B. E., D. R. Van Harken, G. H. Hottendorf, J. T. Doluisio, W. O. Griffen, Jr., D. W. A. Bourne, and L. W. Dittert. "The role of the kidney in the elimination of cephapirin in man." *J. Pharmacokinet. Biopharmaceut.*, **3**, 419–438 (1975).

Chiou, W. L. "Quantitation of hepatic and pulmonary first-pass effect and its implications in pharmacokinetic study. I. Pharmacokinetics of chloroform in man." *J. Pharmacokinet. Biopharmaceut.*, **3**, 193–201 (1975).

Collander, R. and H. Bärlund. "Permeabilitätsstudien an *Chara ceratophylla.*" *Acta Bot. Fenn.*, **11**, 1–114 (1933).

Collander, R. "The permeability of *Nitella* cells to non-electrolytes." *Physiol. Plant.*, **7**, 420–445 (1954).

Cotler, S., A. Holazo, H. G. Boxenbaum, and S. A. Kaplan. "Influence of route of administration on physiological availability of levodopa in dogs." *J. Pharm. Sci.*, **65**, 822–827 (1976).

Dobrinska, M. R., and P. G. Welling. "Pharmacokinetics of methsuximide and a major metabolite in dogs." *J. Pharm. Sci.* **66**, 688–692 (1977).

Eagle, H., R. Fleishman, and M. Levy. "On the duration of penicillin action in relation to its concentration in the serum." *J. Lab. Clin. Med.*, **41**, 122–132 (1953).

Enna, S. J., and L. S. Schanker. "Absorption of drugs from the rat lung." *Am. J. Physiol.*, **223**, 1227–1231 (1972).

Enna, S. J., and L. S. Schanker. "Phenol red absorption from the rat lung: Evidence of carrier transport." *Life Sci.*, **12**, 231–239 (1973).

Fry, B. J., T. Taylor, and D. E. Hathway. "Pulmonary elimination of chloroform and its metabolite in man." *Arch. Int. Pharmacodyn.*, **196**, 98–111 (1972).

Gérardin, A. P., F. V. Abadie, J. A. Campestrini, and W. Theobald. "Pharmacokinetics of carbamazepine in normal humans after single and repeated oral doses." *J. Pharmacokinet. Biopharmaceut.*, **4**, 521–535 (1976).

Ginsburg, J. "Placental drug transfer." *Annu. Rev. Pharmacol.*, **11**, 387–408 (1971).

Gryns, G. "Über den Einfluss Gelöster Stoffe auf die roten Blutzellen, in Verbindung mit den Erscheinungen der Osmose und Diffusion." *Pflügers Arch. Ges. Physiol.*, **63**, 86–119 (1896).

Gunnison, A. F. and E. D. Palmes. "A model for the metabolism of sulfite in mammals." *Toxicol. Appl. Pharmacol.*, **38**, 111–126 (1976).

Hartley, H. O. "The modified Gauss-Newton method for the fitting of non-linear regression functions by least squares." *Technometrics*, **3**, 269–280 (1961).

Hedin, S. G. "Über die Permeabilität der Blutkörperchen." *Pflügers Arch. Ges. Physiol.*, **68**, 229–338 (1897).

Hinderling, P. H. and E. R. Garrett. "Pharmacokinetics of the antiarrhythmic disopyramide in healthy humans." *J. Pharmacokinet. Biopharmaceut.*, **4**, 199–230 (1976).

Hogben, C. A. M. "The alimentary tract." *Annu. Rev. Physiol.*, **22**, 381–406 (1960).

Hogben, C. A. M., L. S. Schanker, D. J. Tocco, and B. B. Brodie. "Absorption of drugs from the stomach. II. The human." *J. Pharmacol. Exp. Ther.*, **120**, 540–545 (1957).

Hogben, C. A. M., D. J. Tocco, B. B. Brodie, and L. S. Schanker. "On the mechanism of intestinal absorption of drugs." *J. Pharmacol. Exp. Ther.*, **125**, 275–282 (1959).

Houston, J. B. and G. Levy. "Effect of route of administration on competitive drug biotransformation interaction. Salicylamide–ascorbic acid interaction in rats." *J. Pharmacol. Exp. Ther.*, **198**, 284–294 (1976).

Hucker, H. B., J. K. Miller, A. Hochberg, R. D. Brobyn, F. H. Riordan, and B. Calesnick. "Studies on the absorption, excretion and metabolism of dimethylsulfoxide (DMSO) in man." *J. Pharmacol. Exp. Ther.*, **155**, 309–317 (1967).

Jacobs, H. and H. N. Glassman. "Further comparative studies on the permeability of the erythrocyte." *Biol. Bull.*, **73**, 387 (1937).

Jusko, W. J., and M. Gibaldi. "Effects of change in elimination on various parameters of the two-compartment open model." *J. Pharm. Sci.*, **61**, 1270–1273 (1972).

Kaplan, S. A. "Pharmacokinetic profile of coumermycin A." *J. Pharm. Sci.*, **59**, 309–313 (1970).

Klaassen, C. D. "Studies on the mechanism of spironolactone protection against indomethacin toxicity." *Toxicol. Appl. Pharmacol.*, **38**, 127–135 (1976).

Lalka, D., M. B. Meyer, B. R. Duce, and A. T. Elvin. "Kinetics of the oral antiarrhythmic lidocaine congener, tocainide." *Clin. Pharmacol. Ther.*, **19**, 757–766 (1976).

Loo, J. C. K., and S. Riegelman. "New method for calculating the intrinsic absorption rate of drugs." *J. Pharm. Sci.*, **57**, 918–928 (1968).

Mayer, S., R. P. Maickel, and B. B. Brodie. "Kinetics of penetration of drugs and other foreign compounds into cerebrospinal fluid and brain." *J. Pharmacol. Exp. Ther.*, **127**, 205–211 (1959).

Meijer, D. K. F, J. G. Weitering, and R. J. Vonk. "Hepatic uptake and biliary excretion of D-tubocurarine and trimethyltubocurarine in the rat *in vivo* and in isolated perfused rat livers." *J. Pharmacol. Exp. Ther.*, **198**, 229–239 (1976).

Meshali, M. M. and C. H. Nightingale. "Effect of alpha tocopherol (vitamin E) deficiency on intestinal transport of passively absorbed drugs." *J. Pharm. Sci.*, **65**, 344–349 (1976).

Metzler, C. M. "A User's Manual for NONLIN," Technical Report No. 7292/69/7293/005, Upjohn Company, Kalamazoo, Mich., 1969.

Mischler, T. W., A. A. Sugerman, D. A. Willard, L. J. Brannick, and E. S. Neiss. "Influence of probenecid and food on the bioavailability of cephradine in normal male subjects." *J. Clin. Pharmacol.* **14**, 604–611 (1974).

Mroszczak, E. J. and S. Riegelman. "Disposition of diethylstilbestrol in the rhesus monkey." *J. Pharmacokinet. Biopharmaceut.*, **3**, 303–327 (1975).

Nagashima, R., G. Levy, and R. A. O'Reilly. "Comparative pharmacokinetics of coumarin anticoagulants. IV. Application of a three-compartmental model to the analysis of the dose-dependent kinetics of bishydroxycoumarin elimination ." *J. Pharm. Sci.*, **57**, 1888–1895 (1968).

Nayak, R. K., R. D. Smyth, J. H. Chamberlain, A. Polk, A. F. DeLong, T. Herezeg, P. B. Chemburkar, R. S. Joslin, and N. H. Reavey-Cantwell. "Methaqualone pharmacokinetics after single- and multiple-dose administration in man." *J. Pharmacokinet. Biopharmaceut.*, **2**, 107–121 (1974).

Nelson, E. and I. O'Reilly. "Kinetics of sulfisoxazole acetylation and excretion in humans." *J. Pharmacol. Exp. Ther.*, **129**, 368–372 (1960).

Nichols, R. L., W. F. Jones, Jr., and M. Finland. "Plasma penicillin levels from oral penicillins V and G and intramuscular penicillin G." *Proc. Soc. Exp. Biol. Med.*, **90**, 688–694 (1955).

Olson, F. C. and E. J. Massaro. "Pharmacodynamics of methyl mercury in the murine maternal/embryo: fetal unit." *Toxicol. Appl. Pharmacol.*, **39**, 263–273 (1977).

Osterhout, W. J. V. "Is living protoplasm permeable to ions?" *J. Gen. Physiol.*, **8**, 131–146 (1925).

Osterhout, W. J. V., S. E. Kamerling, and W. M. Stanley. "Kinetics of penetration. VII. Molecular versus ionic transport." *J. Gen. Physiol.*, **17**, 469–480 (1933).

Pappenheimer, J. R., E. M. Renkin, and L. M. Borrero. "Filtration, diffusion and molecular sieving through peripheral capillary membranes: A contribution to the pore theory of capillary permeability." *Am. J. Physiol.*, **167**, 13–46 (1951).

Pappenheimer, J. R. "Passage of molecules through capillary walls." *Physiol. Rev.*, **33**, 387–423 (1953).

Perrier, D. and M. Gibaldi. "Drug clearance in multicompartment systems". *Can. J. Pharm. Sci.* **9**, 11–13 (1974).

Poole, J. W. "Effect of sex on penicillin blood levels in dogs." *J. Pharm. Sci.*, **59**, 1255–1258 (1970).

Regårdh, C. G., K. O. Borg, R. Johansson, G. Johnsson, and L. Palmer. "Pharmacokinetic studies on the selective $\beta_1$-receptor antagonist metoprolol in man." *J. Pharmacokinet. Biopharmaceut.*, **2**, 347–364 (1974).

Renkin, E. M. "Transport of large molecules across capillary walls." *Physiologist*, **7**, 13–28 (1964).

Rowland, M., L. Z. Benet, and S. Riegelman. "Two-compartment model for a drug and its metabolite: Application to acetylsalicylic acid pharmacokinetics." *J. Pharm. Sci.* **59**, 364–367 (1970).

Schanker, L. S. "Absorption of drugs from the rat colon." *J. Pharmacol. Exp. Ther.*, **126**, 283–290 (1959).

Schanker, L. S. "Passage of drugs across body membranes." *Pharmacol. Rev.*, **14**, 501–530 (1962).

Schanker, L. S. "Physiological transport of drugs." *Adv. Drug Res.*, **1**, 71–106 (1964).

Schanker, L. S. and J. J. Jeffrey. "Active transport of foreign pyrimidines across the intestinal epithelium." *Nature (London)*, **190**, 727–728 (1961).

Schanker, L. S., P. A. Shore, B. B. Brodie, and C. A. M. Hogben. "Absorption of drugs from the stomach. I. The rat." *J. Pharmacol. Exp. Ther.*, **120**, 528–539 (1957).

Schanker, L. S., D. J. Tocco, B. B. Brodie, and C. A. M. Hogben. "Absorption of drugs from the rat small intestine." *J. Pharmacol. Exp. Ther.*, **123**, 81–88 (1958).

Schou, J. "Absorption of drugs from subcutaneous connective tissue." *Pharmacol. Rev.*, **13**, 441–464 (1961).

Schwartz, M. A. and J. J. Carbone. "Metabolism of $^{14}$C–medazepam hydrochloride in dog, rat and man." *Biochem. Pharmacol.*, **19**, 343–361 (1970).

Sha'afi, R. I., C. M. Gary-Bobo, and A. K. Solomon. "Permeability of red cell membranes to small hydrophilic and lipophilic solutes." *J. Gen. Physiol.*, **58**, 238–258 (1971).

Shore, P. A., B. B. Brodie, and C. A. M. Hogben. "The gastric secretion of drugs: A pH partition hypothesis." *J. Pharmacol. Exp. Ther.*, **119**, 361–369 (1957).

Sipes, I. G., P. L. Gigon, and G. Krishna. "Biliary excretion of metabolites of bromobenzene." *Biochem. Pharmacol.*, **23**, 451–455 (1974).

Skinner, S. M., R. E. Clark, N. Baker, and R. A. Shipley. "Complete solution of the three-compartment model in steady state after single injection of radioactive tracer." *Am. J. Physiol.*, **196**, 238–244 (1959).

Soberman, R., B. B. Brodie, B. B. Levy, J. Axelrod, V. Hollander, and J. M. Steele. "The use of antipyrine in the measurement of total body water in man." *J. Biol. Chem.*, **179**, 31–42 (1949).

Spendley, W., G. R. Hext, and F. R. Himsworth. "Sequential application of simplex design and optimization and evolutionary operation." *Technometrics*, **4**, 441–461 (1962).

Treherne, J. E. "The permeability of skin to some non-electrolytes." *J. Physiol.*, **133**, 171–180 (1956).

Tucker, W. E., Jr., F. W. Janssen, H. P. K. Agersborg, Jr., E. M. Young, and H. W. Ruelius. "Sex- and species-related nephropathy of 6-(1-aminocyclohexanecarboxamido) penicillanic acid (cyclacillin) and its relationship to the metabolic disposition of the drug." *Toxicol. Appl. Pharmacol.*, **29**, 1–18 (1974).

Vaughan, D. P. and A. Trainor. "Derivation of general equations for linear mammillary models when the drug is administered by different routes." *J. Pharmacokinet. Biopharmaceut.*, **3**, 203–218 (1975).

Wagner, J. G. "Pharmacokinetics. 7. Percent absorbed–time plots and absorption rate." *Drug Intell.*, **2**, 332–338 (1968).

Wagner, J. G. "Application of the Wagner-Nelson absorption method to the two-compartment open model." *J. Pharmacokinet. Biopharmaceut.*, **2**, 469–486 (1974).

Wagner, J. G. "Do you need a pharmacokinetic model, and, if so, which one?" *J. Pharmacokinetic. Biopharmaceut.*, **3**, 457–478 (1975).

Wagner, J. G. *Fundamentals of Clinical Pharmacokinetics*, Drug Intelligence Publications, Hamilton, Ill. 1975a, pp. 173–201.

Wagner, J. G. *Fundamentals of Clinical Pharmacokinetics*, Drug Intelligence Publications, Hamilton, Ill. 1975b, pp. 220–228.

Wagner, J. G. and E. Nelson. "Percent absorbed time plots derived from blood level and/or urinary excretion data." *J. Pharm. Sci.*, **52**, 610–611 (1963).

Weisel, M. K., J. D. Powers, T. E. Powers, and J. D. Baggott. "A pharmacokinetic analysis of tylosin in the normal dog." *Am. J. Vet. Res.*, **38**, 273–275 (1977).

Winkler, K. and C. Gram. "Models for description of the bromsulfalein elimination curves in man after single intravenous injections." *Acta Med. Scand.*, **169**, 263–272 (1961).

Wright, W. W., H. Welch, J. Wilner, and E. F. Roberts. "Body fluid concentrations of penicillin following intramuscular injection of single doses of benzathine penicillin G and/or procaine penicillin G." *Antibio. Med. Clin. Ther.*, **6**, 232–241 (1959).

# 4

# *Acute Exposure with Nonlinear and Mixed Kinetics of Disposition*

**4.1** Kinetic characteristics of linear and nonlinear systems

**4.2** Historical background

**4.3** Physical origins of nonlinearity

**4.4** Nonlinearities introduced by capacity-limited processes

    4.4.1 Binding to plasma or tissue proteins

    4.4.2 Saturable elimination processes

**4.5** The kidney: An organ in which first-order and saturable elimination processes operate simultaneously

**4.6** Nonlinearities introduced by alteration of kinetic parameters

    4.6.1 Alterations in volumes

    4.6.2 Alterations in rates

In the preceding chapter we were concerned only with systems made up of individual absorption, distribution, and elimination steps all of which were first-order processes. However, as we saw in Chapter 2, many biological processes are saturable and therefore are not first order at high substrate concentrations. Probably the most common example of perturbation of linear kinetic behavior is the saturation of an elimination (metabolism or excretion) step. There are also many causes of nonlinearity apart from saturation of a capacity-limited process; and we consider several of them in detail in this chapter as well as explore the impact on kinetic behavior of saturation of one or more of the routes of elimination of a compound. First, however, we examine the kinetic implications of linear models and consider means by which the degree of conformity of a real system to the predictions of a linear model can be determined.

## 4.1   KINETIC CHARACTERISTICS OF LINEAR AND NONLINEAR SYSTEMS

The fundamental assumption governing the kinetics of a linear process is that the rate of that process is at all times proportional to the amount of material being acted on. There are several important consequences of this assumption, two of which were developed and discussed in the preceding chapter. When disposition is first order, both the half-life and the apparent volume of distribution should be independent of dose:

$$t_{1/2} = \frac{\ln 2}{\beta} \tag{4.1}$$

and

$$V_{\text{extrap}} = \frac{D}{B_0} = \frac{V_1(\alpha - \beta)}{k_{21} - \beta} \tag{4.2}$$

for a two-compartment model. Here $\alpha$ and $\beta$ are rate constants and are defined independently of any consideration of dose level, just as the volume $V_1$ is. The slopes of $\ln C$, $t$ graphs at different doses should therefore be parallel, since $\alpha$ and $\beta$ have not changed. The intercepts of the back-extrapolated $\beta$ segments, however, are proportional to dose:

$$B_0 = \frac{D(k_{21} - \beta)}{V_1(\alpha - \beta)}. \tag{4.3}$$

The situation is even simpler for the one-compartment body model, for which

$$t_{1/2} = \frac{\ln 2}{k_e} \quad \text{and} \quad C_0 = \frac{D}{V}. \tag{4.4}$$

Therefore, if the disposition kinetics of a compound have been studied at several different doses, it should be possible to determine almost by inspection whether the system is linear. It is only necessary to establish that the slopes of $\ln C$, $t$ graphs are parallel and the ordinate intercepts are proportional to dose. If, instead of $\ln C$, $\ln C/C_0$ is graphed, all dieaway curves should superimpose. This expectation has led to development of the principle of superposition. It has been discussed in some detail by Thron (1974), who applied it to a number of different kinetic systems. Let us examine its application to experimental data for compounds which are distributed throughout more than one compartment.

Schnelle and Garrett (1973) studied the disposition of sotalol, an adrenergic nerve blocker, in a dog given 1, 2, and 4 mg/kg intravenously on three widely spaced occasions. Figure 4.1 is the authors' semilogarithmic graph of percentage of dose per unit of plasma volume against time for all three doses.

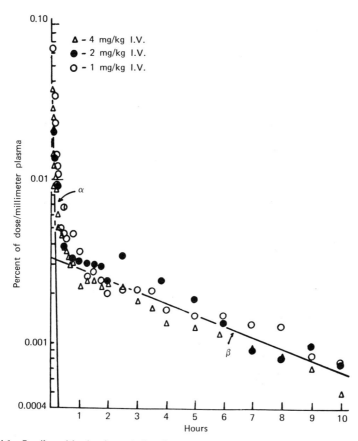

**Figure 4.1** Semilogarithmic plots of the plasma levels as percentage of dose per milliliter of plasma against time following intravenous administration of 4, 2, and 1 mg of sotalol/kg to a 19 kg dog. The data points obtained at the three dose levels could be graphically fitted with one common curve in accordance with a two-compartment open body model. Adapted with permission from Schnelle and Garrett, 1973, Figure 2.

Since all three curves are superimposable throughout, it can be concluded that $\alpha$, $\beta$, and $V_{extrap}$ are independent of dose and that disposition of sotalol is linear in the dog at least up to an intravenous dose of 4 mg/kg.

A dose-related transition from linear to nonlinear kinetic behavior is demonstrated by the kinetics of rose bengal excretion in rats in the dose range studied by Klaassen (1976). Figure 4.2 reproduces the change in plasma concentration with time in rats given five different intravenous doses of the dye rose bengal, from 0.01 to 100 mg/kg. Inspection of Figure 4.2 suggests that the slopes of the curves are parallel and the intercepts roughly proportional to dose up to 10.0 mg/kg but not at 100 mg/kg. This suggestion is confirmed by transforming the data by dividing by the dose and replotting as in Figure 4.3, from which it is clear that the principle of superposition holds

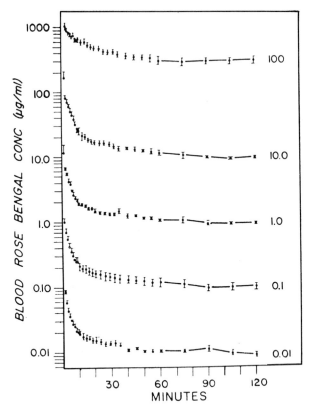

**Figure 4.2**   The concentration of $^{131}I$ in the blood of rats after intravenous administration of the indicated doses of $^{131}I$-labeled rose bengal (mg/kg). Each point represents the mean ± standard error of values from four to seven rats. Reproduced with permission from Klaassen, 1976, Figure 1.

only for doses up to 10.0 mg/kg. The kinetic parameters estimated by analyzing the data in accordance with a two-compartment open model are given in Table 4.1 and show, as expected, that $t_{1/2}$ and $V_{extrap}$ are independent of dose only up to 10.0 mg/kg. In this case the deviation from linearity at 100 mg/kg is attributable at least in part to saturation of rose bengal excretion into the bile, as Figure 4.4 demonstrates.

It is interesting to note that the half-life of excretion into the bile (Figure 4.4) is quite different from the half-life of loss from the plasma (Figure 4.2). Since rose bengal is believed to be excreted unchanged into the bile, it must be supposed that an intrahepatic storage step occurs between the disappearance of rose bengal from the plasma and its appearance in the bile, so that clearance of rose bengal takes place from a compartment other than the plasma.

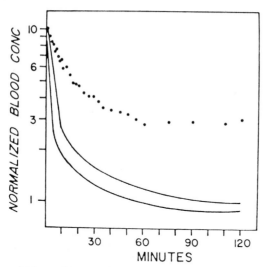

**Figure 4.3** The data of Figure 4.2 normalized by division by the dose. The lines enclose the range of values obtained after 0.01, 0.1, 1.0, and 10 mg of rose bengal per kilogram. The points represent the values obtained after the 100-mg/kg dose. Reproduced with permission from Klaassen, 1976, Figure 2.

It is important to recognize that consideration of the plasma data given for the 100-mg/kg dose of rose bengal alone probably would not have permitted the conclusion that rose bengal kinetics are nonlinear at this dose level. Often, although not always, disposition of a compound at a single dose level will appear to obey first-order kinetics but $t_{1/2}$ or $V_{extrap}$ will be found to be dose dependent. There are many reasons for this behavior: some theoretical, some practical, and all dependent on the source of the nonlinearity. In this particular instance the reason is probably a practical one: variance in the individual plasma data points at 100 mg/kg obscures the distinction between first-order (linear) behavior and zero-order (nonlinear) behavior. Had measurements been extended over a longer time, the nonlinearity might have become apparent. This point is discussed in greater detail in Section 4.4.2. In other instances the biological system may always yield apparent first-order kinetics following a single dose even though $t_{1/2}$ and $V_{extrap}$ are dose dependent. Often both $t_{1/2}$ and $V_{extrap}$ will be found to increase with increasing dose. An example of this kind of behavior is given in Problem 8 at the end of this chapter.

Therefore to determine whether an experimental system obeys first-order kinetic principles throughout a particular dose or exposure range, it is always necessary to examine its kinetic behavior *over the entire range*. The importance of establishing whether $V_{extrap}$ and $t_{1/2}$ are dose dependent cannot be emphasized too strongly. This point is illustrated by several of the examples that follow.

**Table 4.1** Blood pharmacokinetics of rose bengal in the rat.

| Dose (mg/kg) | A (µg/ml)[a] | $\alpha$ (min$^{-1}$)[b] | $t_{1/2}, \alpha$ (min)[c] | B (µg/ml)[d] | $\beta$ (min$^{-1}$)[e] | $t_{1/2}, \beta$ (min)[f] |
|---|---|---|---|---|---|---|
| 0.01 | 0.093 ± 0.006[g] | 0.387 ± 0.026 | 1.85 ± 0.19 | 0.0168 ± 0.0011 | 0.00764 ± 0.00058 | 109 ± 17 |
| 0.1 | 1.13 ± 0.17 | 0.363 ± 0.015 | 1.93 ± 0.09 | 0.185 ± 0.027 | 0.00728 ± 0.00041 | 96.5 ± 5.7 |
| 1.0 | 11.8 ± 0.46 | 0.368 ± 0.024 | 1.93 ± 0.12 | 1.68 ± 0.060 | 0.00667 ± 0.00041 | 106 ± 8 |
| 10.0 | 121 ± 6.8 | 0.256 ± 0.023 | 2.82 ± 0.21 | 18.9 ± 1.21 | 0.00645 ± 0.00082 | 121 ± 19 |
| 100.0 | 717 ± 41 | 0.078 ± 0.008 | 8.85 ± 0.06 | 351 ± 37 | 0.00300 ± 0.00091 | 231 ± 54 |

Reproduced from Klaassen, 1976, Table 1.1

[a] Zero time intercept of the fast or $\alpha$ phase of the blood concentration, time curve.
[b] Exponential time constant of the fast phase of the blood concentration, time curve.
[c] Half-life corresponding to the $\alpha$ phase.
[d] Zero time intercept of the slow or $\beta$ phase of the blood concentration, time curve.
[e] Exponential time constant of the slow phase of the blood concentration, time curve.
[f] Half-life corresponding to the $\beta$ phase.
[g] Each value represents the mean ± SE of four to seven rats.

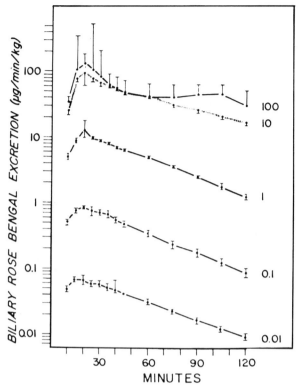

**Figure 4.4** The biliary excretion of rose bengal following intravenous administration of the indicated doses of [131]I-labeled rose bengal (mg/kg). Data from the same rats as in Figure 4.2. Reproduced with permission from Klaassen, 1976, Figure 3.

## 4.2 HISTORICAL BACKGROUND

By the mid-1960s the basic principles of linear kinetic behavior were well established and fairly widely accepted. At about this time a number of original papers began to appear presenting data that suggested that the behavior of many drugs did not conform to linear kinetic principles. Typically the apparent half-life and volume of distribution were observed to be dose dependent. A representative publication is that by Dayton et al. (1967), which provides data on the dose dependency of the half-lives of biscoumacetate, probenecid, diphenylhydantoin, and two analogues of phenylbutazone. For example, at a dose of 20 mg/kg the mean terminal half-life of the plasma level of diphenylhydantoin in a group of three dogs was 2.2 hr. When the dose was increased to 50 mg/kg the mean terminal half-life was markedly increased, to 6.4 hr, while the apparent mean volume of distribution increased somewhat less dramatically, from 8.0 to 12.7 liters.

Actually several publications describing nonlinear kinetic behavior had appeared much earlier. Widmark (1933) had described nonlinearity in ethanol elimination kinetics. Weiner et al. (1950) and Brodie et al. (1952) reported that the half-lives of dicumarol and of biscoumacetate were dose dependent and suggested that the dose dependence was due to saturation of a biochemical mechanism. Lundquist and Wolthers (1958) showed that ethanol elimination data could be fit by the integrated form of the Michaelis-Menten equation.

Krüger-Thiemer (1968) published the mathematical expressions for several nonlinear pharmacokinetic models including saturable metabolism and binding to serum proteins. Pointing out that there are multiple causes of nonlinearity, he considered nonlinearities of absorption, distribution, metabolism, and excretion independently. Wagner (1971) broadened the scope of nonlinear models to include binding to tissue components as well as to plasma proteins. Other authors have developed their own approaches to individual nonlinear kinetics problems.

Wagner (1973b) has tabulated articles in the literature to 1972 which contain evidence of nonlinearities in drug absorption, distribution, metabolism, and renal and biliary excretion.

## 4.3  PHYSICAL ORIGINS OF NONLINEARITY

Since $\alpha$ and $\beta$ are defined in terms of microconstants and since

$$V_{\text{extrap}} = \frac{V_1(\alpha - \beta)}{k_{21} - \beta},$$

where

$$\frac{k_{21}}{k_{12}} = \frac{V_1}{V_2},$$

it is apparent that changes in any of the rate constants or volumes of a two-compartment system will, to a greater or a lesser degree, result in changes in $t_{1/2}$ and $V_{\text{extrap}}$. It is convenient to divide nonlinearities into two general groups on the basis of the origin of the nonlinearity as follows:

1   If one of the processes constituting the system is constrained to operate within a capacity-limited range, the system will not conform to linear kinetic behavior.

2   If the compound itself, or the fact that it is present at excessively high concentration, should alter one or more of the kinetic parameters (rate constants or volumes) of the system, the system will not conform to linear kinetic behavior.

In Sections 4.4 and 4.6 we consider examples of each of these types of nonlinearity.

## 4.4  NONLINEARITIES INTRODUCED BY CAPACITY–LIMITED PROCESSES

### 4.4.1  Binding to Plasma or Tissue Proteins

Many exogenous materials are transported partly in solution in the plasma and partly bound to plasma proteins, primarily to albumin. Since the total number of binding sites on plasma proteins is limited, the amount of a drug or toxicant bound is not always proportional to the total amount of drug or toxicant in the plasma.

Plasma protein binding sites can be thought of as a separate compartment of limited capacity. However, plasma protein binding is usually considered independently of other capacity-limited portions of the systems. When such binding is thought to be potentially important its magnitude is determined in a separate *in vitro* experiment and plasma concentrations corrected for it. The extent of protein binding is usually determined by using equilibrium dialysis, ultrafiltration, or ultracentrifugation to separate protein bound from free drug or toxicant. The first two separation methods may require a correction for binding of the compound to the membrane. Garrett and Hunt (1974) have proposed a technique that avoids the need for physical separation of bound from free compound by using the erythrocyte as a partitioning phase. The red cell–plasma water partition coefficient, which must be known to use this technique, can be determined separately.

Suppose that at a fixed protein concentration $P_{total}$ and a free drug concentration $C$, some fraction of drug is bound to protein in a reversible drug-protein interaction:

$$C + P \underset{k_2}{\overset{k_1}{\rightleftharpoons}} CP;$$

$$k_1(C)(P) = k_2(CP).$$

The dissociation constant of the complex $CP$ is $K$:

$$K = \frac{(C)(P)}{(CP)} = \frac{k_2}{k_1}$$

$$= \frac{(C)(P_{total} - CP)}{(CP)}. \tag{4.5}$$

Equation 4.5 is readily rearranged to solve for $CP$:

$$CP = \frac{(C)(P_{total})}{K+C}.$$

$P_{total}$ is also the maximum possible concentration of complex, or $CP_{max}$. Although it is implicit in this development that there is only one binding site per molecule of protein (see the definition of the dissociation constant $K$), there may in fact be more than one, in which case $CP_{max} = n(P_{total})$, where $n$ is the number of binding sites per molecule of protein. Irrespective of the number of binding sites,

$$CP = \frac{(C)(CP)_{max}}{K+C}. \tag{4.6}$$

Equation 4.6 is the familiar rectangular hyperbola associated with a saturable process. Since the drug-protein complex can break down only in the direction of release of free $C$ and $P$, however, $K$ is a true dissociation constant, not an agglomeration of microconstants. Equation 4.6 can be cast in any of the three linear forms discussed in Chapter 2 to determine $CP_{max}$ and $K$. The most commonly used form is a graph of $CP/(C)(P_{total})$ versus $CP/P_{total}$, called a Scatchard plot. The slope and intercept of a Scatchard plot can be used to estimate $K$ and $n$. A typical Scatchard plot is shown in Figure 4.5, for the binding of a spironolactone derivative to human serum albumin. The value of $CP/P_{total}$ is represented by $\gamma$.

Deviation of any of the linear transforms from linearity suggests that there is more than one class of binding site on the protein molecule. A variety of curve-fitting techniques has been used to determine $n$ and $K$ values for the different classes of binding sites. The various approaches have been applied to experimental data by Vallner et al. (1976) and their relative merits discussed in some detail.

From a kinetic standpoint we are more interested in the fraction of drug bound than in the amount of complex formed. The fraction of drug bound is the ratio of bound to total drug, or

$$\frac{CP}{C+CP} = \frac{1}{1 + \dfrac{K}{CP_{max}} + \dfrac{C}{CP_{max}}}. \tag{4.7}$$

Clearly the fraction of drug bound depends not only on $C$ and on $CP_{max}$ but also on $K$. Goldstein (1949) graphed $CP/(CP+C)$ against $\log(C/CP_{max})$ for different values of $K$ to illustrate the form of this dependence. The graph is reproduced in Figure 4.6. At low and intermediate drug concentrations the fraction free (or bound) is roughly constant. If affinity is high (small $K$) and binding capacity is large (large $CP_{max}$) the fraction bound will approach 1.0.

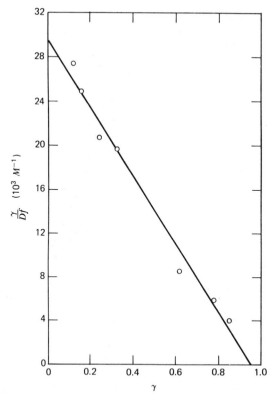

**Figure 4.5** Scatchard plot for spironolactone derivative III binding to human serum albumin at pH 7.4. *Df* represents the absorbed dose; $\gamma = CP/P_{\text{total}}$. From the intercept and slope the values of $n$ and $K$ were calculated to be 0.99 and $3.3 \times 10^{-2}$ m$M$, respectively. Reproduced with permission from Chien et al., 1976, Figure 1.

If affinity is low (large $K$) and binding capacity is limited (small $CP_{\text{max}}$) the fraction bound will be very small. As $C$ approaches $CP_{\text{max}}$, however, the fraction bound begins to drop sharply; when $C$ is about $100(CP_{\text{max}})$, the fraction bound is negligible and $C$ is practically equal to $(C + CP)$.

If the range of drug concentrations studied coincides with the range within which the fraction bound (or free) is roughly constant, protein binding will not introduce nonlinearity into the kinetics of disposition. However, even when the fraction bound is constant, remember that $C + CP$ is always greater than $C$. Since it is the concentration in plasma water that reaches a steady state relationship with the concentration in extracellular and intracellular water, plasma assays must take into account the degree of protein binding. As discussed in Chapter 3, the use of $C + CP$ in graphing dieaway data in the two-compartment system will lead to an overestimation of $B_0$, and therefore to an underestimation of $V_D$.

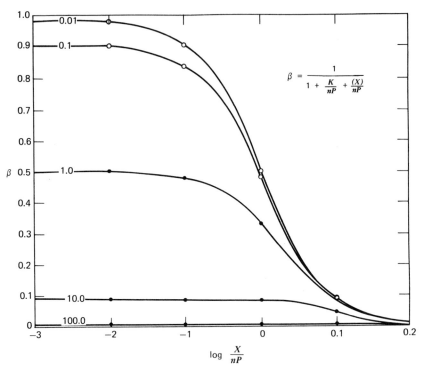

**Figure 4.6**  The fraction of drug bound to protein ($\beta$) as a function of the log of the ratio of the concentration of free drug ($X$) to the total concentration of protein binding sites ($nP$) for different discrete values of $K/nP$, where $K$ is the dissociation constant of the drug-protein complex. Reproduced with permission from Goldstein, 1949, Figure 7, © 1949 by the Williams & Wilkins Co., Baltimore.

Sometimes a drug is sequestered by binding to tissue proteins but remains in a rapidly reestablished steady state relationship with plasma free drug. In this case assays of plasma drug concentration will underestimate the amount of drug available for transport, therefore will overestimate $V_D$.

If within the range of concentrations studied the fraction bound (or free) is not constant, protein binding will introduce nonlinearity into disposition kinetics. To begin with, the fraction of total body drug present in the plasma will be dose dependent. At low doses the drug may be confined largely to the plasma. At higher doses, where $\log C/CP_{max}$ equals or exceeds zero, plasma binding sites will have become saturated and additional dose increments will be distributed to a greater extent into peripheral tissues. As $CP_{max}$ decreases the concentration $C$ of free drug at which plasma sites are saturated becomes correspondingly smaller. For example, Kunin (1965a) showed that the extent of binding of a series of penicillins to plasma proteins was inversely related to the degree of distribution of the antibiotics into peripheral tissues.

A great deal has been written on the impact of plasma protein binding on the pharmacologic activity of drugs. The activities of many antibiotics have been shown to be inversely proportional to their degree of plasma protein binding (Rolinson and Sutherland, 1965). Advantage has been taken of this observation in efforts to potentiate the activity of highly protein bound drugs by coadministering a second drug that will displace the first from its binding sites. Aspirin and certain of the sulfonamides, for example, compete with penicillins for binding sites on human plasma proteins and are capable of displacing the moderately tightly bound penicillin derivatives to a significant extent (Kunin, 1965b). Ordinarily such displacement results in a lower total plasma concentration of the displaced drug but a higher concentration in the tissues and a higher plasma level of unbound drug; consequently there is potentiation of the antimicrobal activity of the penicillin (Kunin, 1964). Generalizations concerning the interaction of two drugs at the protein binding level should be avoided, however. There are instances of a second drug's enhancing the binding of the first.

Whether sequestration of a drug by binding to plasma proteins has a practical effect on its behavior in the body depends partly on its affinity for protein binding sites ($K$ must be of the order of $10^{-4}$ or less for plasma binding to be quantitatively important relative to distribution throughout the tissue water volume) and, in the case of pharmacologically or toxicologically active substances, partly on the location of the receptor sites. If the biophase is part of the central or plasma compartment, the effect of plasma protein binding on the tissue concentration of drug or toxicant may be unimportant. A good review of the effect of plasma protein binding on distribution is that by Meyer and Guttman (1968).

The impact of plasma protein binding on elimination is less well understood than its impact on distribution. It is sometimes stated that passive diffusion is capable of extracting only unbound drug from the plasma. This is true in a sense for static situations in which unbound drug is distributed in a steady state across a membrane. However, dynamic situations such as renal excretion by the purely diffusional mechanism of glomerular filtration are more complex. In this case the relative magnitudes of the rate constant $k_2$ for dissociation of the drug-protein complex and the rate constant $k_3$ for elimination of the compound (Figure 4.7) are of primary importance.

It was pointed out in Chapter 3 that the slowest step in a sequence is the rate-controlling step. If $k_2$ were much less than $k_3$, by analogy with a deep compartment the rate of elimination of the compound would be controlled by $k_2$, not by $k_3$. However, when values of $k_2$ have been determined, they have been found to be of the order of fractions of a second (half-lives of the order of milliseconds) (Froese, 1962), and it is unlikely that $k_2$ is rate determining

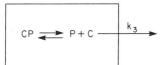

**Figure 4.7** Model for elimination of a protein bound compound: *P*, protein concentration; *C*, concentration of free compound; *CP*, concentration of complex.

for most drugs (Gillette, 1973). Therefore it appears that at least a small part of the bound fraction of drugs is probably available to glomerular filtration. Certainly the bound fraction is available to active elimination processes such as metabolism (Evans et al., 1973). When elimination is particularly efficient, plasma protein binding, by increasing the amount of drug presented to elimination mechanisms per unit of time, may actually accelerate rather than retard elimination. Gillette (1973, 1977) has simulated the effect of protein binding on elimination for a range of combinations of $k_2$ and $k_3$ values, but there has been little or no experimental work in this area.

### 4.4.2 Saturable Elimination Processes

Saturable processes were discussed in detail in Chapter 2. By analogy with the development given there, it is apparent that if a compound is eliminated from the body by a single saturable process (metabolism or active transport), the dependence of its rate of loss on its plasma concentration can be expressed as

$$-\frac{dC}{dt} = \left(\frac{V_m}{K_m + C}\right)(C). \tag{4.8}$$

The quantity $V_m/K_m + C$ is the apparent rate constant of elimination $k_{app}$. Clearly $k_{app}$ is dependent on concentration $C$ and a graph of $\ln C$ versus $t$ will not approach linearity until $C$ has declined to a level at which $C \ll K_m$ and $k_{app} \approx V_m/K_m$. However, as illustrated by the rose bengal example given at the beginning of this chapter, nonlinearity can be difficult to distinguish from experimental variability within a limited concentration range. As a result $k_{app}$ may be estimated from a series of data points at a specific time interval after injection of a compound and found to be dependent on dose in such a way that it becomes smaller as dose becomes larger. This dose dependence results because at each time point the concentration term in the numerator of the expression for $k_{app}$ is larger as the dose is increased. In consequence, of course, the half-life also increases and may even appear to be approaching an infinitely large value as the dose becomes very large.

In a one-compartment system $V_{extrap}$ is a real volume, is not a function of $k_e$, and will not depend on dose. But in a multicompartment system both $V_{extrap}$ and the slopes of the feathered dieaway curve will appear to depend on dose whenever the elimination mechanism is saturable but the data are treated as if it were not. To see why this is so, we will need to integrate Equation 4.8 to obtain the relationship of concentration to time:

$$\frac{C_0 - C}{K_m} + \ln\frac{C_0}{C} = \left(\frac{V_m}{K_m}\right)t, \tag{4.9}$$

where $C = C_0$ when $t = 0$. Since the integral form of Equation 4.9 contains $C$ in both linear and logarithmic terms, it cannot be solved explicitly for $C$ as a

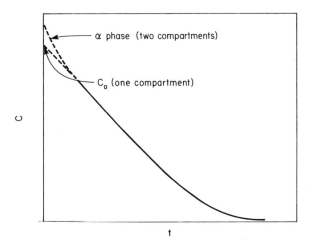

**Figure 4.8** The appearance of a $C, t$ plot following acute administration of a compound eliminated by a saturable mechanism.

function of time. However there is nothing to prevent us from graphing $C$ against $t$. Figure 4.8 is such a graph of Equation 4.9.

Curves of the form shown in Figure 4.8 have been described as having a "hockey stick" shape. As long as $C$ is reasonably close to $C_0$, the $\ln C_0 / C$ term in Equation 4.9 is much less important than the $(C_0 - C)/K_m$ term, and the relationship between $C$ and $t$ is pseudolinear (the handle of the hockey stick). Wagner (1973b) estimated that the $\ln C_0 / C$ term begins to make a significant contribution to Equation 4.9 at about $\ln C_0 / C = 1$. When $\ln C_0 / C > 1$ the $C, t$ graph begins to deviate from pseudolinearity.

When $\ln C_0 / C = 1$, $\ln C_0 / C = \ln e$, and $C = C_0 / e$, where $e$ is the base of natural logarithms. At this time point then, substituting the identity $C = C_0 / e$ into Equation 4.9 to obtain the value $t^*$ of $t$ when $C = C_0 / e$ and calculating the negative slope $k_0$ of the pseudolinear segment from $t = 0$ to $t = t^*$,

$$k_0 = \frac{V_m C_0}{C_0 + K_m / (1 - 1/e)}$$

At very large doses, when $C_0 \gg K_m / (1 - 1/e)$, $k_0$ approaches $V_m$.

Ethanol is the classic example of a compound eliminated by saturable metabolic transformation. It is generally considered that the negative slope of the pseudolinear phase of alcohol elimination is $V_m$ for alcohol dehydrogenase under physiological conditions; but Wagner et al. (1976) have demonstrated that ethanol elimination kinetic data are better fit instead by Equation 4.9. Their data are reproduced in Figure 4.9.

The log of the concentration may also be graphed against time as in Figure 4.10. At later times after administration, when $C$ has become small

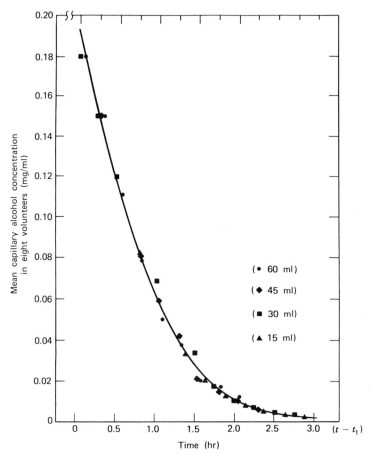

**Figure 4.9** The results of a simultaneous nonlinear least squares fit to Equation 4.9 of blood ethanol concentrations in eight subjects given four different doses of ethanol. The solid line gives the model-predicted concentrations. Times have been adjusted so that data from different doses are superimposed. Reproduced with permission from Wagner et al., 1976, Figure 2.

relative to $K_m$,

$$\frac{dC}{dt} \approx \left( \frac{-V_m}{K_m} \right) C \qquad (4.10)$$

and

$$\ln C \approx \left( \ln C_0 + \frac{C_0}{K_m} \right) - \left( \frac{V_m}{K_m} \right) t, \qquad (4.11)$$

so that a graph of $\ln C$ against $t$ should have a terminal linear segment whose slope is $- V_m / K_m$. Of course, when sufficiently low doses are given it is to be expected that only this terminal first-order phase will be seen, since as long as

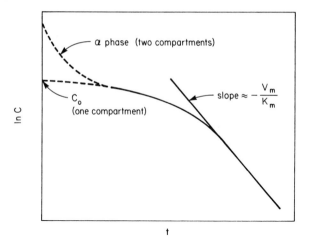

**Figure 4.10** The appearance of a plot of $\ln C$ versus $t$ following acute administration of a compound eliminated by a saturable mechanism.

the saturable process is not saturated, the kinetic behavior of the system should approximate that of a first-order system.

As an example of this behavior consider the study by Sauerhoff et al. (1976) of the pharmacokinetics of 2, 4, 5-T, a plant growth regulator and herbicide. The salts of this compound are readily absorbed by rats and are eliminated primarily by the kidneys. The half-life is dose dependent. To investigate this dose dependency, Sauerhoff et al. gave single intravenous doses of either 5 or 100 mg of radiolabeled 2, 4, 5-T per kilogram of rat body weight and followed the decline of radioactivity as a function of time. Their results, reproduced in Figure 4.11, are consistent with the concept that the renal elimination mechanism is saturable. By applying Equation 4.11 to the data determining curve $A$, the authors estimated that $V_m = 16.6$ $\mu$g/ml/hr and $K_m = 127.6$ $\mu$g/ml. The half-life of 2, 4, 5-T after the 5-mg/kg dose is 5.3 hr. Therefore $k_e$ from curve $B$ is 0.13 hr$^{-1}$, which is equal to $V_m/K_m$ from curve $A$.

Note especially that curve $A$ is linear and parallel to curve $B$ throughout the range of concentrations represented by curve $B$. Whenever saturation of an elimination mechanism is responsible for kinetic nonlinearity, the rate of loss of material from the plasma is dictated by the amount available to the saturable process at that time. Therefore the rate of loss at any given concentration should be independent of the amount originally administered. Irrespective of the dose, all $\ln C$, $t$ graphs should revert to linearity at about the same concentration. We can take advantage of this observation to estimate the dose of 2, 4, 5-T above which nonlinear behavior may be expected to occur. Curve $A$ reverts to first-order kinetics when plasma concentrations of 2, 4, 5-T are below about 100 $\mu$g eq/g. Since a dose of 5 mg/kg gives an initial plasma concentration of about 30$\mu$g eq/g, doses of 15

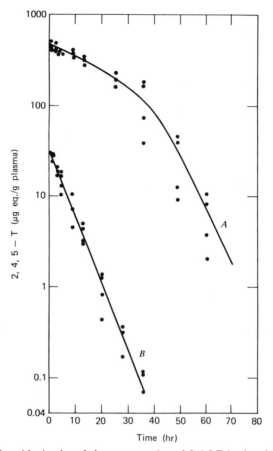

**Figure 4.11** Semilogarithmic plot of the concentration of 2,4,5-T in the plasma of rats as a function of time following a single intravenous administration of $^{14}$C-labeled 2,4,5-T at 5 mg/kg (*B*) and 100 mg/kg (*A*) as determined from the concentration of $^{14}$C activity. Each point represents one rat. Reproduced with permission from Sauerhoff et al., 1976, Figure 1.

mg/kg and above will give initial plasma concentrations of about 100 μg eq/g and more. Nonlinear kinetic behavior should begin to appear above doses of about 15 mg of 2, 4, 5-T/kg.

By inspection of curve *A* it is easy to see that if the analysis had not been carried beyond 30 or 35 hr, the data would have suggested a linear one-compartment system in which the half-life of 2, 4, 5-T was as much as 20 hr. Similarly, by applying a two-compartment linear kinetic analysis to the rose bengal data of Figure 4.2, Klaassen calculated that the apparent half-life of a 100-mg dose of rose bengal per kilogram was twice the apparent half-life when lower doses were given (Table 4.1). The rose bengal data differ from the 2, 4, 5-T data only in that a distributional phase is also apparent.

The most important point to remember is that when the elimination process is saturable (and approaching saturation) a $\ln C$, $t$ graph is not linear after distribution is complete but, instead, falls off with time. Therefore the apparent half-life measured either late on the curve or at very low doses is smaller than that measured early on a saturated curve.

Saturation of elimination mechanisms is particularly likely at the high concentrations associated with toxicity studies in animals or with cases of overexposure in humans. It is therefore very important in high dose studies to extend the observation period to five or six apparent biological half-lives, to prevent the mistaking of either a distributional segment of the dieaway curve or a zero-order segment for the terminal segment representing first-order whole body loss.

If the saturable elimination process is in parallel with a first-order elimination process, then

$$-\frac{dC}{dt} = \frac{V_m C}{K_m + C} + k_e C. \tag{4.12}$$

The integral form of this equation is implicit with respect to $C$. When graphed it closely resembles Figure 4.10. Van Ginneken et al. (1974) have discussed techniques for obtaining estimates of $k_e$, $V_m$, and $K_m$ from dieaway data when elimination is by parallel first-order and saturable processes. However, it has been pointed out by Wagner (1975) that even reasonably thorough analysis of a dieaway curve ordinarily will not permit the researcher to determine whether a first-order elimination process exists in parallel with the more obvious saturable process. In complex systems such as these, where dieaway kinetics indicate a saturated elimination process, it usually is necessary to examine the elimination processes individually to characterize the system fully.

For example, conclusive evidence of a saturable metabolic step can be obtained if the appearance of metabolite can be monitored in the central compartment. If the plasma level of metabolite approaches a plateau, and holds that plateau longer after larger doses of parent compound (see Figure 4.14, below), the mechanism for metabolite production is saturable (and saturated). In experimental animal models, further information on saturable metabolism can often be obtained by inducing or inhibiting the microsomal oxidizing enzyme systems responsible for metabolism. Inhibition should result in a lower and more prolonged plateau level of metabolite; induction, in a briefer plateau or even in its disappearance entirely.

As an illustration of several of the points made in this section consider the study by Garrett et al. (1974) of the pharmacokinetics of amobarbital, a barbiturate that is extensively metabolized by hydroxylation prior to its elimination in the urine. Earlier studies in humans, in which plasma levels of amobarbital were followed for not more than two half-lives, had led to the conclusion that amobarbital pharmacokinetics were first order and describable by a two-compartment open model with an apparent biological half-life of about 21 hr (Balasubramaniam, 1970). Garrett et al. recorded the time course of changes in plasma levels of amobarbital and of its major metabolite hydroxyamobarbital for six apparent half-lives following intravenous administration of amobarbital to dogs. The pattern of amobarbital metabolism is essentially the same in the dog and in man.

Within the plasma amobarbital concentration range studied, about 40% of the amobarbital was found to be bound to plasma proteins. This figure, which was independent of the amobarbital concentration within this range, was used to correct observed plasma levels for pharmacokinetic calculations. Following a rapid distribution phase, loss of amobarbital from the plasma demonstrated the pattern characteristic of a saturable elimination process (Figure 4.12). It was noted that if the plasma dieaway of amobarbital had been followed for only two half-lives and the data analyzed in accordance with the assumptions of first-order kinetics, the apparent biological half-lives would have been found to be dose dependent and about 18, 10, and 7 hr for the 40, 10, and 5 mg/kg doses, respectively. Instead the curves were fit by computer techniques in accordance with the model in Figure 4.13.

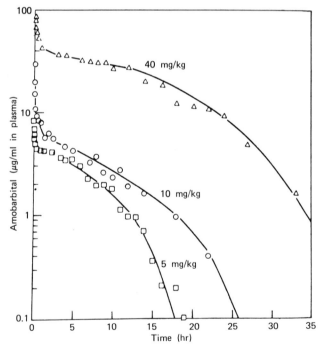

**Figure 4.12** Semilogarithmic plot of amobarbital plasma levels following intravenous administration of 5, 10, and 40 mg/kg to the same dog at different times. Reproduced with permission from Garrett et al., 1974, Figure 3.

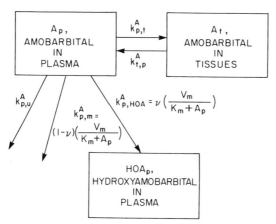

**Figure 4.13** Model for amobarbital disposition. Redrawn with permission from Garrett et al., 1974, Scheme I.

Note that the authors assumed that $K_m$ and $V_m$ for the transformation of amobarbital (A) to hydroxyamobarbital (HOA) and for its transformation to other metabolites (M) were identical. This simplification was justified by the observation that the percentage recovery of amobarbital as hydroxyamobarbital in the urine was independent of dose, so that formation of other metabolites must bear the same kinetic relationship to plasma amobarbital as formation of hydroxyamobarbital. Computer analysis of the data gave mean $K_m$ and $V_m$ estimates in a group of six dogs of $6.4 \times 10^3$ $\mu$g of total plasma amobarbital and 4.6 $\mu$g of total drug per second, respectively. Therefore $V_m/K_m$ is $0.72 \times 10^{-3}$ sec$^{-1}$ or 2.6 hr$^{-1}$, the apparent first-order rate constant for amobarbital metabolism at low plasma concentrations when the metabolic processes are not saturated. The rate constant $k_{p,u}$ for the direct transfer of amobarbital from plasma into the urine was $0.31 \times 10^{-5}$ sec$^{-1}$ or 0.011 hr$^{-1}$, so it is to be expected that only a small amount of amobarbital will appear in the urine unchanged. The measured urinary excretion of amobarbital was 2.4% of the 5-mg/kg dose, 3.0% of the 10-mg/kg dose, and 5.0% of the 40-mg/kg dose. Even less amobarbital was excreted in the bile.

The terminal half-life of amobarbital in the plasma therefore should be about $0.693/(2.6 + 0.01)$ hr$^{-1}$, or about 0.26 hr, irrespective of dose. Note the vast difference between 0.26 and 18 hr, the apparent half-life calculated from early points on the 40-mg/kg curve by treating the data as if they were adequately represented by a simple first-order model.

In this study hydroxyamobarbital levels were also monitored in the plasma, both after the administration of amobarbital and after the administration of hydroxyamobarbital (HOA) itself. The data are shown in Figure 4.14. It is apparent that after amobarbital administration the plasma level of HOA establishes a plateau that persists for a longer time as the dose of parent compound is increased. The parallel terminal HOA line segments observed

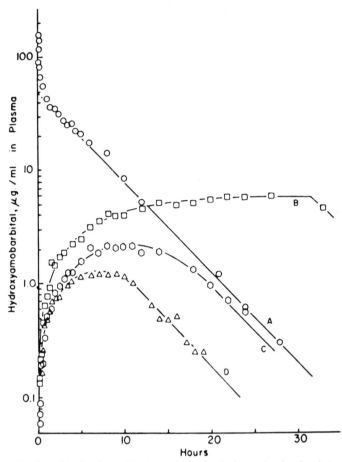

**Figure 4.14** Semilogarithmic plots of hydroxyamobarbital plasma levels after intravenous administration of amobarbital sodium, 5 mg/kg ($\triangle$), 10 mg/kg ($\bigcirc$), and 40 mg/kg ($\square$); and of hydroxyamobarbital itself, 39 mg/kg ($O$), to the same dog at different times. Adapted with permission from Garrett et al., 1974, Figure 4.

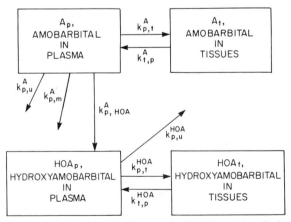

**Figure 4.15** Model for amobarbital and hydroxyamobarbital disposition. Redrawn with permission from Garrett et al., 1974, Scheme II.

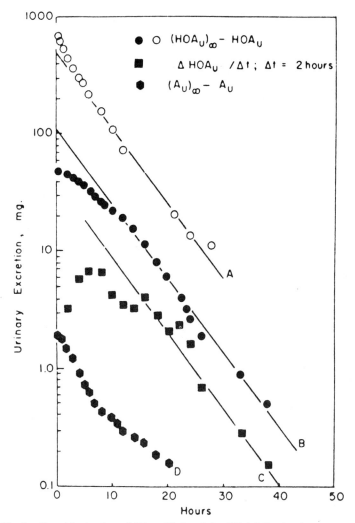

**Figure 4.16**  Semilogarithmic plots of $(U_\infty - U)$ $(O, \bullet)$ for HOA following intravenous administration of either A ($\bullet$, 5 mg/kg) or HOA (O, 39 mg/kg); of $(U_\infty - U)$ ($\bullet$) for A following
intravenous administration of A (5 mg/kg); and of $\Delta U / \Delta t$ ($\blacksquare$) for HOA following intravenous
administration of A (5 mg/kg). Curves *B*, *C*, and *D* were obtained in one dog and curve *A* in
another. Reproduced with permission from Garrett et al., 1974, Figure 11.

after amobarbital administration indicate that the mechanism for metabolite
elimination is not itself saturated. Direct administration of HOA not only
confirms that its elimination kinetics, at least at a dose of 39 mg/kg, are first
order but also demonstrates that HOA is distributed into a peripheral
compartment. Therefore the model of Figure 4.13 must be modified to
incorporate HOA disposition, as shown in Figure 4.15.

$k_{p,u}^{HOA}$ was estimated in three ways after HOA administration: from the
slope of the terminal portion of a ln plasma *C*, *t* plot; from the terminal slope

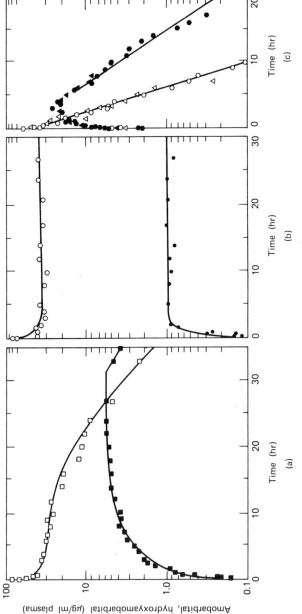

**Figure 4.17** Semilogarithmic plots of A (open symbols) and HOA (solid symbols) plasma levels versus time following intravenous administration of amobarbital sodium, 40 mg/kg, to (*a*) a normal dog; (*b*) a dog 30 min after intraperitoneal administration of SKF 525A, 40 mg/kg; and (*c*) two dogs (△▲ and ○● ● ) pretreated with phenobarbital, 16 mg/kg/day, for 30 days. Reproduced with permission from Garrett et al., 1974, Figure 5.

of a $\ln(U_\infty - U)$, $t$ plot; and from the terminal slope of a $\ln(\Delta U/\Delta t)$, $t$ plot. The estimates in all six dogs agreed well; their mean was $3.8 \times 10^{-5}$ sec$^{-1}$, or 0.14 hr$^{-1}$. The half-life of HOA is therefore about 5 hr (Figure 4.16).

Finally, Garrett et al. administrated phenobarbital, an inducer of microsomal enzyme activity, and SKF 525A, an inhibitor of microsomal enzyme activity, to two different dogs and determined the consequent change in the kinetics of amobarbital metabolism. As Figure 4.17 shows, SKF 525A sharply inhibited amobarbital metabolism, lowering and lengthening the hydroxy-amobarbital plateau and, in general, so emphasizing the zero-order nature of high dose amobarbital metabolism that it appeared almost to abolish metabolism and loss. On the other hand, by inducing the metabolizing enzymes, phenobarbital completely eliminated any evidence of nonlinearity even at 40 mg/kg. Note that there is no evidence for a hydroxyamobarbital distribution phase whenever amobarbital has been administered. Being very rapid (see Figure 4.14), hydroxyamobarbital distribution is buried in the slower transformation or appearance phase.

## 4.5   THE KIDNEY: AN ORGAN IN WHICH FIRST–ORDER AND SATURABLE ELIMINATION PROCESSES OPERATE SIMULTANEOUSLY

The kidney is an important excretory organ for many foreign compounds. It is also kinetically interesting because it contains first-order and saturable excretory mechanisms that function in parallel.

The kidney is a complex organ admirably designed for its dual function of excreting waste metabolic products while retaining key metabolites whose supply must be conserved. These activities take place along the nephrons, the structural and functional units of the kidney.

The nephron can be visualized as a microscopic funnel with a long, narrow stem or tubule. The renal tubule conducts urine from the funnel, or Bowman's capsule, to a larger collecting tubule that empties into the ureters. The renal tubule is made up of several structurally and functionally distinguishable segments lined with epithelial cells. The cells of two of these segments, the proximal and distal convoluted tubules, possess active transport mechanisms both for secretion (transfer from blood plasma to urine) and for reabsorption (return from urine to blood plasma). These active transport mechanisms, by controlling the excretion of specific compounds, either directly or indirectly regulate the volume and the solute content of the urine. They are therefore essential to maintenance of homeostasis.

The first part of the nephron encountered by the blood as it flows through the renal capillaries is the glomerulus, a knot of twisted capillaries almost completely encased by the Bowman's capsule, a double layer of epithelial cells separated by a space or lumen. Plasma water and solutes moving through the glomerulus are filtered into the lumen of the surrounding Bowman's capsule. This filtration process is driven largely by a pressure gradient across the epithelial membrane. In the normal human adult male it results in transfer of about 20% of the plasma water and solutes traversing the glomerulus in a single pass. It is completely nonselective with regard to all solutes small enough to pass through the large pores in the glomerular membrane. Only solutes with molecular weights greater than about 70,000 (this cutoff point is influenced to some extent also by molecular shape and charge) are excluded from the filtration process; this group includes the plasma proteins.

Since the glomerular filtration rate is independent of any concentration measure, the *fraction* of a solute cleared from the plasma during one pass through the glomerulus is also independent of concentration or dose. The *amount* cleared, of course, is proportional to the amount present. Therefore glomerular filtration is a first-order process.

Blood leaving the glomerular capillaries passes into the peributular capillaries surrounding the proximal convoluted renal tubule as filtrate leaving the lumen of the Bowman's capsule moves into the tubular lumen. Here essential nutrients such as glucose and amino acids are actively reabsorbed from the tubular lumen into the blood, and much of the filtered water follows to maintain osmotic balance. As forming urine moves along the tubule, its composition is subject to continual adjustment by active and passive exchange of its water and solute content with peritubular blood.

Like all solutes that are not excessively large, foreign compounds and their metabolites are filtered at the glomerulus. In addition many substances, in particular organic acids and bases, are actively secreted into the tubular lumen. Foreign compounds may also be passively reabsorbed across the tubular wall in accordance with their lipid solubility characteristics. Whether foreign compounds are often actively reabsorbed is not certain, although some at least are known to be (Chremos et al., 1976).

Renal tubular secretory mechanisms are more efficient than glomerular filtration as long as their maximum transport rates have not been exceeded. As discussed in Section 4.4.1, the accessibilities of plasma protein bound materials in general to passive excretory processes such as glomerular filtration and to active excretory processes such as tubular secretion are not well defined. As far as is known, the distinction is not a qualitative but rather a quantitative one. The difference lies in the degree to which the excretory process is able to perturb the equilibrium established between free and protein bound drug in the plasma. Given sufficient time, even a highly protein bound drug would be cleared by glomerular filtration. It is not, however, cleared in one pass through the kidney. To see why this is so, let us consider a simplified example. We assume that fractional protein binding is independent of plasma concentration and that the equilibrium between bound and free drug is adjusted with sufficient rapidity that it is not the controlling process determining excretion rate.

If our drug is 80% bound to plasma proteins, then during a single very small unit of time—say one-fourth of the transit time through the glomerulus —filtration will remove about one-twentieth of the 20% of drug that is unbound. Only 1% of the bound drug will have shifted to the unbound fraction during the same time interval to compensate for drug lost. If, on the other hand, a secretory process can remove all the free drug during the same small time unit, 20% of the bound drug will have shifted to the unbound fraction. For less extensively bound drugs the percentage displacement of drug to compensate for efficient clearance is even larger. It is not difficult to see why actively secreted compounds can be cleared from the plasma during one pass through the kidney even though they may be bound to plasma proteins.

Total clearance represents the volume of plasma cleared of the solute by all elimination mechanisms together during the time unit of choice. Clearance through a specific organ or by a specific mechanism represents the volume of plasma cleared of the solute by that organ or mechanism during the time unit of choice. From another point of view, renal clearance is renal plasma flow rate times the extraction efficiency. Filtration extraction efficiency is a constant independent of dose. Since about 20% of the total renal plasma flow (RPF) of 600–700 ml/min in the adult human can be cleared completely by glomerular filtration, the glomerular filtration rate (GFR) is about 125 ml/min. For materials cleared solely by glomerular filtration, renal clearance is equal to the GFR. Model compounds such as inulin, a large molecular weight polysaccharide of plant origin that is eliminated from the body by glomerular filtration only, are used clinically and experimentally to measure the GFR.

In Section 3.13 it was shown that for compounds eliminated entirely by first-order kinetic processes such as filtration a $(\Delta U/\Delta t)$, $C$ graph should be linear. Its slope is an estimate of $k_u V_D$, or renal clearance. In ordinary clinical and even in experimental practice the renal clearance is commonly calculated from a single assay of $C_u$ and $C_p$, the urine and plasma concentrations, respectively, and a single urine volume by using the standard formula

$$\text{Cl}_{\text{renal}} = \frac{(C_u)(\text{rate of urine flow})}{C_p \text{ at midpoint of urine collection}}. \tag{4.13}$$

The assumption that a $(\Delta U/\Delta t)$, $C_p$ graph would be linear with its intercept at the origin is implicit in the application of this formula. In other words, Equation 4.13 defines the slope of a straight line drawn from one experimental point through the origin. For compounds eliminated by glomerular filtration alone, this procedure is justified, as illustrated by curve

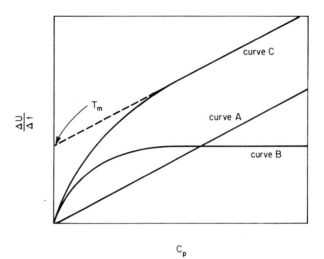

**Figure 4.18** Renal excretion rate as a function of plasma concentration. Curve *A*, glomerular filtration only. Curve *C*, glomerular filtration plus saturable tubular secretion. Curve *B*, curve *C* minus curve *A*: isolation of the tubular secretion process.

A of Figure 4.18. Any single point on the line can be used to estimate the slope.

But Equation 4.13 applies only to the special case of first-order elimination. It does not apply to saturable elimination processes. To begin with, $Cl_{total}$ is not equal to $k_e V_D$ for compounds eliminated by saturable mechanisms. It will be recalled from Section 3.13 that total clearance is defined as

$$Cl_{total} = \frac{D}{(AUC)_\infty} \qquad (4.14)$$

or, more generally,

$$Cl_{total\ to\ time\ t} = \frac{amount\ eliminated\ by\ time\ t}{(AUC)_t}. \qquad (4.15)$$

The corresponding definitions of renal clearance, when renal excretion is not the only elimination mechanism, are

$$Cl_{renal} = \frac{U_\infty}{(AUC)_\infty} \qquad (4.16)$$

and

$$Cl_{renal\ to\ time\ t} = \frac{amount\ eliminated\ in\ urine\ by\ time\ t}{(AUC)_t}. \qquad (4.17)$$

For compounds eliminated by saturable mechanisms such as tubular secretion, $(AUC)_t$ and $(AUC)_\infty$ are not proportional to dose. Wagner (1973) has shown that for a compound eliminated by a single saturable mechanism characterized by a maximum rate $V_m$ and a half-saturation constant $K_m$,

$$(AUC)_t = \frac{1}{V_m}\left[\frac{C_0^2}{2} + \frac{C_p^2}{2} - C_0 C_p + K_m\left\{C_0 - C_p - (C_p)\left(\ln\frac{C_0}{C_p}\right)\right\}\right] + C_p t$$

and

$$(AUC)_\infty = \frac{C_0}{V_m}\left[\frac{C_0}{2} + K_m\right]$$

$$= \frac{D^2}{2V_m V_D^2} + \frac{K_m D}{V_m V_D}. \tag{4.18}$$

$(AUC)_\infty$ increases sharply as $D$ is increased. It is apparent that $Cl_{total}$ for a compound eliminated by a single saturable mechanism is dose dependent. From Equation 4.18 expressing $(AUC)_\infty$ as a function of dose, together with the definition of $Cl_{total}$ given in Equation 4.14, it is easily shown that for the case of saturable elimination

$$Cl_{total} = \frac{2V_m V_D^2}{D + 2K_m V_D}. \tag{4.19}$$

In the kidney, the first-order filtration mechanism is always present in parallel with any saturable secretion mechanism. The rate of excretion due to the secretion mechanism alone would be

$$\frac{dU}{dt} = \frac{V_m C_p V_D}{K_m + C_p},$$

as shown by curve B of Figure 4.18. But the total rate of excretion from the kidney is

$$\frac{dU}{dt} = k_u V_D C_p + \frac{V_m C_p V_D}{K_m + C_p},$$

illustrated by curve C of Figure 4.18. Therefore renal clearance calculated by means of Equation 4.13 is

$$\frac{\frac{dU}{dt}}{C_p} = k_u V_D + \frac{V_m V_D}{K_m + C_p},$$

and the slope of a $(\Delta U/\Delta t)$, $C_p$ graph is a constantly decreasing function of $C_p$. Clearance estimated by using Equation 4.13 will be dependent on the plasma concentration during the particular interval of measurement. Except at values of $D$ so small that the elimination mechanism is not near saturation, clearance estimated from Equation 4.13 will not be equal to the value of $Cl_{renal \text{ to time } t}$ as defined by Equation 4.17. When $C_p \gg K_m$

$$\frac{dU}{dt} \cong k_u V_D C_p + V_m V_D$$

and, as shown by the extrapolation of curve C in Figure 4.18, it may be possible to estimate $V_m$ if experimental determinations of excretion rate can be made at concentrations greatly exceeding $K_m$.

If a compound is eliminated by both glomerular filtration and tubular secretion with no reabsorption, its renal clearance will be larger than the glomerular filtration rate and may approach the total renal plasma flow. Therefore in the adult human as much as 600–700 ml of plasma can be cleared per minute by the two processes combined.

If a compound is actively or passively reabsorbed its renal clearance will, of course, be smaller than it would be in the absence of reabsorption. It is not always possible to infer the existence of a reabsorption mechanism when clearance is estimated by using Equation 4.13, although obviously if renal clearance is less than the GFR, some reabsorption must be taking place. When reabsorption is superimposed on filtration and secretion the relationship of $dU/dt$ to $C_p$ may be very complex, especially if the reabsorption mechanism is saturable. Garrett (1978) outlines methods for analyzing complex renal clearance curves to obtain the kinetic parameters for the component saturable excretion and reabsorption processes.

Irrespective of the mechanism or mechanisms of renal excretion, clearance calculated by dividing $U_\infty$ by $(AUC)_\infty$ is the most accurate estimate of the contribution of renal clearance to the total clearance of a compound. $U_\infty / (AUC)_\infty$ can be viewed as a sort of average clearance over the entire time course of elimination. Use of the expression

$$\frac{(C_u)(\text{rate of urine flow})}{(C_p)}$$

is perfectly acceptable provided the potential dependence of $Cl_{renal}$ calculated in this way on $C_p$ is recognized and understood and, if necessary, characterized. Wagner (1968) has discussed the relationships among various measures of urinary clearance in some detail.

## 4.6 NONLINEARITIES INTRODUCED BY ALTERATION OF KINETIC PARAMETERS

Throughout the foregoing discussion it has been tacitly assumed that physiological determinants of the kinetic parameters (volumes and rate constants) of the system have not changed during the course of exposure. This is not always true, particularly when the material under consideration is toxic.

Strictly speaking, consideration of nonlinearities should be confined to the effects of the compound itself on the kinetics of its absorption and disposition. In some of the discussion that follows, the effects of other factors— specifically, microsomal enzyme inducers and inhibitors and physical factors controlling blood flow—on kinetic parameters are introduced to illustrate the impact of common adaptive or homeostatic physiological and biochemical mechanisms on absorption and disposition kinetics.

### 4.6.1 Alterations in Volumes

Expansion of peripheral volumes with an increase in concentration or dose is physiologically reasonable. Secondary binding sites on plasma or tissue proteins may be activated. Generally such secondary complexes are non-specific rather than specific. Volumes of distribution may become larger as a material "overflows" natural barriers at higher concentration levels.

Compartments may also expand physically to accommodate a compound. For example, exposure of rats to hexane vapors results within a few hours in the appearance of newly deposited liver lipid that serves as a compartment of flexible size to accommodate the highly lipid-soluble absorbed hexane (Figure 4.19). Repeated exposure to many lipid-soluble materials such as ethanol or chloroform induces fatty liver, a condition that may be followed by the

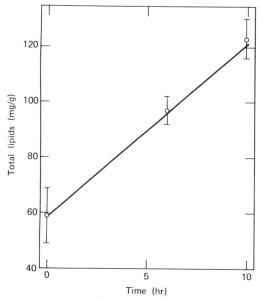

**Figure 4.19** The effect of hexane on liver lipid content as a function of the length of exposure of rats to hexane vapors (170 g/m$^3$). The points represent the mean ± standard deviation of values from four animals. Reproduced with permission from Böhlen et al., 1973, Figure 2.

development of hepatic necrosis (Drill, 1952; Isselbacher and Greenberger, 1964).

### 4.6.2 Alterations in rates

Frequently metabolic rate constants are altered in response to the presence of an exogenous compound. Metabolizing enzymes are induced by a wide variety of materials including polycyclic aromatic hydrocarbons and many of the chlorinated hydrocarbons. Induction is more likely to be an important factor after repeated exposures than during the time course of a single exposure. Even following a single exposure, however, measured metabolic rate constants may vary. For example, in one study, sixteen hours after a single intramuscular dose of 10 mg of *o, p*'-DDT per 100 g of body weight, rat uterine glycolytic and hexose monophosphate shunt enzymes were 2–3 times as active as they had been before exposure (Singhal et al., 1970).

Other compounds may have even more striking effects. The activities of rat hepatic microsomal enzymes were increased by factors of as much as 3200 by a single intraperitoneal injection of 15 mg of a commercial mixture of polybrominated biphenyls per 100 g of body weight. For several of the enzymes monitored, elevation of activity persisted at least until the last sampling time—336 hr (2 weeks) (Dent et al., 1976). Degree of induction is dependent on dose as well as on the identity of the inducer (Breckenridge et al., 1973). That alterations in the levels of metabolizing enzymes can have a significant effect on the half-life of a drug is demonstrated by the effects of the microsomal enzyme inducer phenobarbital and the microsomal enzyme inhibitor SKF 525A on the half-life of phenazone in the dog. Pretreatment of dogs with phenobarbital reduced the half-life of phenazone from a mean of 78.6 days to a mean of 32.4 days. Pretreatment with SKF 525A lengthened it to 246.7 days (Kampffmeyer et al., 1974).

Certain of the microsomal mixed function oxidases require the presence of an oxidizable cosubstrate such as a metabolite for optimum enzyme activity. Whether such a requirement is likely to introduce kinetic nonlinearity into a system is uncertain, however, since ordinarily other reducing agents such as ascorbate can substitute for the metabolite cosubstrate.

Other mixed function oxidases appear to be subject to competitive feedback inhibition by the metabolite formed. Elimination of phenylbutazone is inhibited by coadministration of its metabolite oxyphenbutazone (Jähnchen and Levy, 1972). Elimination of diphenylhydantoin is similarly inhibited by concomitant administration of its primary metabolite (Ashley and Levy, 1972). The effect of product inhibition on drug elimination kinetics is qualitatively different from the effect of a saturable elimination mechanism (Perrier et al., 1973). Substrate activation of metabolizing enzymes is also potentially a cause of kinetic nonlinearity.

Alternatively not metabolizing enzyme activity but the hepatic plasma flow rate may be altered, effectively reducing (or increasing) the amount of

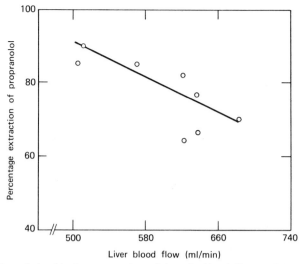

**Figure 4.20** The relationship between estimated hepatic blood flow and hepatic extraction efficiency of propranolol in eight dogs. Reproduced with permission from George et al., 1976, Figure 1.

material available for metabolism during a unit of time. The $\beta$-adrenergic blocking agent propranolol is cleared from the body primarily by extraction and metabolism in the liver. Hepatic extraction efficiency of propranolol in a series of eight dogs ranged from 69 to 92% and was negatively correlated with hepatic blood flow (Figure 4.20). It is probable that whole body clearance of propranol is determined largely by the rate of hepatic blood flow (George et al., 1976). Any factor operating to alter hepatic plasma flow rate would alter the rate of elimination of propranolol; hepatic blood flow rate is sensitive to a number of influences such as heat and exercise (Rowell et al., 1964), as well as to the effects of vasodilating and vasoconstricting drugs.

A reduction in plasma flow rate through other excretory organs such as the kidney or lung could also affect the amount of a drug or toxicant excreted by these routes. Alterations in blood flow rate may also affect absorption (Crouthamel et al., 1975) and would almost certainly affect distribution.

Not only blood flow rate but bile or urine flow rate may be altered. Problem 18 at the end of Chapter 3 demonstrated the effects of phenobarbital and SKF 525A on bile flow rate. The enhancement of bile flow rate by phenobarbital has been studied in detail (Klaassen, 1971). Whether a change in bile flow rate affects clearance in the bile depends on which is the rate-determining step in the elimination sequence. It is quite possible that bile or urine flow rate may be rate determining in some circumstances but not in others. For example, the chlorinated hydrocarbon insecticides kepone and mirex enhance bile flow rate, but although their metabolites are excreted in the bile, the rate of excretion is independent of the bile flow rate (Mehendale, 1977). On the other hand, although phenobarbital induces microsomal metabolizing enzymes as well as increasing bile flow rate, it enhances the rates of excretion of a number of organic compounds that are not metabolized prior to excretion. For example, the rates of biliary excretion in rats of the free (unconjugated) base procaine amide ethyl bromide, the organic acid phenol-3, 6-dibromphthalein disulfonate, and the neutral compound ouabain are enhanced by pretreatment of the animals with phenobarbital. Phenobarbital does not promote the rates of biliary excretion of all unmetabolized organic compounds, however (Klaassen, 1970).

By impairing kidney function, nephrotoxic compounds effectively lower $k_e$, the overall microscopic rate constant of elimination, for any compound eliminated wholly or in part by the kidney. The situation is analogous to that which occurs when alterations in metabolizing enzyme activity affect the half-lives of compounds eliminated primarily or partly by metabolism. Jusko and Gibaldi (1972) showed (see Problem 13 of Chapter 3) that the biological half life $\ln 2 / \beta$ for a two-compartment model does not increase in proportion to the decrease in $k_e$, however. If excretion is only moderately impaired, $\beta$ will be only slightly affected. Only when renal elimination is severely impaired will the biological half-life increase significantly. This natural protective mechanism is illustrated by the half-lives of penicillin and of other antibiotics in functionally anephric patients and in subjects given probenecid, which inhibits renal tubular transport of organic acids. Gibaldi and Schwartz (1968) showed that in spite of a sharp reduction in $k_e$ due to treatment, the biological half-life of nafcillin in subjects receiving probenecid was the same as the biological half-life of nafcillin in control subjects. An additional illustration is provided by the studies of Jusko et al. (1970) on the behavior of riboflavin, which is eliminated primarily by renal excretion. As Figure 4.21 demonstrates, the values of $\beta$ for a normal subject and for a patient with less than 3% of normal renal function were essentially identical.

Riboflavin excretion kinetics are more complex than Figure 4.21 suggests. They are both dose and species dependent. Absorption from the gut is capacity limited in man (Levy and Jusko, 1966) but apparently not in the rat (Axelson and Gibaldi, 1972). Excretion into the urine is linear in man but nonlinear in the rat; excretion into the bile is also nonlinear in the rat (Axelson and Gibaldi, 1972). It has been proposed that saturable tubular reabsorption is the cause of the nonlinearity of rat renal clearance of riboflavin (Jusko and Levy, 1970) but that limited-capacity tissue binding is responsible for the nonlinearity of biliary excretion (Axelson and Gibaldi, 1972).

Riboflavin kinetics have been studied with unusual thoroughness. Frequently detailed kinetic investigations have led to the discovery of complexities and dose dependencies such as those described for riboflavin. The many papers chronicling development of understanding of the complex kinetics of acetylsalicylic acid, reviewed by Levy et al. (1972), are an excellent illustration of this process.

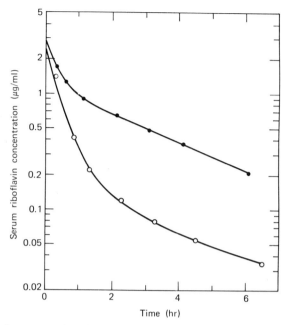

**Figure 4.21** The time course of total riboflavin plasma concentration in an anephric subject (●) after intravenous injection of 38.9 mg of riboflavin as riboflavin-5-phosphate (FMN). Also shown for comparison is riboflavin plasma concentration in a normal subject (O) who received an intravenous dose of 31 mg of FMN. Adapted with persmission from Jusko et al., 1970, Figure 1.

Of course a detailed and thorough kinetic study will not necessarily reveal nonlinearities. But it is safe to say that relatively few nonlinear kinetic systems are known not because so few of them exist but rather because they have not yet been identified. Study of kinetic nonlinearities has been called the "frontier" (Garrett, 1974). It is the point at which classical kinetics yields to the particular peculiarities of specific systems. It is one of the most challenging, exciting, and rapidly developing areas of kinetic investigation today.

### PROBLEMS

1 Show by rearranging the appropriate equations that the principle of superposition applies to disposition in linear one-compartment and two-compartment models with either instantaneous or first-order input.

2 Show that from a Scatchard plot, constructed with $CP/P_{total}$ as the independent variable and $CP/(C)(P_{total})$ as the dependent variable, the number of binding sites $n$ on the protein molecule can be determined. How is $K$ estimated from the graph?

**3** Equation 4.12 expresses the rate of decay of plasma concentration when loss from the plasma takes place by parallel first-order and saturable processes. To what form does this equation reduce if (*a*) the saturable process is saturated at very low *C*; (*b*) the saturable process is saturated only at very high *C*?

**4** For the example of amobarbital pharmacokinetics given in this chapter, can you provide a plausible explanation for the dose dependence of the percentage of amobarbital excreted directly into the urine?

**5** Show that for a compound eliminated entirely by first-order mechanisms, clearance is independent not only of dose but also of the time interval during which the experimental measurements were made. (This property is of course implicit in the linearity of a $\Delta U/\Delta t$, $C_p$ graph). Begin with the definition of clearance to time *t*:

$$\text{Cl}_{\text{total to time } t} = \frac{\text{amount eliminated by time } t}{(\text{AUC})_t}$$

**6** Figure 4.22 shows several dieaway curves for formate obtained in a study of methanol acidosis (Clay et al., 1975). Is the simplest model for this

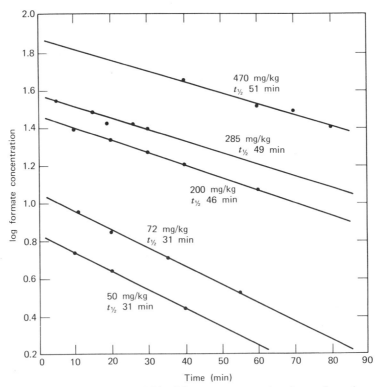

**Figure 4.22** Semilogarithmic plots of blood formate concentrations in monkeys given sodium formate, 100 mg/ml, intravenously in the indicated doses. Curves were fit by linear regression. Reproduced with permission from Clay et al., 1975, Figure 3.

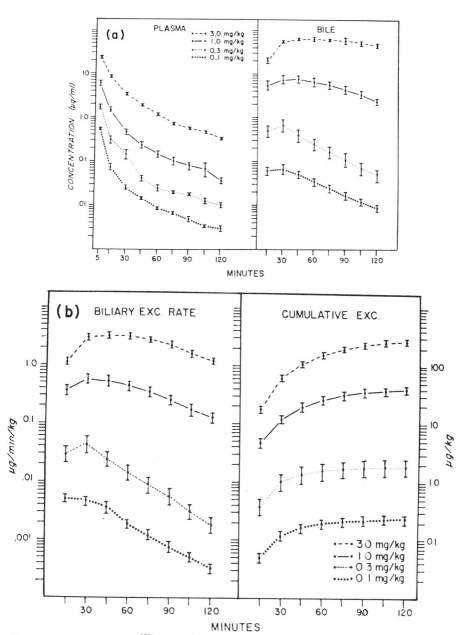

**Figure 4.23** The kinetics of [109]Cd after intravenous administration to rats of 3.0, 1.0, 0.3, or 0.1 mg/kg. Each point represents the mean ±standard error of seven or eight rats. (*a*) Plasma and biliary concentration. (*b*) Biliary excretion rate and cumulative excretion of [109]Cd in the bile. Reproduced with permission from Klaassen and Kotsonis, 1977, Figures 2 and 3.

system single- or multicompartment? Why? Is it linear or nonlinear? Why?

7   Consider Figures 4.23$a$ and 4.23$b$. Are the kinetics of $^{109}$Cd disposition linear or nonlinear within the dose range represented? List four observations that support your conclusion.

8   DiSanto and Wagner (1972) administered four different doses of methylene blue intravenously to an 11.2-kg dog at widely spaced times. After each dose samples of venous blood were drawn at convenient time intervals, and the concentration of methylene blue was determined in extracts of the deproteinized plasma. The data are given in Table 4.2.

Methylene blue is distributed and eliminated in accordance with the behavior predicted by a nonlinear open model.

  (a)   Estimate from suitable graphs the parameters $\alpha$ and $\beta$, the half-life of methylene blue, and the volume of distribution determined by back-extrapolating the $\beta$ segment of the curve for each of the four data sets.

  (b)   Is the half-life a biological half-life or a half-life of elimination from the plasma? Why?

  (c)   Graph $V_{extrap}$ and $t_{1/2}$ against dose. Suggest at least one reasonable physical or biochemical mechanism that would confer nonlinearity of this kind on the methylene blue system.

9   The kinetics of drug elimination by the newborn often differ from those of the adult because of relative differences in the degree of maturity of different elimination pathways. For example, not all renal excretory mechanisms are fully developed in the newborn. These differences are of concern whenever the mother has ingested large amounts of a drug.

A careful study of salicylic acid elimination by the newborn was reported by Garrettson et al. (1975). The mother had taken 6.5 g of aspirin daily for arthritis during her pregnancy. Her infant weighed 3.1 kg and was born with a plasma concentration of 25 mg salicylic acid (SA)/dl in a distribution volume of 300 ml/kg body weight. The mother's plasma SA concentration at delivery was less than 16 mg/dl in a distribution volume of 200 ml/kg body weight. The infant's elimination of SA was assessed by graphing $\ln(U_\infty - U)$ versus $t$ (Figure 4.24) and was compared with those of normal adults and of an intoxicated newborn infant, not chronically exposed *in utero* to aspirin, whose mother had attempted suicide by taking aspirin 27 hr before delivery (Figure 4.25). The ability of the infant under study to convert SA to salicyluric acid was also measured (Figure 4.26). Assume that SA is eliminated by three parallel mechanisms (there are also minor pathways, which you need not consider): conversion to salicyluric acid, glucuronide formation, and direct

**Table 4.2** The time course of methylene blue plasma concentrations following intravenous administration of four different doses at different times to an 11.2-kg dog.

| Dose | Time (hr) | Plasma Concentration of Methylene Blue ($\mu$g/ml) |
|---|---|---|
| 2 mg/kg | 0.046 | 0.941 |
| | 0.175 | 0.365 |
| | 0.325 | 0.275 |
| | 0.493 | 0.199 |
| | 0.997 | 0.124 |
| | 2.20 | 0.0640 |
| | 3.11 | 0.0424 |
| | 4.22 | 0.0310 |
| 5 mg/kg | 0.054 | 2.60 |
| | 0.165 | 0.715 |
| | 0.337 | 0.438 |
| | 0.497 | 0.403 |
| | 1.01 | 0.230 |
| | 2.03 | 0.130 |
| | 4.07 | 0.071 |
| | 5.05 | 0.052 |
| | 6.005 | 0.034 |
| 10 mg/kg | 0.079 | 21.68 |
| | 0.273 | 7.22 |
| | 0.320 | 2.18 |
| | 0.567 | 0.965 |
| | 1.013 | 0.471 |
| | 2.030 | 0.163 |
| | 4.020 | 0.141 |
| | 6.220 | 0.077 |
| 15 mg/kg | 0.046 | 31.2 |
| | 0.163 | 15.01 |
| | 0.323 | 2.45 |
| | 0.491 | 1.44 |
| | 1.01 | 0.396 |
| | 2.01 | 0.238 |
| | 4.01 | 0.189 |
| | 4.99 | 0.152 |
| | 6.03 | 0.122 |
| | 7.25 | 0.085 |

Reproduced from Di Santo and Wagner, 1972, Table 1.

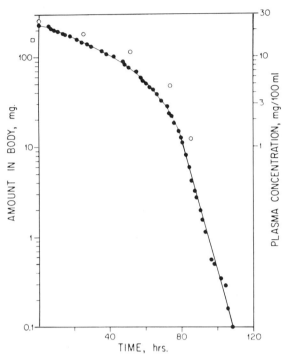

**Figure 4.24**  Time course of salicylate elimination. ●, by a newborn infant of a mother who took 6.5 g of aspirin daily during her pregnancy; total amount in body, calculated as $(U_{5 \text{ days}} - U(t))$; O, by the same infant; plasma concentration. The time scale represents the age of the infant. Salicylate concentration in the mother's plasma 3.5 hr before delivery is shown by square. Reproduced with permission from Garrettson et al., 1975, Figure 1.

renal excretion of SA. Conversion to salicyluric acid is quantitatively the most important; it is an enzymically catalyzed process for which $K_m \approx 4.6$ mg/kg and $V_m \approx 0.82$ mg/kg/hr in the adult. In the previously unexposed intoxicated infant, $K_m$ for the conversion of SA to salicyluric acid was 0.6 mg/kg and $V_m$ was 0.08 mg/kg/hr.

(a)  How does the ability of the infant under study to form salicyluric acid compare with the abilities of a normal adult and of the normal (not chronically exposed) newborn?

(b)  Why wasn't the infant's overall elimination of SA as efficient as her mother's? Why was it more efficient than that of the intoxicated newborn?

(c)  From the kinetic evidence, which of the three elimination pathways in the infant can you identify as saturable? Which as not saturable (or as not saturated at these concentrations)?

(d)  Which of the three pathways is probably the dominant one during the terminal linear dieaway phase in both adult and infant? Why?

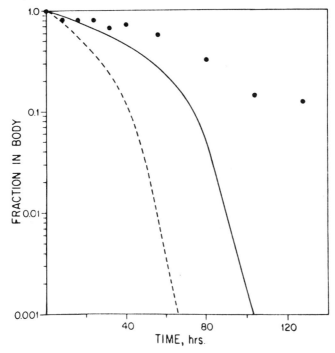

**Figure 4.25** Comparative time course of salicylate elimination by the newborn infant of Figure 4.24 (solid curve), by normal adults (dashed curve), and by an intoxicated newborn not chronically exposed *in utero*, after an exchange transfusion (●). The fraction of salicylate in the body was calculated as $(U_{5\ days} - U(t))$, and normalized to the initial amount of drug in the body or to the initial concentration of salicylate in the plasma (for the intoxicated newborn infant after exchange transfusion). Reproduced with permission from Garrettson et al., 1975, Figure 4.

**10** In Problem 15 of Chapter 3 you were asked to analyze plasma dieaway data for cyclacillin, a penicillin, and for its principal metabolite ACHC. Urinary excretion data for the two compounds, from the same study by Tucker et al. (1974), are given in Table 4.3. What do these additional data suggest about the kinetics of cyclacillin metabolism and/or excretion that is not apparent from the plasma data? Why is your conclusion not clearly apparent from plasma data alone?

Recall that the dose of cyclacillin was 400 mg/kg. Assume that $U_\infty$ for ACHC is 40 mg/kg.

**11** Bloedow and Hayton (1976) studied the metabolism of acetylsulfisoxazole in rats. In one experiment they measured the urinary recovery of free and conjugated sulfisoxazole after oral and intravenous administration of three different doses of acetylsulfisoxazole. No acetylsulfisoxazole was detected in the urine, but it is assumed that both the acetylated and the free forms can be conjugated. What do their data, reproduced in Table 4.4, suggest about the kinetics of acetylsulfisoxazole metabolism?

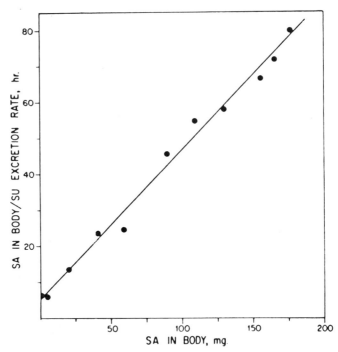

**Figure 4.26** Hanes plot for the excretion of salicyluric acid (SU) by the newborn infant of Figure 4.24. Least squares regression analysis of the data gave the following values for the *in vivo* apparent $K_m$ and $V_m$, respectively: 3.9 mg/kg and 0.8 mg/kg/hr, in terms of salicylic acid (SA). Reproduced with permission from Garrettson et al., 1975, Figure 3.

**Table 4.3** Cumulative urinary excretion of cyclacillin and of its metabolite ACHC at intervals after oral administration of cyclacillin to male and female rats; means of values from 3 animals per sex.

| Time (hr) | Cumulative Renal Excretion of Cyclacillin after 100 mg/kg Orally (mg/kg) | |
| | Males | Females |
| --- | --- | --- |
| 0.5 | 0 | 4 |
| 1.0 | 12 | 12 |
| 1.5 | 20 | 28 |
| 2.0 | 30 | 34 |
| 3.0 | 58 | 56 |
| 4.0 | 80 | 72 |
| 6.0 | 84 | 82 |
| 8.0 | 84 | 84 |

**Table 4.3** (*continued*)

| Time (days) | Cumulative Renal Excretion of ACHC after 400 mg of Cyclacillin Orally (mg/kg) | |
| | Males | Females |
|---|---|---|
| 0.25 | 0.4 | 3.0 |
| 0.5 | 1.0 | 6.0 |
| 1 | 2.0 | 13.0 |
| 2 | 3.0 | 21.0 |
| 3 | 4.0 | 27.0 |
| 4 | 5.0 | 32.0 |
| 5 | 7.0 | 34.0 |
| 6 | 7.0 | 35.0 |
| 7 | 8.0 | 36.0 |

From Tucker et al., 1974, data read from Figures 10 and 11.

**Table 4.4** Urinary recovery of sulfisoxazole following oral and intravenous administration of 10, 25, and 100 mg/kg of acetylsulfisoxazole.

| Dose (mg/kg) | Cumulative Percent[a] of Dose Recovered at 96 hr | | | Fraction[c] Conjugated |
| | Free Drug | $N^4$-Conjugate[b] | Total | |
|---|---|---|---|---|
| | *Oral Administration as Solution in Polysorbate 80* | | | |
| 10 | 88.68 ± 2.34 | 26.15 | 114.83 ± 5.06 | 0.228 |
| 25 | 85.75 ± 3.67 | 18.97 | 104.72 ± 2.79 | 0.181 |
| 100 | 99.27 ± 14.54 | 12.52 | 111.79 ± 22.08 | 0.112 |
| | *Intravenous Administration as Solution in Polyethylene Glycol 400 Containing 10% Water* | | | |
| 10 | 101.15 ± 5.91 | 9.32 | 110.49 ± 4.94 | 0.085 |
| 25 | 99.81 ± 2.89 | 10.36 | 110.67 ± 3.29 | 0.098 |
| 100 | 95.02 ± 8.70 | 8.42 | 103.44 ± 9.13 | 0.081 |

Reproduced from Bloedow and Hayton, 1976, Table IV.
[a] On a molar basis; average of six animals ± SD for each dose.
[b] Difference between total and free drug.
[c] Ratio of $N^4$-conjugate to total.

**12** The renal clearance of riboflavin in man is plotted in Figure 4.27 as a function of the logarithm of the serum riboflavin concentration (Jusko and Levy, 1970). Renal clearance values were calculated by dividing the urinary excretion rate by the midinterval serum concentration. The creatinine clearances also shown in the graph are a measure of the glomerular filtration rate.

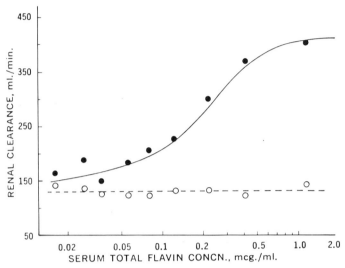

**Figure 4.27**   Renal clearance of total riboflavin (●) in a human subject plotted as a function of serum total riboflavin concentration. Simultaneously determined creatinine clearances are also shown (○). Reproduced with permission from Jusko and Levy, 1970, Figure 4.

By what mechanism(s) (glomerular filtration, tubular secretion, tubular reabsorption) is riboflavin handled in the human kidney? Give your reasoning.

13   Para-aminosalicylic acid (PAS) is a bacteriostatic drug that is used together with other drugs in the treatment of tuberulosis. Wagner et al. (1973) undertook a study of several commercially available dosage forms of PAS because there were reports that PAS was not fully available to the systemic circulation from all dosage forms.

Adult male volunteers served as subjects. Four dosage forms were given, each containing 1 g of PAS: a water solution of a PAS salt, a water suspension of PAS powder, a tablet, and an enteric-coated tablet designed to maximize the amount of PAS reaching the intestine. PAS, the active bacteriostat, is partially metabolized to *N*-acetyl PAS, and both parent and metabolite are excreted in the urine.

Figure 4.28 shows the areas under the plasma concentration, time curves for both PAS and *N*-acetyl PAS after each dosage form. From these data, what would you conclude about the relative availability of the four dosage forms? Is there any evidence of nonlinearity in this system?

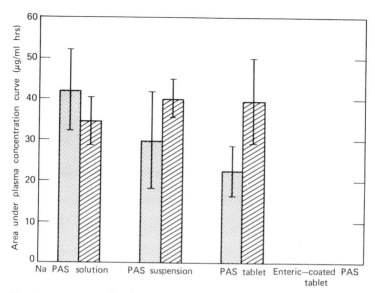

**Figure 4.28** Average areas under plasma concentration, time curves for PAS (stippled bars) and *N*-acetyl PAS (lined bars) following oral administration of four dosage forms, each containing 1 g of PAS, to human volunteers. The standard deviations are also given. Adapted with permission from Wagner et al., 1973, Figure 2.

**14** Pentikainen et al. (1973) also studied the bioavailability of PAS. They administered a 2-g and a 4-g dose of PAS (tablet form) to adult human volunteers and measured the areas under the plasma PAS concentration, time curves. The AUC for the 2-g dose was 89 $\mu$g hr/ml; AUC for the 4-g dose was 271 $\mu$g hr/ml. Are these results consistent with the data of Wagner et al. (Problem 13)?

## REFERENCES

Ashley, J. J. and G. Levy. "Inhibition of diphenylhydantoin elimination by its major metabolite." *Res. Commun. Chem. Pathol. Pharmacol.*, **4**, 297–306 (1972).

Axelson, J. E. and M. Gibaldi. "Absorption and excretion of riboflavin in the rat: An unusual example of nonlinear pharmacokinetics." *J. Pharm. Sci.*, **61**, 404–407 (1972).

Balasubramaniam, K., S. B. Lucas, G. E. Mawer, and P. J. Simons. "The kinetics of amylobarbitone metabolism in healthy men and women." *Br. J. Pharmacol.*, **39**, 564–572 (1970).

Bloedow, D. C. and W. L. Hayton. "Saturable first-pass metabolism of sulfisoxazole *N'*-acetyl in rats." *J. Pharm. Sci.*, **65**, 334–338 (1976).

Böhlen, P., U. P. Schlunegger, and E. Läuppi. "Uptake and distribution of hexane in rat tissues." *Toxicol. Appl. Pharmacol.*, **25**, 242–249 (1973).

Breckenridge, A., M. l'E. Orme, L. Davies, S. S. Thorgeirsson, and D. S. Davies. "Dose-dependent enzyme induction." *Clin. Pharmacol. Ther.*, **14**, 514–520 (1973).

Brodie, B. B., M. Weiner, J. J. Burns, G. Simson, and E. K. Yale. "The physiological disposition of ethyl biscoumacetate (Tromexan) in man and a method for its estimation in biological material." *J. Pharmacol. Exp. Ther.*, **106**, 453–463 (1952).

Chien, Y. W., L. M. Hofmann, H. J. Lambert, and L. C. Tao. "Binding of spironolactones to human plasma proteins." *J. Pharm. Sci.*, **65**, 1337–1340 (1976).

Chremos, A. N., D. Shen, M. Gibaldi, J. D. Proctor, and J. H. Newman. "Time-dependent change in renal clearance of bethanidine in humans." *J. Pharm. Sci.*, **65**, 140–142 (1976).

Christensen, S. "Studies on riboflavin metabolism in the rat. I. Urinary and faecal excretion after oral administration of riboflavin-5'-phosphate." *Acta Pharmacol. Toxicol.*, **27**, 27–33 (1969).

Clay, K. L., R. C. Murphy, and W. D. Watkins. "Experimental methanol toxicity in the primate: Analysis of metabolic acidosis." *Toxicol. Appl. Pharmacol.*, **34**, 49–61 (1975).

Crouthamel, W. G., L. Diamond, L. W. Dittert, and J. T. Doluisio. "Drug absorption. VII. Influence of mesenteric blood flow on intestinal drug absorption in dogs." *J. Pharm. Sci.*, **64**, 664–671 (1975).

Dayton, P. G., S. A. Cucinell, M. Weiss, and J. M. Perel. "Dose-dependence of drug plasma level decline in dogs." *J. Pharmacol. Exp. Ther.*, **158**, 305–316 (1967).

Dent, J. G., K. J. Netter, and J. E. Gibson. "The induction of hepatic microsomal metabolism in rats following acute administration of a mixture of polybrominated biphenyls." *Toxicol. Appl. Pharmacol.*, **38**, 237–249 (1976).

DiSanto, A. R. and J. G. Wagner. "Pharmacokinetics of highly ionized drugs. III. Methylene blue–blood levels in the dog and tissue levels in the rat following intravenous administration." *J. Pharm. Sci.*, **61**, 1090–1094 (1972).

Drill, V. A. "Hepatotoxic agents: Mechanism of action and dietary interrelationship." *Pharmacol. Rev.*, **4**, 1–42 (1952).

Evans, G. H., and D. G. Shand. "Disposition of propranolol. VI. Independent variation in steady state circulating drug concentrations and half-life as a result of plasma drug binding in man." *Clin. Pharmacol. Ther.*, **14**, 494–500 (1973).

Froese, A., A. H. Sehon, and M. Eigen. "Kinetic studies of protein-dye and antibody-hapten interactions with the temperature-jump method." *Can. J. Chem.*, **40**, 1786–1797 (1962).

Gallaher, E. J. and T. A. Loomis, "Metabolism of ethyl acetate in the rat: Hydrolysis to ethyl alcohol *in vitro* and *in vivo*." *Toxicol. Appl. Pharmacol.*, **34**, 309–313 (1975).

Garrett, E. R. "Classical pharmacokinetics to the frontier," in *Pharmacology and Pharmacokinetics*, T. Teorell, R. S. Dedrick, and P. G. Condliffe, Eds., Plenum Press, New York, 1974, pp. 3–25.

Garrett, E. R. "Pharmacokinetics and clearances related to renal processes." *Int. J. Clin. Pharmacol.*, **16**, 155–172 (1978).

Garrett, E. R., J. Bres, K. Schnelle, and L. L. Rolf., Jr. "Pharmacokinetics of saturably metabolized amobarbital." *J. Pharmacokinet. Biopharmaceut.*, **2**, 43–103 (1974).

Garrett, E. R. and C. A. Hunt. "Physiocochemical properties, solubility, and protein binding of $\Delta^9$-tetrahydrocannabinol." *J. Pharm. Sci.*, **63**, 1056–1064 (1974).

Garrettson, L. K., J. A. Procknal, and G. Levy. "Fetal acquisition and neonatal elimination of a large amount of salicylate: Study of a neonate whose mother regularly took therapeutic doses of aspirin during pregnancy." *Clin. Pharmacol. Ther.*, **17**, 98–103 (1975).

George, C. F., M. l'E. Orme, P. Buranapong, D. Macerlean, A. M. Breckenridge, and C. T. Dollery. "Contribution of the liver to overall elimination of propranolol." *J. Pharmacokinet. Biopharmaceut.*, **4**, 17–27 (1976).

Gérardin, A. P., F. V. Abadie, J. A. Campestrini, and W. Theobald. "Pharmacokinetics of carbamazepine in normal humans after single and repeated oral doses." *J. Pharmacokinet. Biopharmaceut.*, **4**, 521–535 (1976).

Gibaldi, M. and M. A. Schwartz. "Apparent effect of probenecid on the distribution of penicillins in man." *Clin. Pharm. Ther.*, **9**, 345–349 (1968).

Gillette, J. R. "Overview of drug-protein binding." *Ann. N.Y. Acad. Sci.*, **226**, 6–17 (1973).

Gillette, J. R. and K. S. Pang. "Theoretic aspects of pharmacokinetic drug interactions." *Clin. Pharmacol. Ther.*, **22**, 623–639 (1977).

Goldstein, A. "The interactions of drugs and plasma proteins." *Pharmacol. Rev.*, **1**, 102–165 (1949).

Isselbacher, K. J. and N. J. Greenberger. "Metabolic effects of alcohol on the liver." *New Engl. J. Med.*, **270**, 402–409 (1964).

Jähnchen, E. and G. Levy. "Inhibition of phenylbutazone elimination by its metabolite oxyphenbutazone." *Proc. Soc. Exp. Biol. Med.*, **141**, 963–965 (1972).

Jusko, W. J. and M. Gibaldi. "Effects of change in elimination on various parameters of the two-compartment open model." *J. Pharm. Sci.*, **61**, 1270–1273 (1972).

Jusko, W. J. and G. Levy. "Pharmacokinetic evidence for saturable renal tubular reabsorption of riboflavin." *J. Pharm. Sci.*, **59**, 765–772 (1970).

Jusko, W. J., J. R. Leonards, and G. Levy. "Riboflavin distribution and elimination in two functionally anephric human patients." *J. Pharm. Sci.*, **59**, 566–567 (1970).

Kampffmeyer, H. G. "Metabolic rate of phenacetin and of paracetamol in dogs before and after treatment with phenobarbital or SKF 525A." *Biochem. Pharmacol.*, **23**, 713–724 (1974).

Klaassen, C. D. "Effects of phenobarbital on the plasma disappearance and biliary excretion of drugs in rats." *J. Pharmacol. Exp. Ther.*, **175**, 289–300 (1970).

Klaassen, C. D. "Studies on the increased biliary flow produced by phenobarbital in rats." *J. Pharmacol. Exp. Ther.*, **176**, 743–751, (1971).

Klaassen, C. D. "Pharmacokinetics of rose bengal in the rat, rabbit, dog and guinea pig." *Toxicol. Appl. Pharmacol.*, **38**, 85–100 (1976).

Klaassen, C. D. and F. N. Kotsonis. "Biliary excretion of cadmium in the rat, rabbit and dog." *Toxicol. Appl. Pharmacol.*, **41**, 101–112 (1977).

Kunin, C. M. "Enhancement of antimicrobial activity of penicillins and other antibiotics in human serum by competitive serum binding inhibitors." *Proc Soc. Exp. Biol. Med.*, **117**, 69–73 (1964).

Kunin, C. M. "Effect of serum binding on the distribution of penicillins in the rabbit." *J. Lab. Clin. Med.*, **65**, 406–415 (1965a).

Kunin, C. M. "Inhibitors of penicillin binding to serum proteins." *J. Lab. Clin. Med.*, **65**, 416–431 (1965b).

Krüger-Thiemer, E. "Nonlinear dose-concentration relationships." *Farmaco, Ed. Sci.*, **8**, 717–756 (1968).

Levy, G. and W. J. Jusko. "Factors affecting the absorption of riboflavin in man." *J. Pharm. Sci.*, **55**, 285–289 (1966).

Levy, G., T. Tsuchiya, and L. P. Amsel. "Limited capacity for salicyl phenolic glucuronide formation and its effect on the kinetics of salicylate elimination in man." *Clin. Pharmacol. Ther.,* **13**, 258–268 (1972).

Lundquist, F. and H. Wolthers. "The kinetics of alcohol elimination in man." *Acta Pharmacol. Toxicol.,* **14**, 265–289 (1958).

Mehendale, H. M. "Effect of preexposure to Kepone on the biliary excretion of imipramine and sulfobromophthalein." *Toxicol. Appl. Pharmacol.,* **40**, 247–259 (1977).

Meyer, M. C. and D. E. Guttman. "The binding of drugs by plasma proteins." *J. Pharm. Sci.,* **57**, 895–918 (1968).

Pentikainen, P., S. H. Wan, and D. L. Azarnoff. "Bioavailability studies on *p*-aminosalicylic acid and its various salts in man. II. Comparison of Parasal and Pascorbic." *Am. Rev. Respir. Dis.,* **108**, 1340–1347 (1973).

Perrier, D., J. J. Ashley, and G. Levy. "Effect of product inhibition on kinetics of drug elimination." *J. Pharmacokinet. Biopharmaceut.,* **1**, 231–242 (1973).

Rolinson, G. N. and R. Sutherland. "The binding of antibiotics to serum proteins." *Br. J. Pharmacol.,* **25**, 638–650 (1965).

Rowell, L. B., J. R. Blackmon, and R. A. Bruce. "Indocyanine green clearance and estimated hepatic blood flow during mild to maximal exercise in upright man." *J. Clin. Invest.,* **43**, 1677–1690 (1964).

Sauerhoff, M. W., W. H. Braun, G. E. Blau, and P. J. Gehring. "The dose-dependent pharmaco-kinetic profile of 2, 4, 5-trichlorophenoxy acetic acid following intravenous administration to rats." *Toxicol. Appl. Pharmacol.,* **36**, 491–501 (1976).

Schnelle, K. and E. R. Garrett. "Pharmacokinetics of the $\beta$-adrenergic blocker sotalol in dogs." *J. Pharm. Sci.,* **62**, 362–375 (1973).

Singhal, R. L., J. R. E. Valadares, and W. S. Schwark. "Metabolic control mechanisms in mammalian systems. IX. Estrogen-like stimulation of uterine enzymes by *o-p'*-1,1,1-trichloro-2-2-bis( *p*-chlorophenyl)ethane." *Biochem. Pharmacol.,* **19**, 2145–2155 (1970).

Thron, C. D. "Linearity and superposition in pharmacokinetics." *Pharmacol. Rev.,* **26**, 3–31 (1974).

Tucker, W. E., Jr., F. W. Janssen, H. P. K. Agersborg, Jr., E. M. Young, and H. W. Ruelius. "Sex- and species-related nephropathy of 6-(1-aminocyclohexanecarboxamido)-penicillanic acid (cyclacillin) and its relationship to the metabolic disposition of the drug." *Toxicol. Appl. Pharmacol.,* **29**, 1–18 (1974).

Vallner, J. J., J. H. Perrin, and S. Wold. "Comparison of graphical and computerized methods for calculating binding parameters for two strongly bound drugs to human serum albumin." *J. Pharm. Sci.,* **65**, 1182–1187 (1976).

van Ginneken, C. A. M., J. M. van Rossum, and H. L. J. M. Fleuren. "Linear and nonlinear kinetics of drug elimination. I. Kinetics on the basis of a single capacity-limited pathway of elimination with or without simultaneous supply-limited elimination." *J. Pharmacokinet. Bio-pharmaceut.,* **2**, 395–415 (1974).

Wagner, J. G. "Pharmacokinetics. 2. The kidney and urinary excretion." *Drug Intell.,* **2**, 95–99 (1968).

Wagner, J. G. "A new generalized nonlinear pharmacokinetic model and its implications," in *Biopharmaceutics and Relevant Pharmacokinetics,* Drug Intelligence Publications, Hamilton, Ill., 1971, pp. 302–317.

Wagner, J. G. "Properties of the Michaelis-Menten equation and its integrated form which are useful in pharmacokinetics." *J. Pharmacokinet. Biopharmaceut.,* **1**, 103–121 (1973a).

Wagner, J. G. "A modern view of pharmacokinetics." *J. Pharmacokinet. Biopharmaceut.*, **1**, 363–401 (1973b).

Wagner, J. G. *Fundamentals of Clinical Pharmacokinetics*. Drug Intelligence Publications, Hamilton, Ill., 1975, pp. 265–267.

Wagner, J. G., P. K. Wilkinson, A. J. Sedman, D. R. Kay, and D. J. Weidler. "Elimination of alcohol from human blood." *J. Pharm. Sci.*, **65**, 152–154 (1976).

Wagner, J. G., P. D. Holmes, P. K. Wilkinson, D. C. Blair, and R. G. Stoll. "Importance of the type of dosage form and saturable acetylation in determining the bioactivity of *p*-aminosalicylic acid." *Am. Rev. Respir. Dis.*, **108**, 536–546 (1973).

Weiner, M., S. Shapiro, J. Axelrod, J. R. Cooper, and B. B. Brodie. "The physiological disposition of dicumarol in man." *J. Pharmacol. Exp. Ther.*, **99**, 409–420 (1950).

Widmark, E. M. P. "Verteilung und Umwandlung des Athylalkohols im Organismus des Hundes." *Biochem. Z.*, **267**, 128–134 (1933).

# 5

# *Chronic Exposure*

**5.1** The kinetic consequences of chronic exposure: Demonstration of the plateau principle

    **5.1.1** Constant absorption

    **5.1.2** Repeated exposure

**5.2** Development of the plateau principle

    **5.2.1** Repeated equally spaced administrations

    **5.2.2** Constant infusion

**5.3** Half-life of approach to steady state and volume of distribution at steady state

**5.4** Steady state in a multicompartment model

**5.5** Comparison of the general statements of the plateau principle and their proper applications

**5.6** Practical uses of the plateau principle

    **5.6.1** Clinical applications

    **5.6.2** Experimental applications

    **5.6.3** Industrial applications

    **5.6.4** Toxicologic applications

The previous chapters have dealt exclusively with acute exposures. Understanding of the kinetics of absorption and disposition of single doses is essential in instances of accidental poisoning or attempted suicide, or in industrial accidents. It is also important in experimental work, where an acute study can provide useful information about the disposition of a drug or a toxicant even though the usual mode of administration or exposure is chronic. But it is equally important that the relationship of acute kinetic parameters to the behavior of the drug or toxicant on repeated or continuous administration be well understood, since few clinical, industrial, or environmental exposures occur singly.

Increasing numbers and quantities of natural and synthetic compounds are making their way into the environment. Some, such as food additives, are introduced under controlled conditions for a specific purpose. Others, such as industrial by-products or waste products, are introduced into the environment often in large amounts and under less well controlled conditions. These may become widely disseminated through air, water, or soil systems, providing a relatively constant and continuous source of exposure.

Environmental exposures are chronic exposures. There are other kinds of chronic exposure: regular ingestion of a drug tablet or repeated ingestion in food or in drinking water may represent chronic exposure. But these experiences also may simply represent repeated acute exposure. What is the distinction between multiple acute exposure and chronic exposure?

> If administration is repeated at intervals that are shorter than the time required to clear all the drug or toxicant from the body, then exposure is chronic.

## 5.1 THE KINETIC CONSEQUENCES OF CHRONIC EXPOSURE: DEMONSTRATION OF THE PLATEAU PRINCIPLE

### 5.1.1 Constant Absorption

During chronic exposure the rate of absorption may be constant. An experimental example of constant absorption is the slow intravenous infusion of a test compound that is too locally toxic or irritating to be given as a single large injection. Continuous inhalation of a gaseous or particulate pollutant widely dispersed in ambient air is an example of absorption occurring at a nearly constant rate in an environmental situation.

As defined in Chapter 1 and explored in some detail in Chapters 2 and 4, processes occurring at constant rates are zero-order processes. It is intuitively reasonable that as long as elimination is first order there should be some concentration at which the zero-order rate into a compartment is equal to the first-order rate out of the compartment. This concentration is the plateau level, $C(t_\infty)$. For the simple one-compartment model shown schematically in Figure 5.1,

$$Vk_eC(t_\infty)=A,$$

where $A$ is the constant entry rate and $k_e$ is the first-order elimination rate constant.

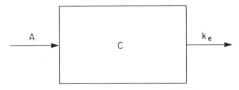

**Figure 5.1**  The linear one-compartment open model with constant rate input.

The plateau level exists because the rate $Vk_eC(t_\infty)$ is infinitely adjustable up or down (provided of course that it remains first order) to equal the absorption rate $A$. At concentrations less than the plateau level, $A$ will exceed $Vk_eC(t_\infty)$ and accumulation will continue until the plateau level is reached. Should the concentration for some reason momentarily exceed the plateau level, $Vk_eC(t_\infty)$ will exceed $A$ and there will be a net loss from the compartment until the concentration has decayed again to the plateau level.

### 5.1.2 Repeated Exposure

Alternatively the rate of absorption during chronic exposure may vary in a cyclic fashion around a constant mean. There are many examples of this type of chronic exposure. The administration of a drug in liquid, capsule, or tablet form in accordance with a predetermined dose regimen is one. In some regimens the period of all cycles is the same; in others it is not—for example, the drug may be taken three times a day with the meals but not at all during the night. Other examples of cyclic absorption are ingestion in the food or drinking water. Generally such ingestion occurs in a semiregular or irregular pattern.

It is less obvious intuitively that a concentration plateau is also established when chronic exposure is repetitive rather than continuous. The simplest and best demonstration of the existence of a plateau in such an exposure situation is a graphic demonstration.

To demonstrate the plateau principle graphically, the blood level curves for each time interval are summed by drawing them on semilogarithmic graph paper. Linear graph paper may be used but semilog paper simplifies the process because it allows parallel straight lines to be drawn to simulate the dieaway phases in all intervals. The following procedure is illustrated in Figure 5.2 for the one-compartment body model with regularly repeated administration of the same dose $D$. The reader is urged to try the same procedure with another exposure pattern, such as one of the common clinical regimens with several equal intervals during the day and a longer interval overnight.

1  Select arbitrary values for the dose $D$, the time interval $\Delta t$, the volume of distribution $V$, and the rate constant for elimination $k_e$.

2  Assume that absorption of the dose $D$ at the beginning of each time interval $\Delta t$ is instantaneous, with homogeneous mixing within the volume $V$. On semilogarithmic graph paper plot $C(1) = D/V$ at the beginning of the first time interval (Figure 5.2).

3  Draw a line from $C(1)$ with slope $-k_e$ to the beginning of the second time interval. To the point terminating this line add $C(1)$ and plot the total, $C(2)$, at the beginning of the second time interval.

4  Draw a line from this new point with slope $-k_e$ to the beginning of the third time interval.

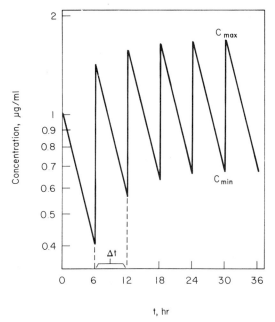

**Figure 5.2** Graphic demonstration of the plateau principle in the one-compartment open model: $D = 200$ mg every 6 hr, $V = 200$ liters, and $k_e = 0.15$ hr$^{-1}$ ($t_{1/2} = 4.6$ hr).

**5** Continue as in 3 and 4 until $C(n) = C(n-1)$ as in Figure 5.2. When this happens the blood levels will have taken on the character of a constantly repeated cycle whose period is the time interval between doses. If the time interval between doses is not constant but varies in accordance with a regularly repeated pattern, the blood levels at steady state will follow the same pattern. In other words, rather than a single cycle repeating itself, a cluster of cycles will recur repeatedly.

Graphic demonstration of the plateau principle can satisfy the reader that the existence of a plateau level is a natural consequence of either constant or constantly repeated absorption and first-order elimination acting in concert. It does not enable prediction of either the magnitude of the plateau level or the rapidity of its establishment. Full understanding and application of the plateau principle require its formulation in explicit mathematical terms.

## 5.2 DEVELOPMENT OF THE PLATEAU PRINCIPLE

The plateau principle was first stated explicitly by Widmark and Tandberg (1924) for the one-compartment open model with either repeated instantaneous administration or continuous administration. Krüger-Thiemer (1966) generalized earlier approaches to the design of drug dose regimens in a comprehensive treatment that includes the concept of a loading dose (Section 5.6.1). Van Rossum (1968) published simple equations describing the approach to and achievement of a plateau in the one-compartment open model with repeated first-order administration and first-order elimination. A review by Levy (1974) provides a succinct and simple conceptual summary of much of the material presented in this and in the following sections.

### 5.2.1 Repeated Equally Spaced Administrations

What follows is a logical progression from consideration of what happens during the first dose interval to consideration of events during the $n$th dose interval. We develop the plateau principle first for equally spaced instantaneous administrations, and then consider the case in which absorption is first order rather than instantaneous. Constant absorption is really a special limiting case of repeated administration, approached as the time interval between doses approaches zero. It is considered in Section 5.2.2.

As was done for graphical demonstration of the plateau principle, assume that a regularly repeated constant dose $D$ distributes itself instantaneously and homogeneously in a volume of distribution $V$ so that $D/V = C(1)$, the plasma concentration at $t_1$, the beginning of the first time interval. Then $C(2)$ is the plasma concentration at $t_2$, and so on (Figure 5.2).

Now $\Delta t = t_2 - t_1 = t_3 - t_2 = t_n - t_{n-1}$.

Let $k_e$ be the rate constant for (first-order) elimination. Then

$$C(2) = C(1) + C(1)e^{-k_e \Delta t},$$

$$C(3) = C(1) + C(1)e^{-k_e \Delta t} + C(1)e^{-2k_e \Delta t},$$

$$C(n) = C(1)(1 + e^{-k_e \Delta t} + e^{-2k_e \Delta t} + \cdots + e^{-(n-1)k_e \Delta t}). \qquad (5.1)$$

Multiplying both sides of Equation 5.1 by the expression $1 - e^{-k_e \Delta t}$,

$$C(n)(1 - e^{-k_e \Delta t}) = C(1)(1 - e^{-k_e \Delta t} + e^{-k_e \Delta t} - e^{-2k_e \Delta t} + e^{-2k_e \Delta t} - \cdots$$
$$- e^{-(n-1)k_e \Delta t} + e^{-(n-1)k_e \Delta t} - e^{-nk_e \Delta t}),$$

or

$$C(n)(1 - e^{-k_e \Delta t}) = C(1)(1 - e^{-nk_e \Delta t}). \qquad (5.2)$$

As the number of doses grows very large ($n$ approaches infinity) with the interval between doses remaining constant, $e^{-nk_e \Delta t}$ approaches zero and

$$C(n)(1 - e^{-k_e \Delta t}) \to C(1) = \frac{D}{V}, \qquad (5.3)$$

or

$$C(n_\infty) = \frac{D}{V(1 - e^{-k_e \Delta t})} = C_{max},$$ (5.4)

where $C(n_\infty)$ is the plasma level at the beginning of the $\infty$th dose interval. It is also the maximum plasma level within this dose interval.

Equation 5.4 is the statement of the plateau principle for a large number of individual doses $D$ spaced at equal time intervals $\Delta t$. $D$, $V$, $k_e$, and $\Delta t$ are all constant. Therefore $C_{max}$, the plasma level at the beginning of the $\infty$th dose interval, is a constant, and so is $C_{min}$, the plasma level at the end of the $\infty$th dose interval:

$$\begin{aligned} C_{min} &= C_{max} e^{-k_e \Delta t} \\ &= \frac{D e^{-k_e \Delta t}}{V(1 - e^{-k_e \Delta t})}. \end{aligned}$$ (5.5)

The magnitude of the difference between the maximum and minimum plasma levels at steady state is dependent only on the dose and the volume of distribution:

$$C_{max} - C_{min} = \frac{D}{V},$$ (5.6)

but the *fraction* of $C_{max}$ that is lost in one time interval is

$$\frac{C_{max} - C_{min}}{C_{max}} = 1 - e^{-k_e \Delta t}.$$ (5.7)

The expression $1 - e^{-k_e \Delta t}$, therefore, represents the fractional fluctuation in concentration during one time interval, while $D/V$ is the absolute value of that fluctuation. Since the system is at steady state once the plateau has been achieved, it is intuitively reasonable that the amount lost during each subsequent time interval should be equal to the amount entering, the dose $D$. Once a steady state has been established, the plasma concentration cycles between the limits $C_{max}$ and $C_{min}$ until the dose regimen is altered.

An additional concentration measure is useful in consideration of the way in which steady state concentrations cycle around a constant mean during repeated administration. The average concentration in the $n$th dose interval was defined by Wagner et al. (1965) as

$$\bar{C}(n) = \frac{1}{\Delta t} \int_{t_n}^{t_{n+1}} C(n, t)\, dt.$$ (5.8)

Now

$$C(n,t)=C(n)e^{-k_e(t-t_n)}=\left(\frac{D}{V}\right)\left(\frac{1-e^{-nk_e\Delta t}}{1-e^{-k_e\Delta t}}\right)e^{-k_e(t-t_n)}, \qquad (5.9)$$

so that

$$\bar{C}(n)=\left(\frac{D}{V\Delta t}\right)\left(\frac{1-e^{-nk_e\Delta t}}{1-e^{-k_e\Delta t}}\right)\int_{t_n}^{t_{n+1}}e^{-k_e(t-t_n)}\,dt. \qquad (5.10)$$

The value of the integral in Equation 5.10 is (Van Rossum and Tomey, 1968)

$$\Big|_{t_n}^{t_{n+1}}\left(-\frac{e^{-k_e(t-t_n)}}{k_e}\right)=\frac{1-e^{-k_e(t_{n+1}-t_n)}}{k_e}=\frac{1-e^{-k_e\Delta t}}{k_e}.$$

Therefore

$$\bar{C}(n)=\left(\frac{D}{V\Delta t}\right)\left(\frac{1-e^{-nk_e\Delta t}}{k_e}\right). \qquad (5.11)$$

As $n$ approaches $\infty$ with the interval between doses remaining constant, $\bar{C}(n)$ approaches $D/k_eV\Delta t$, or

$$\bar{C}(\infty)=\frac{D}{k_eV\Delta t}, \qquad (5.12)$$

where $\bar{C}(\infty)$ is the average concentration during the $\infty$th dose interval.

At what time $t=t^*$ during the $n$th dose interval does $C(n,t)$ equal $\bar{C}(n)$? From Equations 5.9 and 5.11 the measured concentration should be the average concentration when

$$\frac{e^{-k_e(t-t_n)}}{1-e^{-k_e\Delta t}}=\frac{1}{k_e\Delta t},$$

or

$$t^*=t_n+\left(\frac{1}{k_e}\right)\ln\left(\frac{k_e\Delta t}{1-e^{-k_e\Delta t}}\right),$$

or

$$t^*=t_n+\left(\frac{1}{k_e}\right)\left(\ln\frac{k_e\Delta tC_{max}}{C_{max}-C_{min}}\right). \qquad (5.13)$$

$t^*-t_n$ is independent of $n$; that is, the measured concentration should be equal to the average concentration at times corresponding to a constant fraction of each dose interval.

The value of $\bar{C}(\infty)$ can be estimated by using Equation 5.12. Alternatively it may be calculated from the experimental area under the $C(t),t$ curve from

$t_0$ to $t_\infty$ after an acute administration. Since this area is equal to $D/k_eV$ (Section 3.12), it follows from Equation 5.12 that the average concentration $\bar{C}(\infty)$ at steady state may be predicted directly from experimental acute dose data:

$$\bar{C}(\infty) = \frac{1}{\Delta t} \int_{t_0}^{t_\infty} C(t)\, dt. \tag{5.14}$$

From the definition of $\bar{C}(n)$ (Equation 5.8) it is apparent that at steady state

$$\bar{C}(\infty) = \frac{1}{\Delta t} \int_{t_n}^{t_{n+1}} C(n, t)\, dt.$$

Therefore the area under the $C(t), t$ curve from $t_0$ to $t_\infty$ after an acute administration is equal to the area under the $C(t_\infty), t$ curve from $t_n$ to $t_{n+1}$ during steady state on repetitive dosing. Partly because of the simplicity of the expressions for $\bar{C}(\infty)$, the average concentration is often useful in steady state calculations, as will be seen in Section 5.6.1. Another reason for the importance of the concept of an average concentration will become apparent in Section 5.2.2.

Figure 5.3a shows the kinetic behavior of the antibiotic minocycline when it was given to human patients on a multidose regimen. The data are taken from Macdonald et al. (1973). Minocycline, which was found to conform to a one-compartment body model in this study, was given 3 times as a daily dose of 200 mg infused intravenously over a 60-min period. The maximum plasma concentration within each dose interval was observed at the end of the infusion period, after which the plasma concentration declined at a rate determined by the first-order elimination rate constant $k_e$, 0.043 hr$^{-1}$. (Compare Figure 5.3a with the idealized Figure 5.2.)

Oral dosage with 100 mg of minocycline every 12 hr gave $C_{max}$ and $C_{min}$ values of 3.5 and 2.3 $\mu g/ml$ at steady state, suggesting (Equation 5.6) that $D/V = 1.2\ \mu g/ml$ and $V = 100\ mg/1.2\ mg/l = 83$ liters. From these values of $V$ and $k_e$ it should be possible to predict the concentrations of minocycline at the end of each infusion and at the end of each dose interval in Figure 5.3a, using Equations 5.4 and 5.6:

$$C_{max} = \frac{D}{V(1 - e^{-k_e \Delta t})} = \frac{200\ mg}{(83\ \text{liters})(1 - e^{-(0.043\ \text{hr}^{-1})(24\ \text{hr})})}$$

$$= 3.7\ \mu g/ml;$$

$$C_{min} = C_{max} - \frac{200\ mg}{83\ \text{liters}}$$

$$= 3.7\ \mu g/ml - 2.4\ \mu g/ml$$

$$= 1.3\ \mu g/ml.$$

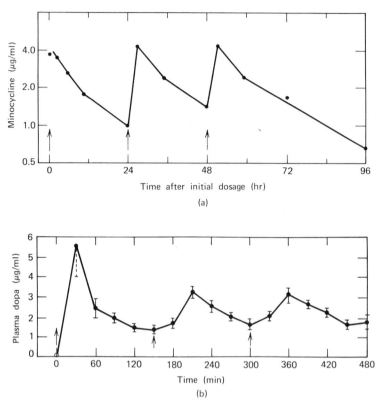

**Figure 5.3** Observed behavior of drugs given repeatedly. (*a*) By intravenous infusion. Average levels of minocycline in serum of three human subjects during a 3-day period with 200 mg of minocycline infused daily. Arrows indicate times of infusion. Reproduced with permission from Macdonald et al., 1973, Figure 2. (*b*) By oral administration. Average levels of dopa in plasma of seven parkinsonian patients receiving sequential oral doses of levodopa in combination with carbidopa. Arrows indicate the times of levodopa administration at the following average doses: $211 \pm 40$ mg, $179 \pm 33$ mg, and $161 \pm 34$ mg, given sequentially. Reproduced with permission from Shoulson et al., 1975, Figure 1.

These predicted values correspond reasonably well with those actually observed (Figure 5.3*a*). Slight discrepancies exist because the minocycline was infused over a period of time rather than injected instantaneously, and the predictions were based on data from an oral rather than an intravenous dose schedule.

Drugs are more commonly given orally in solution, capsule, or tablet form than by intravenous injection or infusion. It can be shown by a procedure analogous to the one used above, beginning with Equation 3.42 rather than with the expression for instantaneous and homogeneous distribution in one compartment, that drugs that are absorbed and eliminated exclusively by first-order processes will also reach steady state levels in the plasma upon repetitive administration of the same dose $D$. For drugs given orally or absorbed by a first-order process from some other depot,

$$C(n_\infty) = \frac{C(2)}{(1 - e^{-k_e \Delta t})(1 - e^{-k_a \Delta t})} \tag{5.15}$$

or

$$C(n_\infty) = \frac{D k_a}{V(k_a - k_e)} \frac{e^{-k_e \Delta t} - e^{-k_a \Delta t}}{(1 - e^{-k_e \Delta t})(1 - e^{-k_a \Delta t})}, \tag{5.16}$$

where $C(2)$ is the concentration at the end of the first interval (and also the concentration at the beginning of the second interval), $C(n_\infty)$ is the concentration at the beginning and at the end of the $\infty$th interval, $k_a$ is the absorption rate constant, and $D$, $V$, $k_e$, and $\Delta t$ are as previously defined.

In Chapter 3, $t_{max}$ for the one-compartment model with first-order absorption and elimination was defined as the time at which the plasma concentration is at its maximum value. Depending on whether $t_{max}$ is less than or greater than $\Delta t$, plasma concentrations within the $(n-1)$th dose interval may or may not reach a maximum greater than $C(n)$, the concentration at the end of the interval. Usually drug absorption is sufficiently rapid and the time interval between doses sufficiently long that drug concentration peaks relatively early in the interval. Instead of being abrupt and nearly instantaneous like the peaks characteristic of intravenous administration, however, the peaks associated with oral administration are delayed and have the curvilinear shape characteristic of first-order absorption, as shown in Figure 5.3b for plasma dopa levels during the oral administration of levodopa to patients with Parkinson's disease (Shoulson et al., 1975).

As $k_a$ becomes very large relative to $k_e$, Equation 5.16 approaches Equation 5.5 for the concentration at the end of the $\infty$th interval when absorption is instantaneous. Often, if $k_a$ is large, Equations 5.4 and 5.5 may be used as reasonable approximations of the maximum and final concentrations within the $\infty$th interval even though administration was oral, not intravenous. The condition that $k_a$ be large is met if the plasma concentration peaks early in the dose interval. It is common practice to approximate oral administration by the expressions for intravenous administration. When there is clear experimental evidence that this approximation is not justified, however, the expressions that incorporate a first-order absorption step should be applied.

It is worthwhile to see what the status of the system will be after only $n$ dose intervals, each $\Delta t$ in length. Consider the instantaneous absorption model. Divide Equation 5.2 by Equation 5.4 or Equation 5.11 by Equation 5.12:

$$\frac{\bar{C}(n)}{\bar{C}(\infty)} = \frac{C(n)}{C(n_\infty)} = 1 - e^{-n k_e \Delta t}. \tag{5.17}$$

Equation 5.17 may be used to estimate either the number $n$ of doses required to reach a predetermined fraction of the plateau level or the appropriate dosage interval $\Delta t$, whenever the other is known or fixed by convenience. Note that the *fraction* of the plateau level reached after $n$ doses is independent of the magnitude of the dose. Like the fractional fluctuation at steady state, it is dependent on $k_e$ and $\Delta t$; it is also dependent on $n$. The *concentration* $C(n)$ reached after $n$ doses, like the magnitude of the fluctuation at steady state, is of course dependent on the dose. For the first-order absorption model, the expression for $C(n)/C(n_\infty)$ states the same conclusion: that the fraction of the plateau level reached after $n$ doses is independent of the dose rate.

### 5.2.2 Constant Infusion

Equation 5.7 states that $1-e^{-k_e\Delta t}$ is the fraction lost during one dose interval $\Delta t$. It can be shown that if $\Delta t$ is very small, $1-e^{-k_e\Delta t}$ is approximately equal to $k_e\Delta t$:

$$\frac{dC}{dt}=-k_eC(1) \quad \text{and} \quad \frac{\Delta C}{\Delta t}=\frac{C(2)-C(1)}{t_2-t_1}.$$

If $\Delta t$ is very small so that $dC/dt\approx\Delta C/\Delta t$, then

$$k_eC(1)\approx\frac{-(C(2)-C(1))}{t_2-t_1} \quad \text{and} \quad \frac{C(1)-C(2)}{C(1)}\approx k_e(t_2-t_1).$$

But $C(2)=C(1)e^{-k_e(t_2-t_1)}$, so

$$C(1)-C(2)=C(1)\left[1-e^{-k_e(t_2-t_1)}\right]$$

and

$$\frac{C(1)-C(2)}{C(1)}=1-e^{-k_e\Delta t}\approx k_e\Delta t.$$

Therefore, from Equation 5.2, when $\Delta t$ is very small,

$$C(n)\approx\frac{D}{k_eV\Delta t}(1-e^{-nk_e\Delta t}). \tag{5.18}$$

Now $n\Delta t$ is the real time $t$, or the elapsed time since administration of the first dose. If we allow $n$ to become very large while at the same time $\Delta t$ becomes infinitesimally small—in other words, if $n$ approaches infinity as $\Delta t$ approaches zero—the repeated doses merge into a constant infusion rate

$D/\Delta t$ or $A$ and

$$C(t) = \frac{A}{k_e V}(1 - e^{-k_e t}). \tag{5.19}$$

As $t$ approaches $\infty$,

$$C(t) \text{ approaches } C(t_\infty) = \frac{A}{k_e V}. \tag{5.20}$$

Equation 5.20 is the statement of the plateau principle for true zero-order or continuous and constant absorption. The correspondence between Equation 5.20 and Equation 5.12, and between Equation 5.18 and Equation 5.11, demonstrates why the concept of average concentration at steady state during repetitive exposure is important. The average concentration is the concentration that would be measured during repetitive exposure at times

$$t^* = t_n + \left(\frac{1}{k_e}\right)\left(\ln \frac{k_e \Delta t\, C_{max}}{C_{max} - C_{min}}\right)$$

if administration were actually continuous and taking place at a rate $D/\Delta t$. In other words, the times $t^*$ are the times at which the hypothetical curves for repetitive exposure to dose $D$ at time intervals $\Delta t$ and for continuous exposure to dose rate $D/\Delta t$ cross each other, as shown in Figure 5.4.

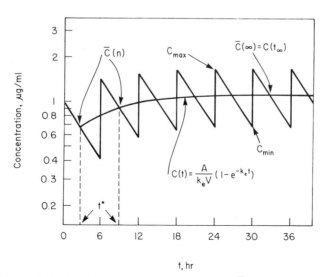

**Figure 5.4** The relationship between average concentration $\bar{C}(n)$, calculated for repetitive administration, and the time course of concentration change during continuous administration of the hypothetical compound of Figure 5.2, where $D/\Delta t = 200$ mg/6 hr.

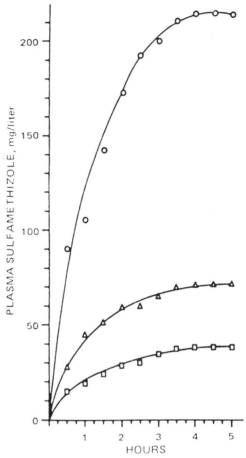

**Figure 5.5** Plasma concentration of sulfamethizole in a dog during constant intravenous infusion of 68 (□), 141 (△), and 385 (○) mg/hr for 5 hr on three separate occasions. Reproduced with permission from Kowarski et al., 1976, Figure 1.

**Table 5.1** Plasma sulfamethizole concentration after 5 hr infusion into the jugular vein of a dog

| Infusion Rate, $a$ (mg/hr) | Steady State Plasma Concentration, $b$ (mg/l) | Proportionality Constant, $c = \dfrac{a}{b}$ (l/hr) |
|---|---|---|
| 68.0 | 36.2 | 1.88 |
| 140.8 | 72.8 | 1.93 |
| 385.0 | 214.0 | 1.80 |

From Kowarski et al., 1976, Table 1.

Figure 5.5 is taken from a study by Kowarski et al. (1976). It shows the plasma concentration of sulfamethizole as a function of time during a 5-hr infusion of sulfamethizole into the jugular vein of a dog at three different constant rates. The authors concluded that a plateau was reached in all cases by the end of the third hour of infusion. That this plateau is proportional to the infusion rate, as predicted by Equation 5.20, is shown by presenting the data as in Table 5.1. The proportionality constant calculated is, of course, $k_e V$ or the clearance of sulfamethizole in the dog.

What will be the status of the infusion system at an arbitrary time $t$ prior to the attainment of infusion steady state? Divide Equation 5.19 by Equation 5.20:

$$\frac{C(t)}{C(t_\infty)} = 1 - e^{-k_e t}. \tag{5.21}$$

The fraction of the plateau level achieved at any time point should be independent of the rate of infusion, just as the fraction of the plateau level achieved after an arbitrary number of repeated doses is independent of the magnitude of the dose. It is suggested that the reader illustrate this point for himself by referring again to Figure 5.5. Select an arbitrary time and determine the fraction of each of the three plateaus achieved by this time. For example, after 45 min about 0.50, 0.49, and 0.48 of the final plateau had been achieved at infusion rates of 68, 141, and 385 mg/hr, respectively.

## 5.3 HALF–LIFE OF APPROACH TO A STEADY STATE AND VOLUME OF DISTRIBUTION AT STEADY STATE

What kind of process is the attainment of steady state on continuous constant administration of a drug or a toxicant? This question was addressed by Van Rossum (1968).

From Equations 5.19 and 5.20, $C(t_\infty) - C(t) = C(t_\infty)e^{-k_e t}$;

$$\frac{d(C(t_\infty) - C(t))}{dt} = -k_e C(t_\infty)e^{-k_e t} = -k_e(C(t_\infty) - C(t)). \tag{5.22}$$

Equation 5.22 states that the attainment of steady state is a first-order process whose rate is a function of $k_e$ but not of $A$. When the accumulation is half completed, $C(t) = C(t_\infty)/2$ and from either Equation 5.21 or 5.22 it follows that $t_{1/2} = \ln 2/k_e$. Therefore the half-life of approach to a steady state is fixed only by the rate constant of *elimination* from the system.

Similar treatment of Equations 5.2 and 5.4 or Equations 5.11 and 5.12 shows that in the case of repetitive administration also, the approach to a steady state is a first-order process whose rate is controlled only by $k_e$ and whose half-life is the half-life of elimination. Because of the fluctuations in plasma concentration, however, the time at which the measured concentration should be equal to $C(n_\infty)/2$ may not represent an integral multiple of $\Delta t$; in other words, $C(n_\infty)/2$ may lie between $C(n)$ and $C(n+1)$, or $\overline{C}(\infty)/2$ between $\overline{C}(n)$ and $\overline{C}(n+1)$. With many drug dose regimens $C(n_\infty)/2$ is actually less than $C(1)$ (see Figures 5.2 and 5.3).

The concept that the half-life of approach to a steady state is the half-life of elimination is intuitively difficult to grasp. It is not immediately apparent why the time course of the establishment of a steady state should be determined by the elimination rate constant alone. It may help to consider that when the administration rate $A$ is doubled with no change in $k_e$, the plasma level has twice as far to go (to $2A/k_eV$); but since the compound is also entering twice as fast ($2A$), there is no change in the time required to achieve any designated fraction of the expected plateau level. If, on the other hand, $k_e$ is halved with no change in $A$, the plasma level still has twice as far to go [to $(A/V)/(k_e/2)=2A/k_eV$]; but now there is no compensatory change in the entering rate $A$, so that the time required to reach any specified fraction of the expected plateau is doubled.

Figure 5.6 shows the kinetic behavior of $N$-desmethyldiazepam, a metabolite of chlordiazepoxide, during and after chronic administration of chlordiazepoxide for 36 days to a human subject (Dixon et al., 1976). Plasma $N$-desmethyldiazepam levels were determined at intervals throughout a 46-day period. It can be seen from Figure 5.6 that during both the postadministration phase and the buildup to steady state the half-life is about 4 days, or $k_e \cong 0.17$ day$^{-1}$.

Once the half-life has been estimated, the volume of distribution may be calculated from the relationship $V = A/k_e C(t_\infty)$.

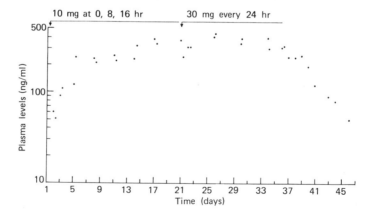

**Figure 5.6** A typical plasma level profile of $N$-desmethyldiazepam in man following chronic administration of chlordiazepoxide HCl. Reproduced with permission from Dixon et al., 1976, Figure 5.

## 5.4   STEADY STATE IN A MULTICOMPARTMENT MODEL

If $C(t_\infty)$ in a single compartment is equal to $A/k_e V$, what happens at infusion steady state in a multicompartment system?

Consider the peripheral compartment of a two-compartment open model as an independent single compartment. At infusion steady state the concentration in the peripheral compartment is $C_2(t_\infty)$. From the plateau principle we know that

$$C_2(t_\infty) = \frac{k_{12} V_1(C_1(t_\infty))}{k_{21} V_2},$$

where $k_{12} V_1(C_1(t_\infty))$ is the rate of entry of material into the peripheral compartment from the central compartment containing an amount $V_1(C_1(t_\infty))$. The rate of entry is zero order because infusion steady state has been achieved; $C_1(t_\infty)$ is a constant.

But from Section 3.7 we know that $V_1/V_2 = k_{21}/k_{12}$, so that

$$C_2(t_\infty) = C_1(t_\infty). \tag{5.23}$$

At infusion equilibrium the concentrations in the central compartment and in all peripheral compartments should be equal. This dynamic steady state is different from the state that obtains during dieaway, when concentrations in peripheral tissues are greater than that in the plasma.

Although based on the infusion steady state model, this demonstration applies also to the intermittent administration model. Irrespective of its precise nature, chronic exposure is associated with equal steady state concentrations in all body compartments.

Two additional general points should be made at this time. First, establishment of a plateau or steady state level of a compound in a particular body fluid is in no way related to saturation of the body fluid by that compound. It has been assumed throughout this development that linear kinetics apply: that steady state concentrations in the body are proportional to dose throughout the entire dose range considered, as illustrated by the data in Table 5.1. Saturation is an independent phenomenon.

Second, concentration must be related to the volume of the phase in which the compound is actually dissolved. For lipophilic materials this phase may be the lipid subfraction of the blood or of other tissues rather than whole blood or tissue fluid volumes. Lindström et al. (1974) simulated the kinetic behavior of dieldrin, a highly lipophilic chlorinated hydrocarbon pesticide, in adipose tissue and blood of a 68-kg man. Concentrations for the simulations were referenced to the lipid phases of adipose tissue and blood; it was assumed that identical plateau concentrations would be reached in all body lipid compartments. Predicted concentrations were compared with reported values (Hunter and Robinson, 1967) in three adult men. The agreement

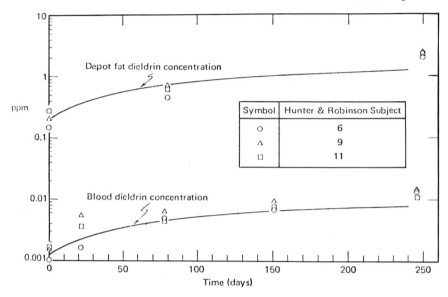

**Figure 5.7** Typical simulated curves for dieldrin levels in depot fat and arterial blood based on feeding rates, flows, and compartment sizes for a 68-kg man. Reproduced with permission from Lindström et al., 1974, Figure 6. Data points plotted are from Hunter and Robinson (1967).

between expectation and observation is excellent (Figure 5.7), demonstrating that identical plateau levels were achieved in the lipid subfractions of the two tissues (Table 5.2).

In a multicompartment model, $C_1(t_\infty) = A/k_eV_1$. To express the infusion steady state concentration $C_1(t_\infty)$ in terms of the parameter $\beta$ of the two-compartment model, it will be necessary to return to the distribution volume $V_\beta$ defined in Chapter 3. It was shown in Section 3.8 that $\beta V_\beta = k_eV_1$, so that

$$C_1(t_\infty) = \frac{A}{k_eV_1} = \frac{A}{\beta V_\beta}. \qquad (5.24)$$

Let us examine the volume parameter $V_\beta$ in greater detail.

**Table 5.2** Dependence of dieldrin plateau level on tissue lipid content in the adult male

| Tissue | Dieldrin Plateau Level in Tissue ($\mu$g/g) | Lipid Content of Tissue as Fraction of Tissue Weight | Dieldrin Plateau Level in Tissue Lipid ($\mu$g/g) |
|---|---|---|---|
| Blood | 0.008 | 0.004 | 2 |
| Depot fat | 1.3 | 0.637 | 2 |

Dieldrin data from Hunter and Robinson, 1967; fractional tissue lipid content from Lindström et al., 1974, Table VII.

All volumes of distribution relate an amount to a concentration, usually to concentration in the plasma. Useful volumes of distribution relate the total amount in the body to concentration in the plasma. For the two-compartment open model, in general

$$V = \frac{(C_1(t))V_1 + (C_2(t))V_2}{C_1(t)},$$

and since $V_2 = k_{12}V_1/k_{21}$,

$$V = V_1\left(1 + \frac{(k_{12})(C_2(t))}{(k_{21})(C_1(t))}\right). \tag{5.25}$$

Therefore different volumes of distribution may be defined for different relationships of $C_2(t)$ to $C_1(t)$.

$V_\beta$ relates plasma concentration to total body burden during the $\beta$ phase of dieaway after an acute exposure when

$$\frac{C_2(t)}{C_1(t)} = \frac{k_{21}}{k_{21} - \beta},$$

as shown in Section 3.7. Therefore,

$$V_\beta = V_1\left(1 + \frac{k_{12}}{k_{21} - \beta}\right). \tag{5.26}$$

$V_\beta$ is sometimes designated $V_{area}$; since $(AUC)_\infty = D/k_e V_1 = D/\beta V_\beta$, $V_\beta = D/\beta(AUC)_\infty = V_{area}$ (Gibaldi et al., 1969).

On the other hand, at infusion steady state $C_1(t) = C_2(t) = C_1(t_\infty) = C_2(t_\infty)$. Thus it is convenient to define yet another proportionality factor having the dimensions of volume: $V_{ss}$ is defined as the proportionality factor (or volume of distribution) that relates plasma concentration to body burden at infusion steady state:

$$V_{ss} = V_1\left(1 + \frac{k_{12}}{k_{21}}\right) \tag{5.27}$$

and, since $V_2 = k_{21}V_1/k_{21}$,

$$V_{ss} = V_1 + V_2.$$

$V_{ss}$ is an accurate estimate of the real volume of the system. It is the only appropriate proportionality factor to use to estimate body burden from infusion steady state plasma concentration; and this is so even though $C(t_\infty)$ itself is related to $V_\beta$ and not directly to $V_{ss}$ (Perrier and Gibaldi, 1973). $V_{ss}$

**Table 5.3** Interrelationships among various kinetically determined volumes of distribution for drugs having different kinetic characteristics

| Drug | $\alpha$ (hr$^{-1}$) | $\beta$ (hr$^{-1}$) | $k_{12}$ (hr$^{-1}$) | $k_{21}$ (hr$^{-1}$) | $k_{10}$ (hr$^{-1}$) | $\dfrac{V_\beta}{V_{ss}}$ | $\dfrac{V_{extrap}}{V_{ss}}$ | $\dfrac{k_{21}}{\beta}$ | $\dfrac{V_{ss}}{V_1}$ |
|---|---|---|---|---|---|---|---|---|---|
| Theophylline (Mitenko and Ogilvie, 1973) | 5.81 | 0.159 | 2.72 | 2.94 | 0.314 | 1.03 | 1.06 | 18.5 | 1.92 |
| Sulfisoxazole (Loo and Riegelman, 1970) | 7.44 | 0.660 | 3.17 | 3.55 | 1.38 | 1.11 | 1.24 | 5.38 | 1.89 |
| Sotalol (Schnelle and Garrett, 1973) | 3.91 | 0.209 | 2.31 | 0.886 | 0.944 | 1.21 | 1.51 | 4.24 | 3.61 |
| Oxacillin (Rosenblatt et al., 1968) | 7.62 | 1.62 | 2.22 | 3.60 | 3.42 | 1.32 | 1.89 | 2.22 | 1.61 |
| Quinidine (Isaacs and Schoenwald, 1974) | 23.4[a] | 1.59 | 6.96 | 2.34 | 15.6 | 2.62 | 7.33 | 1.47 | 3.97 |

[a]Average value; see Section 5.6.2.

also relates the plasma concentration after a single dose to the amount in the body at the instant when $dC_2(t)/dt=0$, since at this instant also a steady state obtains at which $C_2=C_1$. $V_{ss}$ may be estimated from experimental areas under the curve (Gibaldi, 1969a), but it is usually calculated from an explicit expression such as Equation 5.27 for the two-compartment model. Values of the ratio $V_{ss}/V_1$ are given in Table 5.3 calculated from their experimental hybrid kinetic rate constants for five drugs whose kinetics conform to a two-compartment open model.

$V_{ss}$ is always smaller than $V_\beta$. The magnitude of the discrepancy between the two proportionality factors is related to the relative magnitudes of $k_{21}$ and $\beta$. If $k_{21}$ is large relative to $\beta$, there will be only a small distributional time lag between the central and the peripheral compartments, and $V_{ss}$ and $V_\beta$ will not be greatly different. In Table 5.3 the ratios $V_\beta/V_{ss}$ are given. For the first four drugs, for all of which $k_{12}$ has about the same value, the ratio $V_\beta/V_{ss}$ increases smoothly as the ratio $k_{21}/\beta$ decreases. For quinidine, $k_{12}$ is larger than for the other four drugs; consequently $V_\beta/V_{ss}$ for quinidine assumes a particularly large value.

Finally, let us compare $V_{ss}$, $V_{\beta}$, and $V_{extrap}$:

$$V_{ss} = V_1\left(1 + \frac{k_{12}}{k_{21}}\right) = V_1\frac{k_{12} + k_{21}}{k_{21}}. \tag{5.27}$$

$$V_{\beta} = V_1\left(1 + \frac{k_{12}}{k_{21} - \beta}\right) = V_1\frac{(k_{21} + k_{12}) - \beta}{k_{21} - \beta} = V_1\frac{\alpha - k_e}{k_{21} - \beta}. \tag{5.26}$$

$$V_{extrap} = V_1\frac{\alpha - \beta}{k_{21} - \beta}. \tag{5.28}$$

Values of the ratios $V_{extrap}/V_{ss}$ are given in Table 5.3. Since $\beta$ is always smaller than $k_e$, $V_{extrap}$ is always larger than $V_{\beta}$ and, in fact, is the largest of the three volume parameters. More important, however, $V_{extrap}$ does not relate $C_1(t)$ to total body burden at any time, whereas $V_{\beta}$ and $V_{ss}$ may be used to calculate body burden from measurements of $C_1(t)$ during dieaway pseudo-steady state and during infusion steady state, respectively.

## 5.5  COMPARISON OF THE GENERAL STATEMENTS OF THE PLATEAU PRINCIPLE AND THEIR PROPER APPLICATIONS

$$\bar{C}(n) = \left(\frac{D}{V\Delta t}\right)\left(\frac{1 - e^{-nk_e\Delta t}}{k_e}\right) \tag{5.11}$$

$$\bar{C}(n_\infty) = \frac{D}{k_e V\Delta t} \tag{5.12}$$

$$C(t) = \frac{A}{k_e V}(1 - e^{-k_e t}) \tag{5.19}$$

$$C(t_\infty) = \frac{A}{k_e V} \tag{5.20}$$

Equations 5.11 and 5.12 relate average plasma concentrations after a finite and after an infinite number of equally spaced repetitive doses to the magnitude of the dose, the volume of distribution, the dose interval, and the elimination rate constant. Equations 5.19 and 5.20 relate plasma concentrations at time $t$ and at infinite time during continuous exposure to the magnitude of the dose rate, the volume of distribution, and the elimination rate constant.

The only example of continuous controlled zero-order absorption is an intravenous infusion. But most environmental exposures are also assumed to be roughly continuous rather than intermittent. Excursions above and below some practical mean absorption rate are considered to be insignificant over a long time period. In part this treatment is dictated by the lack of information that would allow absorption to be precisely quantitated. There is nearly always unresolvable uncertainty over actual absorption or exposure rates in retrospective studies involving lengthy exposure periods leading up to the time of sampling. Therefore it is fortunate that Equations 5.11 and 5.12 for average concentration are completely equivalent to Equations 5.19 and 5.20. Equations 5.19 and 5.20 are commonly applied to environmental exposures. Based on the average steady state plasma level and known values of $k_e$ and $V$ (or on average body burden and a known value of $k_e$), the absorption process is assigned a single constant rate that, considered over the entire exposure period, is presumed to yield the total amount actually absorbed during that period.

When the pattern of exposure is known, it may be taken into account. Intermittent continuous exposures occur in industrial situations. In such cases the length and magnitude of exposure can usually be fairly well defined. Estimates of industrial exposure on which recommendations for the setting of industrial standards are based commonly incorporate the 8-hr day, 5-day work week exposure pattern. Data are generally handled by applying Equation 5.19 in an on-off fashion together with the appropriate expression for dieaway during the periods of absence from the workplace, since it cannot be assumed a priori either that $C(t)$ approximates $C(t_\infty)$ during the 8-hr working day or that all absorbed material is eliminated either overnight or during the weekends.

Equations 5.11 and 5.12 are used in the design of drug dose regimens together with Equations 5.4 and 5.5 for $C_{max}$ and $C_{min}$ at the beginning and end of the $\infty$th dose interval:

$$C(n_\infty) = C_{max} = \frac{D}{V(1 - e^{-k_e \Delta t})}, \tag{5.4}$$

and

$$C_{min} = \frac{D e^{-k_e \Delta t}}{V(1 - e^{-k_e \Delta t})}. \tag{5.5}$$

The amplitudes of the excursions above and below the average plasma level are important in consideration of drug dose regimens for several reasons: the drug may cause undesirable side effects or be overtly toxic at concentrations not greatly above the average plasma level, or it may be ineffective at concentrations not greatly below it.

Equations 5.2 through 5.20 can be exploited in a number of ways. Any of the parameters $A$ (or $D$), $V$, $k_e$, or $n$ or $\Delta t$ can be calculated from the appropriate form of the plateau expression when the other parameters are known. For example, if the absorption rate $A$ is known or can be controlled as an independent variable, values of $V$ and $k_e$ obtained from an acute kinetic study can be used to predict the steady state or plateau level in the plasma on chronic exposure. Because they differ in their emphases and in the kind of information that is usually at hand, clinical, experimental, industrial, and toxicologic applications of the plateau principle are considered separately in the next section.

## 5.6 PRACTICAL USES OF THE PLATEAU PRINCIPLE

### 5.6.1 Clinical Applications

The plateau principle, stated for repetitive equal doses at constant intervals (Equations 5.4, 5.5, and 5.12), is used in the calculation of dose regimens. Usually the size of the dose is restricted by the standard form or forms in which the drug is commercially available. The volume of distribution is estimated on the basis of body weight. The value of the overall elimination rate constant $k_e$ must be available from a separate dieaway study; ordinarily a mean $k_e$ value for normal persons is chosen, but the patient's clinical condition may dictate an adjustment in the $k_e$ value used. For example, if the drug is eliminated wholly or in part in the urine and the patient is known or suspected to have impaired renal function, a $k_e$ appropriate to the patient's actual excretory efficiency must be used to avoid excessive drug accumulation.

The effective drug concentration or therapeutic range must also be known. The therapeutic range is the range of plasma drug concentrations that is associated with a therapeutic effect on the disease. (The concept of a therapeutic range is based on the assumption that the effect of a drug is proportional to its concentration in the plasma. This relationship does not always hold. The conditions under which it is valid will be discussed in connection with dose, effect relationships in Chapter 7.) Then a dose interval that should confine both $C_{max}$ and $C_{min}$ to this range may be calculated.

Sometimes a drug is toxic at concentrations that do not greatly exceed the effective concentration; in other words, it has a very narrow therapeutic range. Diphenylhydantoin is an example of such a drug. In this case, to minimize fluctuations, it may be desirable to employ a very short dose interval. Then the dose interval may be specified and the size of the required dose may be calculated. On the other hand, if an inappropriately large value of $k_e$ is used to calculate dose regimens for patients with impaired excretory function, the steady state concentration may lie within the range of toxicity even when the therapeutic range is not narrow.

Whenever it is practical, a long dose interval is more convenient, particularly if the patient is ambulatory. Often a drug's half-life is used as a rough index of an appropriate dose interval, and a dose is selected whose magnitude will cause the steady state levels to fall within the therapeutic range. But there is also another consideration associated with the half-life of the drug: how long will it be before the drug begins to act? For drugs such as antihypertensive agents or antiepileptic formulations, which are to be administered repetitively over a long time period to control a chronic disease, this consideration may be unimportant. But for drugs such as analgesics or antibiotics, to which a rapid or reasonably rapid response is either desirable or essential, the time to effect is an important consideration.

It was shown in Section 5.3 that the half-life of approach to steady state is fixed by the rate constant of elimination. For drugs administered repetitively, this half-life is equal to some multiple $n$ of the dose interval $\Delta t$:

$$\frac{\overline{C}(n)}{\overline{C}(\infty)} = \frac{C(n)}{C(n_{\infty})} = \frac{1}{2} = (1 - e^{-nk_e \Delta t}), \qquad nk_e \Delta t = \ln 2,$$

and

$$n \Delta t = \frac{\ln 2}{k_e} = t_{1/2}. \tag{5.29}$$

It follows from Equation 5.29 that the number of doses $n$ required to achieve a plasma concentration that is half the steady-state concentration is directly proportional to the half-life of elimination from the plasma. For any arbitrary dose interval $\Delta t$, the real time $n \Delta t$ at which half the steady state concentration will be achieved is equal to the elimination half-life, or inversely proportional to $k_e$. Similarly, the time required to reach any other specified fraction $C(n)/C(n_{\infty})$ of the steady state plasma level is inversely proportional to $k_e$. Assuming that $C(n_{\infty})$ is slightly larger than the minimum effective drug concentration, time to initial effect is also inversely proportional to $k_e$. If $k_e$ is large, the drug will take effect quickly. But if $k_e$ is small it may be necessary to give an initial loading dose if rapid onset of effect is desired. Use of a loading dose when necessary ensures that effective drug levels will be reached promptly. Alternatively the maintenance dose can be given more frequently initially.

For example, most penicillins have short half-lives and are therefore quick acting, requiring no loading dose. But renal disease prolongs the half-life of penicillins. If the penicillin dose regimen is altered to prevent the development of excessively high plasma penicillin levels at steady state in patients with renal disease, then time to initial effect may be undesirably long and a loading dose may be necessary.

A loading dose larger than the dose required to maintain the steady state level is given to induce rapid achievement of the effective drug concentration. After the effective drug concentration is established, the patient is continued on the maintenance dose. Suppose that we wish the maximum plasma level after a single loading dose $D_l$ to be equal to the maximum steady state plasma level during regular administration of the maintenance dose $D_m$. Then

$$\frac{D_l}{V} = \frac{D_m}{V(1 - e^{-k_e \Delta t})} \qquad \text{or} \qquad 1 - e^{-k_e \Delta t} = \frac{D_m}{D_l}.$$

$$-k_e \Delta t = \ln\left(1 - \frac{D_m}{D_l}\right). \tag{5.30}$$

If the dose interval is chosen to equal the half-life, $\Delta t = t_{1/2} = (\ln 2)/(k_e)$, then

$$-k_e \Delta t = -\ln 2 = \ln\left(1 - \frac{D_m}{D_l}\right), \qquad \frac{D_m}{D_l} = \frac{1}{2}, \qquad \text{and} \qquad D_l = 2D_m,$$

so that the loading dose should be twice the maintenance dose. Assignment of other arbitrary values to $\Delta t$ results in other $D_m/D_l$ ratios.

A practical example of the way in which dosage regimens and loading doses may be calculated from kinetic parameters is provided by Sardemann et al. (1976). Amikacin is a broad spectrum antibiotic whose half-life in infants is dependent on age. (Since amikacin is excreted primarily in the urine, the age dependence of its clearance is presumably related to the immaturity of renal excretory mechanisms in the newborn.) Sardemann and his co-workers measured total body amikacin clearance in 22 infants from 1 to 34 days old; the mean clearance is given in Table 5.4 for each of seven ages.

Amikacin kinetics conform to a two-compartment body model. The volume of distribution was calculated both as $V_{extrap}$ and as $V_\beta$ after intramuscular administration of amikacin; since absorption from the intramuscular depot was complete and very rapid, the error introduced by equating intramuscular to intravenous administration was minimal. $V_\beta$ was

**Table 5.4** Amikacin clearance, half-life, and calculated dose regimen in infants up to 30 days old

| Age (days) | Amikacin Clearance (ml/min/kg) | $\beta$ (min$^{-1}$) | $t_{1/2}$ (hr) | $D_m$, Every 8 hr (mg/kg) | $D_l$ (mg/kg) |
|---|---|---|---|---|---|
| 1 | 0.88 | 0.00138 | 8.4 | 4.2 | 8.7 |
| 5 | 1.09 | 0.00170 | 6.8 | 5.2 | 9.3 |
| 10 | 1.35 | 0.00211 | 5.5 | 6.5 | 10.3 |
| 15 | 1.61 | 0.00252 | 4.6 | 7.7 | 11.0 |
| 20 | 1.87 | 0.00292 | 4.0 | 9.0 | 12.0 |
| 25 | 2.13 | 0.00333 | 3.5 | 10.2 | 12.8 |
| 30 | 2.39 | 0.00373 | 3.1 | 11.5 | 13.8 |

Clearance values were calculated from the regression equation given by Sardemann et al., 1976, with Figure 4.

0.64 1/kg and $V_{\text{extrap}}$ was 1.28 1/kg, in accordance with the observation that $\alpha$ was only about 4 times as large as $\beta$, allowing for substantial excretion during the distribution phase. From the clearances and the volume of distribution $V_\beta$, the values of $\beta$ and the biological half-lives can be calculated, as shown in the third and fourth columns of Table 5.4.

The purpose of this study was to design amikacin dose regimens appropriate for use in infants up to the age of 1 month. An arbitrary average steady state concentration $\bar{C}$ of 10 $\mu$g/ml and a dose interval of 8 hr were chosen (note that this dose interval is of the same order of magnitude as the biological half-life in the youngest infants). The appropriate maintenance dose $D_m$ was calculated for each of the ages in Table 5.4 by using a rearrangement of Equation 5.12, $D = \bar{C}(\infty) \cdot \Delta t \cdot$ clearance. These doses are given in the fifth column. Another advantage of using the average concentration $\bar{C}$ becomes apparent in this example. Since $V_\beta \beta = V_1 k_e$, the average concentration may be calculated when $\alpha$, hence $k_{12}$, $k_{21}$, and $k_e$, are not known. Calculation of either $C_{\max}$ or $C_{\min}$ requires a value of $k_e$.

In addition appropriate loading doses may be calculated for infants of different ages by using Equation 5.30. All the $D_l$ values are given in the last column of Table 5.4. Note that for the 1-day old infant, whose amikacin half-life is approximately equal to the dosage interval, $D_l$ is roughly twice $D_m$. For the 30-day-old infant, $\Delta t = 2.58 t_{1/2}$ and $D_l = 13.8$ mg/kg, only slightly larger than $D_m$. At this dose schedule a loading dose is hardly necessary. The biological half-life is sufficiently short that $D_l \approx D_m$.

More detailed discussion of the design of drug dose regimens and of the ways in which they may be tailored to fit the idiosyncrasies of the drug or the patient, or the patient's clinical condition, is outside the scope of this book. The application of kinetic principles to the design of drug dose regimens has been investigated more fully than many other kinetic applications, and excellent publications on this subject are available. A good basic source is the introductory text by Notari (1975). Consideration of the ways in which disease states may affect the design of dose regimens by altering drug pharmacokinetics is the basis of a more specialized compilation of papers edited by Benet (1976).

### 5.6.2  Experimental Applications

There are many experimental applications of the plateau principle. It may be used to estimate either $V$ or $k_e$, provided the other is known. It may be used to determine whether $V$ or $k_e$ changes with dose, and to suggest possible causes whenever nonlinearity does exist. It may be used to challenge the adequacy of the acute model and to infer the presence or absence of a deep compartment. And it may be resorted to when a material is too toxic or too irritating to be given as a rapid intravenous injection or in a single large oral dose. Examples of these applications are given in this section.

### To Test for Kinetic Linearity

If the infusion rate of a compound is shifted abruptly to a new level and periodic estimates are made of the plasma level of the drug until the plateau level is established (this may also be done at the start of an infusion, of course), the value of $k_e$ can be estimated by analyzing the data in accordance with Equations 5.19 and 5.20 for continuous exposure: subtract Equation 5.19 from Equation 5.20:

$$C(t_\infty) - C(t) = C(t_\infty)e^{-k_e t}, \tag{5.31}$$

$$\ln(C(t_\infty) - C(t)) = \ln C(t_\infty) - k_e t. \tag{5.32}$$

Since $C(t_\infty) = A/k_e V$, the volume of distribution can also be calculated. In fact, if either $V$ or $k_e$ is known, the other can be calculated from a single assay for $C(t_\infty)$, the magnitude of $A$ being an independent variable. Therefore if the compound can be infused over a wide range of rates $A$, it is possible to establish quickly whether $V$ and $k_e$ are indeed constant with dose as is predicted by linear kinetic theory, or whether $V$ and/or $k_e$ are dose dependent.

The quantity $C(t_\infty)/A$ should be constant and independent of dose when disposition is first order, which is another way of saying that $C(t_\infty)$ should be linearly related to $A$. For most drugs the expected relationship is observed at least within the therapeutic concentration range. An example is clonazepam, an anticonvulsant (Figure 5.8a). However, when elimination mechanisms are saturable and approaching saturation, the quantity $C(t_\infty)/A$ increases without bound. Diphenylhydantoin, another anticonvulsant, is typical of compounds in this group (Remmer et al., 1969; Atkinson et al., 1973). The therapeutic plasma concentration range is about 10–20 $\mu$g/ml. At concentrations within and only slightly in excess of this range the steady state plasma level of diphenylhydantoin is not proportional to dose but increases at an accelerating rate as the dose rate is increased (Figure 5.8b) (Bochner et al., 1972).

### To Study the Kinetic Behavior of a Compound That Cannot be Given by Intravenous Injection

Sometimes a compound may be either too acutely toxic or too locally irritating to be injected as a large dose. The plateau principle may be exploited to study the kinetic behavior of compounds that cannot be injected rapidly but may be infused slowly over a period of time until infusion steady state is reached.

When an infusion is terminated after attainment of a steady state, the subsequent kinetic behavior of the compound may be used to determine the same kinetic parameters determined from the kinetic behavior of the compound after acute administration. In other words, dieaway from a plateau in the central compartment of a mammillary system exhibits whatever multiphasic behavior is characteristic of the acute kinetics. For example, the

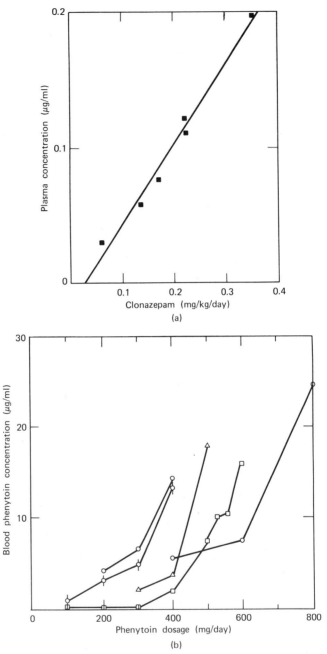

**Figure 5.8** The relationship of $C(t_\infty)$ to dose rate. (*a*) Expected behavior assuming first-order elimination. The relationship of clonazapam dose rate to plasma clonazepam concentration in a patient whose daily intake of other drugs was unaltered throughout the period of observation. Reproduced with permission; after Eadie, M.J., Plasma level monitoring of anticonvulsants, *Clin. Pharmacokinet*, **1**, 52–66, 1976, Figure 3. (*b*) Deviation from expected behavior. The relationship of phenytoin (diphenylhydantoin) dose rate to blood phenytoin concentrations in five patients. Reproduced with permission from Bochner et al., 1972, Figure 1.

dieaway curve describing a two-compartment body model can be resolved into two linear components with slopes $-\alpha$ and $-\beta$. The ordinate intercepts of the $\alpha$ and $\beta$ lines are not, however, identical with the ordinate intercepts of the corresponding $\alpha$ and $\beta$ lines after acute administration. This point is discussed below.

This is another of those kinetic facts that are not particularly obvious intuitively. It is not difficult to understand why, after an intravenous injection, a compound should disappear from the plasma rapidly at first, then more slowly as peripheral reservoirs fill and return from peripheral tissues to the plasma becomes kinetically significant. But when infusion steady state has been achieved, it is to be presumed that all peripheral compartments have already been filled. Why then should the rate of disappearance from the plasma after cessation of infusion exhibit multicompartment kinetic characteristics?

During infusion steady state the concentrations of the compound in all compartments are equal (Section 5.4) and represent the achievement of a balance between the infusion rate and the rate of loss from the system. Once infusion has been terminated, this balance is destroyed. The system will then seek a new steady state in which the concentration in each peripheral compartment is greater than the concentration in the central compartment by a constant factor that is related to the magnitude of the transfer lag time between the compartments. The new steady state relationship between concentration in peripheral and central compartments will be the same as that observed during the pseudo–steady state phase of dieaway after acute administration.

The kinetics of the shift from one kind of steady state to another on termination of an infusion are controlled by the same microconstants that control the acute kinetics of the compound. Only the boundary conditions are different. Therefore it should not be too surprising that the slopes of the linear components of dieaway from a plateau in the central compartment of a mammillary model should be identical to the slopes of the linear components of dieaway in the central compartment of a mammillary model after a single injection. Let us consider in greater detail the kinetic behavior of a compound that has reached infusion steady state in the central compartment and in one peripheral compartment prior to termination of the infusion. The model is shown in Figure 5.9.

The initial conditions are:

$$C_1(t_0) = C_2(t_0) = C_1(t_\infty) = C_2(t_\infty) = \frac{M_1(t_\infty)}{V_1} = \frac{M_2(t_\infty)}{V_2}.$$

The expressions for $C_1$ and $C_2$ are:

$$C_1(t) = \left( \frac{M_1(t_\infty)}{V_1(\alpha - \beta)} \right) \left[ (k_{10} - \beta)e^{-\alpha t} + (\alpha - k_{10})e^{-\beta t} \right] \qquad (5.33)$$

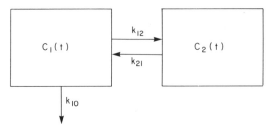

**Figure 5.9** The linear two-compartment open model after completion of infusion to steady state.

and

$$C_2(t) = \left( \frac{M_2(t_\infty)}{V_2(\alpha - \beta)} \right) \left[ \alpha e^{-\beta t} - \beta e^{-\alpha t} \right], \tag{5.34}$$

where $\alpha$ and $\beta$ are defined as they were in Chapter 3 (Equations 3.24 and 3.25). When Equations 5.33 and 5.34 are compared with Equations 3.22 and 3.23 for dieaway after a bolus injection, it can be seen that the corresponding expressions for $C_1(t)$ and $C_2(t)$ are similar in general form and have the same exponents but differ in their coefficients:

$$C_1(t) = \left( \frac{D}{V_1(\alpha - \beta)} \right) \left[ (\alpha - k_{21}) e^{-\alpha t} + (k_{21} - \beta) e^{-\beta t} \right] \tag{3.22}$$

and

$$C_2(t) = \left( \frac{D}{V_2(\alpha - \beta)} \right) \left[ k_{12} e^{-\beta t} - k_{12} e^{-\alpha t} \right]. \tag{3.23}$$

It is the coefficients that are fixed by the boundary conditions of the system. To emphasize the similarities between Equation 3.22 and Equation 5.33, Equation 5.33 may be written in the form $C_1(t) = E_0 e^{-\alpha t} + F_0 e^{-\beta t}$, where

$$E_0 = \frac{(M_1(t_\infty))(k_{10} - \beta)}{V_1(\alpha - \beta)} \quad \text{and} \quad F_0 = \frac{(M_1(t_\infty))(\alpha - k_{10})}{V_1(\alpha - \beta)}.$$

Consider the behavior of $C_1(t)$ as described by Equation 5.33. At early times after cessation of infusion both terms will contribute to the magnitude of $C_1(t)$. Since $\alpha$ is larger than $\beta$, however, the term in $e^{-\alpha t}$ will decay faster than the term in $e^{-\beta t}$. Once the term in $e^{-\alpha t}$ has become negligible relative to the term in $e^{-\beta t}$, the shift to the new dynamic steady state has been accomplished. The system has degenerated into one apparent compartment whose elimination rate constant is $\beta$. When $C_1(t)$ is graphed against time on semilogarithmic paper the plot will terminate in a linear segment defined by the expression

$$C_1(t) \approx \left( \frac{(M_1(t_\infty))(\alpha - k_{10})}{V_1(\alpha - \beta)} \right) e^{-\beta t}, \qquad (5.35)$$

or

$$\ln C_1(t) \approx \ln F_0 - \beta t, \qquad (5.3\ )$$

which was obtained by dropping the term in $e^{-\alpha t}$ from Equation 5.33 for $C_1(t)$.

The concentration of the compound in the peripheral compartment falls continuously after cessation of infusion. The situation in the peripheral compartment is analogous to that in a one-compartment model with first-order absorption and elimination, from the point $C_{max}$, $t_{max}$ onward in time. During the early period of redistribution between the central and the peripheral compartments $C_2(t)$ falls more slowly than $C_1(t)$. Once the new dynamic steady state has been achieved, the term in $e^{-\alpha t}$ can be dropped from Equation 5.34 for $C_2(t)$ and at subsequent times,

$$C_2(t) \approx \left( \frac{(M_2(t_\infty))(\alpha)}{(V_2)(\alpha - \beta)} \right) e^{-\beta t}, \qquad (5.37)$$

or

$$\ln C_2(t) \approx \ln \left( \frac{(M_2(t_\infty))(\alpha)}{V_2(\alpha - \beta)} \right) - \beta t. \qquad (5.38)$$

The slope of the terminal segment of a $\ln C_2(t)$, $t$ graph is therefore $-\beta$, and the antilog of the ordinate intercept of the back-extrapolated terminal segment is $C_2(t_\infty)[\alpha/(\alpha - \beta)]$. Note the analogy with the antilog of the ordinate intercept of the back-extrapolated terminal portion of Equation 3.42 with $k_a > k_e$, which is $(D/V)[k_a/(k_a - k_e)]$ (Equation 3.44.)

During the terminal phase of dieaway from a plateau,

$$\frac{C_2(t)}{C_1(t)} = \frac{(M_2(t_\infty))(\alpha)(V_1)(\alpha - \beta)}{(M_1(t_\infty))(\alpha - k_{10})(V_2)(\alpha - \beta)}$$

or, since

$$\frac{M_2(t_\infty)}{V_2} = \frac{M_1(t_\infty)}{V_1},$$

$$\frac{C_2(t)}{C_1(t)} = \frac{\alpha}{\alpha - k_{10}}.$$

Now $k_{10} = \alpha\beta/k_{21}$ (Section 3.9), so that

$$\frac{C_2(t)}{C_1(t)} = \frac{\alpha}{\alpha(1 - \beta/k_{21})} = \frac{k_{21}}{k_{21} - \beta}.$$

This relationship is identical to that which was calculated for the acute model in Section 3.7. Therefore the pseudo-steady state relationship between peripheral and central compartments during the terminal phase of dieaway is the same irrespective of whether the starting point was an acute administration into the central compartment or equal concentrations in the central and peripheral compartments.

If $\alpha$ is of the same order of magnitude as $\beta$ the central and peripheral compartments may not reach a pseudo-steady state during the time period of measurement. In this case the terminal slopes of the graphs of $\ln C_1(t)$ versus $t$ and $\ln C_2(t)$ versus $t$ will not be constant and will not be equal at any measurement time. (Compare this behavior with the behavior of Equation 3.42 when $k_a \leqslant k_e$.) If $k_{21}$ is less than $k_{10}$, the peripheral compartment is a deep compartment. Reestablishment of a steady state will be very slow after cessation of infusion, and the terminal slopes of the graphs of $\ln C_1(t)$ versus $t$ and $\ln C_2(t)$ versus $t$ will be reflect $k_{21}$ rather than $\beta$.

Assuming that the system is well behaved and that $\alpha \gg \beta$, Equation 5.33 may be feathered to obtain the value of $\alpha$ and the ordinate intercept $E_0$. The microconstants $k_{12}$, $k_{21}$, and $k_{10}$ are estimated as follows:

$$\frac{E_0}{F_0} = \frac{k_{10} - \beta}{\alpha - k_{10}},$$

from which

$$k_{10} = \frac{\alpha E_0 + \beta F_0}{E_0 + F_0}, \tag{5.39}$$

$$k_{21} = \frac{\alpha\beta}{k_{10}}, \tag{5.40}$$

and

$$k_{12} = \alpha + \beta - k_{21} - k_{10}. \tag{5.41}$$

Therefore all the kinetic parameters of a two-compartment model may be estimated from the dieaway behavior of concentration in the central compartment after termination of a steady state intravenous infusion. The initial conditions assumed in this development were those of infusion steady state, and infusion steady state must have been reached before Equations 5.39, 5.40, and 5.41 can be applied to a dieaway analysis. The ordinate intercepts are functions of the concentrations in the central and peripheral compartments at

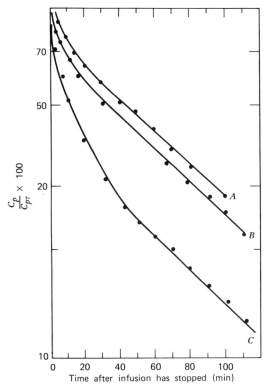

**Figure 5.10** Sulfisoxazole plasma levels after cessation of intravenous infusion in the rabbit. Curve *A*, after a 60-min infusion; curve *B*, after a 30-min infusion; curve *C*, after a 10-sec infusion. $C_p$ =plasma concentration after infusion has stopped; $C_{p\tau}$ =plasma concentration at the end of the infusion. Data are normalized by use of $C_p/C_{p\tau}$. Reproduced with permission from Loo and Riegelman, 1970, Figure 1.

termination of infusion. These concentrations are dependent on the length of the infusion time; consequently the intercepts are always intermediate between $A_0, B_0$ at one extreme (infusion time $= 0$; instantaneous administration) and $E_0, F_0$ at the other (infinitely long infusion time). Figure 5.10 shows sulfisoxazole plasma levels in rabbits after infusions of 60 min, 30 min and 10 sec duration (curves *A*, *B* and *C*, respectively). The 10-sec infusion is essentially an intravenous injection. The authors estimated the hybrid kinetic parameters in Table 5.5 from their experimental data. Note that as the infusion time is lengthened, the differences between the observed intercepts and the intercepts obtained from an instantaneous administration curve increase.

Equations for calculation of the microconstants of a mammillary model from the hybrid kinetic parameters estimated from a postinfusion curve irrespective of whether infusion equilibrium has been achieved were published by Loo and Riegelman (1970) for the general case of *n* compartments.

**Table 5.5** Kinetic parameters describing the postinfusion plasma curves obtained after rapid and prolonged administration of sulfisoxazole intravenously into a male rabbit

| Infusion Time | $\alpha$ (min$^{-1}$) | $\beta$ (min$^{-1}$) | $\alpha$ Intercept, $\dfrac{C(t)}{C(t_\infty)}$ | $\beta$ Intercept, $\dfrac{C(t)}{C(t_\infty)}$ |
|---|---|---|---|---|
| 10 sec | 0.124 | 0.011 | 0.573 | 0.427 |
| 30 min | 0.129 | 0.010 | 0.330 | 0.673 |
| 60 min | 0.134 | 0.010 | 0.228 | 0.772 |

From Loo and Riegelman, 1970, Table I.

The more specialized treatment given in detail in this book, for dieaway from infusion steady state in a two-compartment model, appears in a publication by Gibaldi (1969b).

As a final example of postinfusion dieaway, Figure 5.11 is taken from a study by Isaacs and Schoenwald (1974) in which the kinetics of quinidine, a drug used in the treatment of cardiac arrhythmias, were correlated with the dynamics of intensity of effect of the drug in rabbits given quinidine either by intravenous infusion over a 1-min period or by slow intravenous infusion over a 95-min period. The two curves were computer fit to give the hybrid parameters in Table 5.6. In this case the values of $\beta$ match well; those of $\alpha$ do not. However, note that $\alpha$ is very large (at least 100 times $\beta$); and since the

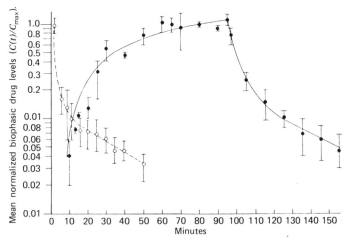

**Figure 5.11** Time course of variation in biophase drug levels following rapidly (○) and slowly infused (●) doses of quinidine. Each open point is an average of eight determinations calculated from response intensities measured in two rabbits given four doses of 2.5, 3.75, 5.0 and 6.25 mg/kg. The solid points represent a slowly infused dose of 0.0145 mg/kg/min to each of two rabbits. Vertical bars represent ± standard deviation. Dashed and solid lines are computer least squares lines of best fit. Reproduced with permission from Isaacs and Schoenwald, 1974, Figure 5.

**Table 5.6** Kinetic parameters describing the postinfusion-derived biophasic drug level curves in two rabbits infused either slowly or rapidly with quinidine

| Curve | $\alpha$ (min$^{-1}$) | $\beta$ (min$^{-1}$) | $\alpha$ Intercept, $\dfrac{C(t)}{C_{\max}}$ | $\beta$ Intercept, $\dfrac{C(t)}{C_{\max}}$ |
|---|---|---|---|---|
| Rapid infusion | 0.687 | 0.0265 | 3.48 | 0.127 |
| Slow infusion | 0.177 | 0.0206 | 0.809 | 0.170 |

From Isaacs and Schoenwald, 1974, Table I.

values of $\alpha$ were obtained using at most four data points, these values are not particularly reliable. Analysis of effect data in this study gave $\alpha$ values of 0.461 and 0.247 min$^{-1}$.

An interesting feature of quinidine kinetics should be apparent on comparison of Figures 5.10 and 5.11. Notice that the $\beta$ intercept of the 60-min postinfusion curve of Figure 5.10 is nearly twice the $\beta$ intercept of the postinjection curve, even though the total infusion time is less than the biological half-life. In contrast, in spite of the rather long infusion period, the $\beta$ intercept of the postinfusion curve of Figure 5.11 is not greatly different from the postinjection curve $\beta$ intercept. This observation suggests that the kinetic microconstants of the quinidine system may be related to one another in a rather unusual way. Since the infusion time was between 3 and 4 times the biological half-life, we can assume that quinidine was very nearly in a steady state at the end of the infusion period, and we can calculate $k_{12}$, $k_{21}$, and $k_{10}$ from the data in Table 5.6 by using Equations 3.33, 3.34, and 3.35 for the postinjection curve and Equations 5.39, 5.40, and 5.41 for the postinfusion curve (Table 5.7).

It is evident that $k_{21} \ll k_{10}$. Quinidine enters a deep compartment from which it returns relatively slowly ($t_{1/2}$ of return is about 22 min). That its entry into the deep compartment is not as slow as its return suggests possible heterogeneous binding to a readily accessible tissue.

### To Probe for Biologic and Kinetic Idiosyncrasies of the Test System

Ultimate proof of the validity of a proposed first-order model is coincidence of the blood levels predicted from acute studies with those actually obtained on chronic exposure. In a multicompartment system during chronic exposure

**Table 5.7** Kinetic microconstants for quinidine calculated from the hybrid constants in Table 5.6

| Curve | $k_{12}$ (min$^{-1}$) | $k_{21}$ (min$^{-1}$) | $k_{10}$ (min$^{-1}$) |
|---|---|---|---|
| Rapid infusion | 0.116 | 0.039 | 0.26 |
| Slow infusion | 0.069 | 0.025 | 0.33 |

the plateau levels in the fluid compartments of all tissues should be equal to the plateau level in the plasma when steady state has been reached. However, different compartments will fill at different rates, the half-time to plateau achievement being in each case reciprocally related to the rate constant of exit from the compartment. If deep compartments exist, they will fill slowly and will achieve a steady state relationship with the plasma later than all other compartments. The observation that the final approach to a plateau in the plasma is very slow suggests that a deep compartment may still be filling. If poorly accessible or deep compartments are sufficiently large, the plateau level in the plasma will be found to be lower than that which was predicted on the basis of acute studies.

For example, if an acute study has given particular values for $V_\beta$ and for $\beta$, it would be predicted that at infusion steady state

$$C_1(t_\infty) = \frac{A}{\beta V_\beta}.$$

However, during an acute study a deep or poorly accessible compartment never achieves a steady state relationship with the plasma; it may not fill to a sufficient extent even to be kinetically observable. The value of $V_\beta$, which relates body burden to plasma level during the $\beta$ phase of dieaway, is always too small whenever there are compartments that have not reached a steady state relationship with the central compartment during the apparent $\beta$ phase of dieaway from an acute exposure. Since the estimated $V_\beta$ value is too small, the actual $C_1(t_\infty)$ value attained on chronic exposure will be found to be smaller than the predicted value. Furthermore, if there is a deep compartment of moderate to high capacity, there can be an enormous difference between the terminal half-life after cessation of chronic exposure and that observed in acute studies. When a chronic exposure during which steady state was achieved is terminated, the rate-determining step during the terminal phase of dieaway is return from the deep compartment to the plasma, for which process the rate constant is less than $k_e$. (This is another example of flip-flop.) Conclusive evidence of the existence of a deep compartment is the finding of a larger terminal half-life in a chronic study than in an acute study, coupled with the observation that actual plateau levels are lower than those predicted.

An alternative explanation for an observed plateau level lower than that predicted on the basis of an acute study is the induction of metabolizing enzymes. As indicated in Chapter 4, induction of metabolizing enzyme activity can be both prompt and massive. In most instances, however, it appears likely that enzyme induction will result in a gradual downward drift of monitored plasma levels after an initial peak rather than in a smooth rise to a plateau that is lower than that expected. A good example is provided by a study by Pitlick and Levy (1977) in which carbamazepine, an anticon-

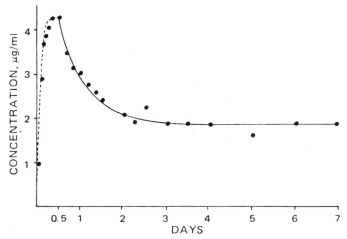

**Figure 5.12** Plot of serum carbamazepine concentration as a function of time for a monkey during a week on long-term carbamazepine infusion at a constant rate of 17.3 mg/hr. Reproduced with permission from Pitlick and Levy, 1977, Figure 1.

vulsant, was continuously infused into a male rhesus monkey for 1 week by means of jugular and femoral catheters (Figure 5.12). Carbamazepine induces its own metabolism in monkeys. Whether the maximum observed serum carbamazepine concentration, 4.32 $\mu$g/ml, represents the plateau that would have been established in the absence of any induction cannot be determined from these data. But it is clear that maximum metabolizing enzyme activity was not reached until the second day. After this time there is no further increase in metabolizing enzyme activity, and the serum carbamazepine concentration remains fixed at its newly established plateau level.

A third explanation for an observed plateau level lower than that predicted could be displacement of plasma protein bound parent drug by its metabolite. This phenomenon has not been studied in any detail.

The plateau level may also drift upward, rather than downward, during an infusion. When this happens, interference with one or more elimination processes is suggested. If the compound is metabolized, approaching saturation of the metabolizing enzymes is the simplest possibility. If the maximum capacity of the metabolizing enzyme system is exceeded by the infusion rate, $C(t)$ will increase continuously and a plateau will never be established.

Alternative explanations also could account for a gradual upward drift in the plateau level. Product inhibition of a metabolic transformation step is one possibility. Substrate inhibition of metabolism can also occur. Drug-associated renal or hepatic damage or changes in blood flow rates could cause progressive impairment of excretion or metabolism, which in turn would cause a gradual plateau shift to a new, higher level reflecting the prolonged half-lives of materials eliminated by the affected mechanisms.

### 5.6.3   Industrial Applications

Chronic industrial exposure is intermittent continuous, provided the material
is present only in the workplace or is present in the workplace in concentrations in excess of those found in the general environment. During the work
day the material will accumulate to some extent in the tissues of exposed
persons; overnight and during the weekend it will be cleared from the body,
wholly or in part, by whatever mechanisms mediate elimination of the
compound.

What kinetic parameters determine the extent of accumulation during the
exposure periods and the completeness of clearance during the times
the worker is away from the workplace? The two important parameters are
the half-life and the exposure level. The half-life is both the half-time of
approach to steady state and the half-time of postexposure dieaway. The
exposure level, in conjunction with the half-life, determines steady state tissue
levels.

After 3 half-lives 87.5% of either the accumulation or the dieaway process
is complete. After 5 half-lives these processes are almost 97% complete, and
after 8 half-lives they are more than 99% complete. It is generally considered
that for practical purposes a steady state is reached after 4–5 half-lives. If the
half-life is very short, relatively low constant plasma levels may be observed
throughout the work day followed by prompt and complete clearance overnight. Each day's concentration, time profile will be the same.

At the other extreme, if the half-life is long, plasma levels may increase
continuously throughout the work day and elimination may not be complete
overnight. In this case each day's profile will be superimposed on the residue
from the previous day, with eventual buildup to a constant (plateau) residue
or baseline level and daily excursions above this plateau.

The length of the weekend period is particularly important because if the
compound can be cleared completely from the body during the weekend,
incomplete elimination during the work week may be unimportant unless the
compound is toxic at the daily levels reached. For this reason the most
important single time to sample plasma residues is Monday morning.

Figure 5.13 shows the rate of loss of pentachlorophenol (PCP) from tissues
of rats given a single acute dose (Hoben et al., 1976). If the half-life of PCP in
humans is approximately the same as it is in rats, should there be significant
quantities of PCP on Monday morning in the tissues of workers exposed only
during the work week? In other words, would PCP be designated a "highly
cumulative substance"? From Figure 5.13, PCP half-life is around 8 hr. The
individual exposed for 8 hr a day, 5 days a week, would probably show some
accumulation during the work week but over the weekend (64 hr = 8 half-lives)
essentially all PCP should be cleared from the body. PCP should not be a
highly cumulative substance.

In this way the degree of accumulation of an industrial compound under
normal industrial exposure conditions can be estimated based on knowledge

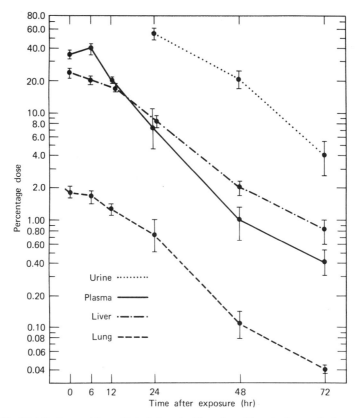

**Figure 5.13** Distribution and loss of inhaled pentachlorophenol in rats given a single acute dose. Reproduced with permission from Hoben et al., 1976, Figure 1.

of its acute kinetic behavior, in particular of its half-life, together with the plateau principle. But it is well to remember, as discussed in the preceding sections, that predicted levels of a compound may not be in agreement with actual levels in the presence of induction or inhibition of metabolizing enzymes, hepatic or renal damage by toxicants eliminated by these routes, tissue binding, or deep compartments.

Corresponding to the increasing number of women entering the work force there is increasing concern over possible fetotoxicity of industrial compounds. There is evidence that the fetus is a deep compartment for certain drugs (Section 5.6.4), but industrial compounds have been little studied in this regard. Exposure of the fetus to compounds for which it is a deep compartment is potentially of much greater magnitude than the mother's exposure. In addition, the experimental situation is complicated by the short gestation periods of the common laboratory animal species, which make them poor models for study of the effects on the fetus of extended low maternal exposure.

Other important considerations in industrial practice do not relate directly to the plateau principle itself but are concerned instead with determinants of the values of kinetic parameters, including the half-life, in a heterogeneous worker population. Acute kinetic parameters, when they have been measured in humans at all, have most commonly been based on study of a subpopulation of young healthy adult males. Such a selected population may not be kinetically representative of the larger worker population, which includes females and males of a wide range of ages, some with organic diseases and some taking pharmaceutical or other drug preparations.

Kinetic differences between females and males are not uncommon. Examples appearing in this text are the more efficient elimination of the metabolites of methadone (Section 3.2) and of cyclacillin (Problem 15, Chapter 3) by females than by males in the species studied. In experimental animals not only have sex differences been observed, but species and even strain differences as well (Quinn et al., 1958). Most commonly these differences have been related to differences in microsomal enzyme activities (Kato et al., 1962; Kato and Gillette, 1965). Sex-related differences in metabolism have been shown in some cases to be linked with sex hormone activity (Murphy and DuBois, 1958; Kato et al., 1962). Inorganic materials such as lead (Kostial et al., 1974) and cadmium (Pence et al., 1977) also exhibit sex-related kinetic behavior and effects. To what extent such differences are to be found in humans is not known, but it is reasonable to suppose that at least some of them exist.

Many clearance mechanisms are age related. Average creatinine clearance in 25-year-old males is about 120 ml/min; in 55-year-old males it is about 80 ml/min. The distribution of a compound may change with age as the percentage and distribution of body fat and the rates of perfusion of different tissues are altered. The effects of age on pharmacokinetics have been reviewed by Triggs and Nation (1975).

The effects of disease states on pharmacokinetics were mentioned briefly in Section 5.6.1; some, particularly the effects of renal and hepatic impairment, have been intensively studied in connection with drug dose regimen design (Benet, 1976; Dettli, 1974). A number of diseases, injuries, and infections alter the proportions of serum proteins. The effect of pregnancy on kinetics has been little studied, but pregnancy is known to lower plasma albumin levels. Cigarette smoking may alter metabolic rates (Conney et al., 1974).

Drugs taken for the control of disease may alter the kinetics of other compounds. Some drugs, such as chloramphenicol or disulfiram, can inhibit metabolism. Others, such as propranolol or lidocaine, alter the rate of perfusion of liver and other tissues and therefore have potential for affecting absorption, distribution, and elimination rates. The barbiturates and many other drugs are inducers of metabolizing enzymes. The magnitude and pattern of alcohol consumption affect both the distribution and the elimination of many other compounds. The kinetics of drug-drug interactions have been reviewed by Rowland (1974); the same principles apply to the kinetics of interaction of drugs with industrial compounds.

In some cases particular individuals or groups of individuals may be genetically distinct from the majority of the population, usually with regard to their ability to metabolize a compound. For example, the tuberculostatic drug isoniazid is acetylated rapidly by about half the United States population and slowly by the other half. Slow acetylation is determined by homozygous inheritance of a recessive gene. Current knowledge of pharmacogenetics has been reviewed by La Du (1974) and by Vesell (1973).

Proper consideration should be given to the age, sex, health, and relevant personal habits of persons comprising the worker population, as well as to pharmacogenetic quirks when these are known, in predicting the likelihood of significant accumulation of a compound in tissues of persons exposed under industrial conditions.

### 5.6.4 Toxicologic Applications

The plateau principle provides a rationale for the use of plasma or tissue levels of a toxicant as indices of exposure, both in single case and in epidemiological studies. More than likely the reader has never considered why tissue or plasma concentration and exposure level should be related at all. It is the plateau principle that states that the concentration measured should reflect the exposure as long as the kinetics of absorption and disposition are first order.

For example, a study by Joselow et al. (1974) reported blood lead levels in children in Honolulu, Hawaii (mean, 17 $\mu$g/100 ml; range, 10–30 $\mu$g/100 ml), and in Newark, New Jersey (mean, 28 $\mu$g/100 ml; range 15–60 $\mu$g/100 ml). Based on the observation that the Hawaiian children had lower blood lead levels than the New Jersey children, it was concluded that lead exposure was lower in Honolulu than in Newark.

In another study (Koirtyohann et al., 1974) the levels of mercury in fish taken from golf course lakes were used to infer the relative levels of mercury in the lake water and, by extension, the intensity of the runoff of organic mercurials used as fungicides on the golf greens.

The plateau principle also states that both the amount that will eventually be stored in a particular tissue and the time required to achieve steady state are directly proportional to the half-life of elimination of the compound from the tissue. Therefore deep compartments, though they fill slowly, have high capacities. This is why cumulative toxicity may develop insidiously with such substances as heavy metals—lead, mercury, or cadmium—that are bound tenaciously within tissue matrices, or with chlorinated hydrocarbon pesticides, which accumulate in body fat depots. Considerable accumulation of toxic materials such as these may have occurred before any manifestations of toxicity appear. Eventually, if the deep compartment has a high capacity, toxicities may be manifested that were not evident on acute exposure, even though the blood level on chronic exposure is less than the maximum level on acute exposure. Additionally, the large time gap between initial exposure and the onset of any symptoms may make it difficult to trace the source of the toxicity.

A few relevant studies suggest that the fetus may be a deep compartment for some compounds. For example, the antineoplastic agent cytosine arabinoside and the antibacterial cephaloridine are both eliminated substantially more slowly from fetal blood than from maternal blood (Krowke and Neubert, 1977; Arthur and Burland, 1969). This behavior is particularly significant in the case of the antineoplastic agent, since antineoplastic agents themselves often have neoplastic activity. Another possibility with regard to fetotoxicity is illustrated by ampicillin, for which the amniotic fluid, rather than the fetus itself, is a deep compartment (Bray et al., 1966; MacAulay et al., 1966). If other drugs are shown to behave in this fashion, it may be necessary to consider the amniotic fluid a potential drug reservoir and continuing source of fetal exposure.

## PROBLEMS

1  Construct a table showing the percentage of the plateau level that will have been reached at the beginning of dosage intervals 1, 2, 3, 4, 5, 6, 7, and 8 when the dosage interval is equal to the half-life of the drug.

2  Using the expression $C_1(t) = A_0 e^{-\alpha t} + B_0 e^{-\beta t}$ for dieaway from instantaneous administration into the central compartment of a two-compartment system and the expression $C_1(t) = E_0 e^{-\alpha t} + F_0 e^{-\beta t}$ for dieaway from infusion steady state in the central compartment of a two-compartment system, together with the relationship $\alpha + \beta = k_{12} + k_{21} + k_{10}$, show that $A_0 > E_0$ and $B_0 < F_0$, provided $D = M_1(t_\infty) + M_2(t_\infty)$. Do the values of $A_0$, $B_0$, $E_0$, and $F_0$ given for the sulfisoxazole example in Section 5.6.2 (Table 5.5) conform to this prediction?

3  Knaus et al. (1976) measured the accumulation of fluoride ion in the blood of rats infused intravenously with solutions containing different concentrations of [$^{18}$F] NaF. They also monitored fluoride during dieaway after cessation of the 6-mg/kg/hr infusion. Some of their results are given in Table 5.8 and Figure 5.14. Do these data obey the plateau principle? Why or why not?

4  Davison et al. (1975) studied the effect of mirex, a chlorinated hydrocarbon insecticide, on eggshell thickness in chickens. In the course of this study mirex residues were determined in eggs and carcasses of chickens that had been fed the insecticide in their diet (Figure 5.15).

(a)  Do these curves obey the plateau principle? Why or why not?

**Table 5.8** The dieaway of exogenous fluoride, measured as $^{18}$F, in the blood of a rat infused for 3 hr at the rate of 6 mg/kg/hr

| Time (hr)[a] | $^{18}$F Concentration ($\mu$g/ml) |
|---|---|
| 0 | 6.1 |
| 1.1 | 3.7 |
| 1.4 | 2.9 |
| 3.1 | 0.9 |

From Knaus et al., 1976, Table 2.
[a]Measured from termination of infusion.

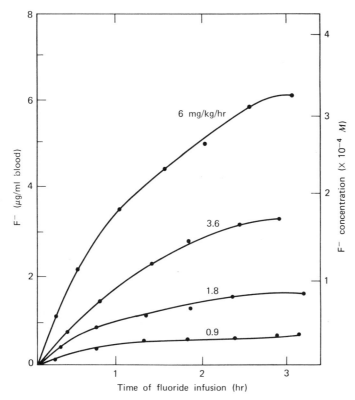

**Figure 5.14** Accumulation of fluoride as $^{18}$F in blood during infusion of [$^{18}$F]NaF into rats at the rates indicated for 3 hr, in each case accompanied by 150 mg of glucose/hr and in a total volume of 0.84 ml/hr. Maximum values reached were 0.8 $\mu$g/g at 0.9 mg/kg/hr; 1.7 $\mu$g/g at 1.8 mg/kg/hr; 3.4 $\mu$g/g at 3.6 mg/kg/hr, and 6.1 $\mu$g/g at 6.0 mg/kg/hr. Reproduced with permission from Knaus et al., 1976, Figure 1.

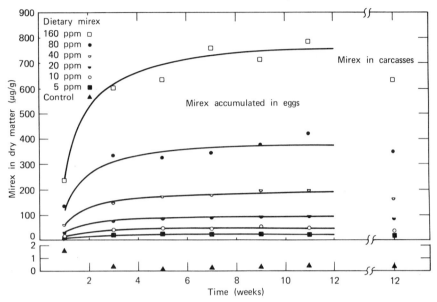

**Figure 5.15** Average mirex residues in dry matter of eggs and carcasses of chickens fed various levels of technical mirex. Reproduced with permission from Davison et al., 1975, Figure 1.

**(b)** Arbitrarily considering the body and (unlaid) eggs to be a single compartment, how long would you expect mirex to persist in the eggs (give the half-life) after it had been withdrawn from the diet?

**5** DiVincenzo et al. (1972) wanted to assess the usefulness of in-plant breath monitoring techniques for the estimation of the magnitude of worker exposure to volatile organic solvents. Using methylene chloride as the experimental solvent, they first established that the dog was a suitable animal model for their purpose; breath dieaway curves in dogs could be used to predict breath dieaway curves in humans. Some of their subsequent dieaway data from dogs are shown in Figures 5.16*a* and 5.16*b*.

**(a)** Does methylene chloride exhibit linear or nonlinear kinetic characteristics? Does it distribute through one or more than one kinetically distinguishable compartment?

**(b)** What do you predict would be the half-time for achievement of plateau levels of methylene chloride in the blood after the onset of exposure?

**(c)** Are the blood and breath in a steady state relationship during the time period of the measurements?

**(d)** Assuming that human kinetic parameters are of the same order of magnitude as the dogs', would you recommend breath monitoring

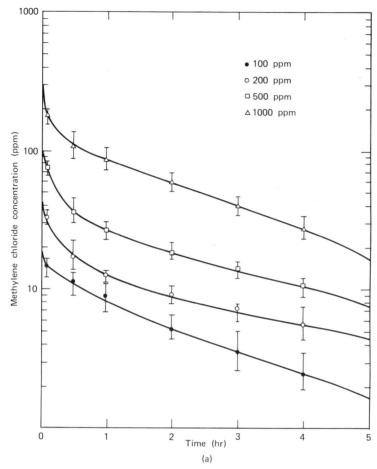

**Figure 5.16** Postexposure data from dogs exposed for 2 hr to methylene chloride vapor concentrations of 100, 200, 500 and 1000 ppm. Each value represents the mean and range of three to five exposures. (*a*) Breath excretion curves. (*b*) Blood levels. Reproduced with permission from DiVincenzo et al., 1972, Figures 7 and 9, courtesy of *American Industrial Hygiene Association Journal*.

(apart from its speed and ease) as an index of exposure to methylene chloride vapor during exposure (e.g., during the work day)? after exposure has ceased and the worker has left the work environment?

Support your answers with statements based on the graphs.

**6** The data in Tables 5.9*a* and 5.9*b* are taken from a study by Blake and Mergner (1974) of the biotransformation and elimination of trichlorofluoromethane and dichlorodifluoromethane in beagles exposed by inhalation. The authors state that "In general, there was a proportional

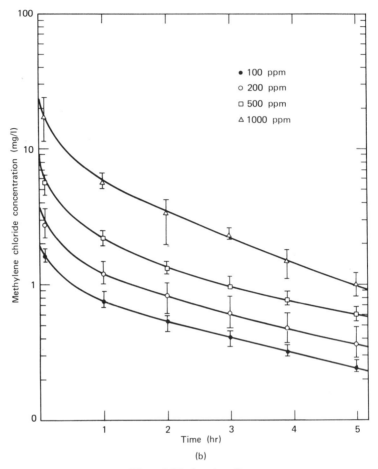

**Figure 5.16**  (*continued*)

relationship between the inhaled concentration and the peak blood concentration with each compound...." Comment briefly on:

**(a)**  The accuracy of this observation.

**(b)**  The reason(s) for expecting such a proportionality under the conditions of this study.

7   Curley et al. (1971) studied the distribution and storage of polychlorinated biphenyls (PCBs) in rats. PCB isomers were fed to rats for 98 days at the level of 1000 ppm in the diet. At the end of the feeding period PCB residues were measured in selected tissues. Some of the results are given in Table 5.10. Do these data obey the plateau principle? In what tissue subcompartment are PCB's dissolved?

**Table 5.9a**  Dosing, recovery, and elimination of [$^{14}$C]trichlorofluoromethane (FC-11) in beagles

| Experiment | Dog | Sex | FC-11 Dose ppm | mg | μCi | Exposure Time (min) | Peak FC-11 in blood (μg/ml) | Exhaled FC-11 | Recovery of Radioactivity (% of inhaled dose) Exhaled $CO_2$ | Urine | Total |
|---|---|---|---|---|---|---|---|---|---|---|---|
| 1 | B | ♂ | 1900 | 410 | 10.0 | 6 | ND[a] | 128.0 | 0.32 | 0.020 | 128.3 |
| 2 | A | ♂ | 1040 | 510 | 17.2 | 14 | ND[a] | 109.1 | 0.51 | 0.008 | 109.6 |
| 3 | B | ♂ | 5300 | 2370 | 25.2 | 20 | 22.6 | 100.9 | 0.25 | 0.012 | 101.1 |
| 4[b] | A | ♂ | 4500 | 1930 | 175.0 | 15 | 17.4 | 96.2 | 0.37 | 0.007 | 96.6 |
| 5[c] | C | ♂ | 5500 | 2700 | 131.0 | 19 | 19.3 | 82.6 | 0.28 | 0.006 | 82.8 |
| 6[c] | D | ♀ | 4700 | 2880 | 178.6 | 23 | 24.7 | 92.7 | 0.09 | 0.004 | 92.8 |
| | | | | | | | Mean±SD | 101.6±14.3 | 0.30±0.13 | 0.0095±0.007 | 101.8±13.8 |

Reproduced from Blake and Mergner, 1974, Table 1.

[a] ND = not determined.

[b] Phenobarbital pretreated, 50 mg/kg for 3 days.

[c] Sacrificed at 24 hr.

Table 5.9b  Dosing, recovery, and elimination of [$^{14}$C]dichlorodifluoromethane (FC-12) in beagles

| Experiment | Dog | Sex | FC-12 Dose ppm | mg | µCi | Exposure Time (min) | Peak FC-12 in Blood (µg/ml) | Recovery of Radioactivity (% of inhaled dose) Exhaled FC-12 | Exhaled $CO_2$ | Urine | Total |
|---|---|---|---|---|---|---|---|---|---|---|---|
| 7 | A | ♂ | 9900 | 4280 | 127.2 | 20 | 12.7 | 95.9 | 0.11 | 0.02 | 96.0 |
| 8 | B | ♂ | 11800 | 4460 | 130.0 | 20 | 14.0 | 98.5 | 0.15 | 0.05 | 98.7 |
| 9[a] | E | ♀ | 8200 | 3230 | 136.9 | 15 | 8.0 | 100.2 | 0.13 | 0.03 | 100.5 |
| 10[a] | F | ♂ | 9800 | 3700 | 117.2 | 12 | 9.3 | 107.4 | 0.10 | 0.03 | 107.6 |
| 11[b] | A | ♂ | 10100 | 4035 | 101.1 | 15 | 9.4 | 112.8 | 0.21 | 0.06 | 113.1 |
| | | | | | | | Mean±SD | 103.0±6.2 | 0.14±0.04 | 0.04±0.02 | 103.2±6.3 |

Reproduced from Blake and Mergner, 1974, Table 2.
[a] Sacrificed at 24 hr.
[b] Phenobarbital pretreated, 50 mg/kg for 3 days.

**Table 5.10** PCB levels in tissues of rats following a 98-day exposure to a dietary level of 1000 ppm Aroclor 1254

| Tissue | Mean PCB Level ($\mu$g/g fresh weight) | Tissue Lipid Content (mg/g fresh weight) |
|---|---|---|
| Plasma | 18 | 10 |
| Liver | 182 | 123 |
| Brain | 102 | 96 |
| Kidney | 55 | 53 |

PCB data are derived from Curley et al., 1971, Table II, by averaging values for male and female rats. Tissue lipid contents are taken from Böhlen et al., 1973.

**8** Ethosuximide is a drug used in the treatment of petit mal epilepsy. It is completely absorbed and its half-life in adults is 53 hr. Given the data in Table 5.11, answer the following questions.

**(a)** What is the volume of distribution of ethosuximide in adults?

**(b)** Do you think it likely that ethosuximide is bound either to plasma or to tissue proteins?

**9** In children the half-life of ethosuximide is only about 30 hr and its volume of distribution is 0.63 l/kg of body weight. The therapeutic range of plasma concentrations of ethosuximide is 40–70 $\mu$g/ml (Buchanan et al., 1976), Suppose that you are a physician. Your patient is a child weighing 20 kg. You can prescribe ethosuximide in multiples of a capsule containing 100 mg of the drug. If possible, you would prefer to have your patient take the drug once rather than twice a day, to increase the likelihood of patient compliance with your instructions.

Will it be possible to prescribe a once-a-day dosage regimen? What dosage regimen will you prescribe?

**Table 5.11** Steady state plasma levels of ethosuximide in adults during chronic dosing

| | Plasma Levels ($\mu$g/ml) | |
|---|---|---|
| | Dose Rate 500 mg/day | Dose Rate 750 mg/day |
| Single daily dose | 35.7 | 51.2 |
| Multiple daily doses | 28.1 | 43.6 |
| | (2 × 250 mg) | (3 × 250 mg) |

Adapted from Goulet et al., 1976, Table II, by taking the means of the measured steady state levels.

**10**  Canrenone is a major metabolite of the diuretic spironolactone. Karim et al. (1976) monitored the maximum (4 hr after dosing) and minimum (just prior to the next dose) steady state plasma levels of canrenone during administration of the parent spironolactone in young male subjects. Spironolactone was given either as one 200-mg dose every 24 hr or as one 50-mg dose every 6 hr. Maximum and minimum plasma levels of canrenone were about 500 and 100 ng/ml on the daily dose regimen, and the minimum plasma level was about 200 ng/ml on the 4-times-daily dose regimen. Assume that the amount of canrenone formed was directly proportional to the amount of spironolactone administered.

The authors also reported that the half-life of canrenone was about 19 hr following 15 days of daily treatment, but only about 12 hr following 15 days of 4-times-daily treatment.

Are the authors' data self-consistent? In answering this question, use the instantaneous absorption model.

**11**  In a study of the uptake and distribution of hexane in rat tissues, Böhlen et al. (1973) reported the data given in Table 5.12 and Figure 5.17. Hexane is generally classified as a lipid-soluble compound, although in the blood it may be bound to plasma proteins as well.

Explain on the basis of the data given why each of the curves in Figure 5.17 rises to the height it does.

**12**  Carbamazepine, an antiepileptic drug, obeys a one-compartment body model. When Gérardin et al. (1976) gave single, oral 200-mg doses of carbamazepine to human volunteers, they found that its half-life was

**Table 5.12**  Tissue hexane content and total lipid after exposure of rats to hexane vapors, 170 g/m$^3$, for 10 hr

| Tissue | Plateau Level (mg/g fresh tissue)[a] | Total Lipids (mg/g fresh tissue) | |
|---|---|---|---|
| | | After 10 hr Exposure | Controls |
| Blood | 0.15 ± 0.01 (29) | 5 ± 1 (3) | 6 ± 1 (3) |
| Liver | — | 123 ± 7 (4) | 59 ± 10 (4) |
| Brain | 0.39 ± 0.05 (27) | 96 ± 6 (3) | 95 ± 5 (3) |
| Adrenals | 0.49 ± 0.12 (23) | 121 ± 24 (7) | 142 ± 5 (3) |
| Kidneys | 0.20 ± 0.03 (23) | 53 ± 3 (3) | 48 ± 4 (3) |
| Spleen | 0.14 ± 0.03 (22) | 30 ± 2 (3) | 29 ± 3 (3) |

From Böhlen et al., 1973, Tables 1 and 2.
[a]Calculated from all values beyond the 4-hr time; see Fig. 5.17. Means ± standard deviations are given; number of animals is in parentheses.

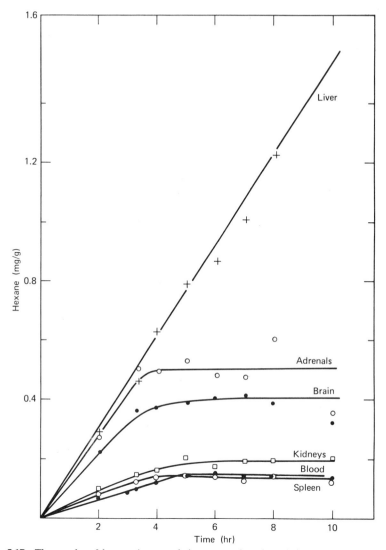

**Figure 5.17** The uptake of hexane in several tissues as a function of the length of exposure of rats to hexane vapors ($170 \text{ g/m}^3$). Each point represents the mean of values from four to six animals. Reproduced with permission from Böhlen et al., 1973, Figure 1.

$37.7 \pm 5.7$ hr and its apparent volume of distribution was 83 liters $\times f$, the fraction of the dose absorbed.

(a) What would you expect the minimum plateau level (in $\mu\text{g/ml}$) to be on chronic administration of 200 mg of carbamazepine/day?

(b) Suggest a kinetic reason for failure to reach this level (see Figure 5.18) when carbamazepine is administered to human volunteers at the rate of 200 mg/day.

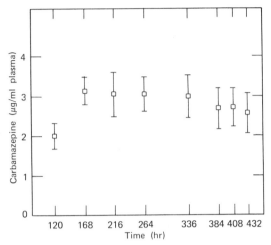

**Figure 5.18** Carbamazepine plasma concentrations at times corresponding to the minima during a 200-mg daily repeated-doses experiment in human volunteers. Adapted with permission from Gérardin et al., 1976, Figure 4.

**13**   Figures 5.19 and 5.20 show the kinetics of ethanol (EtOH) in rats following acute and chronic (zero-order) administration of the EtOH precursor ethyl acetate (EtAc). These data do not obey the plateau principle.

    **(a)**   Point out the discrepancies between these data and the predictions of the plateau principle.

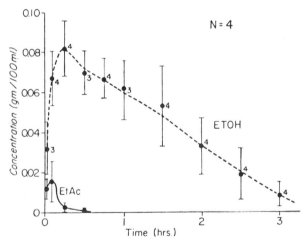

**Figure 5.19** Hydrolysis of ethyl acetate (EtAc) *in vivo*. The concentrations in blood of EtAc and ethanol (EtOH) following the injection of EtAc. Each point represents the mean ± standard deviation of values from the number of rats indicated next to each EtOH point. Reproduced from Gallaher and Loomis, 1975, Figure 2.

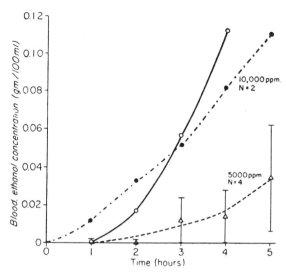

**Figure 5.20** Accumulation of ethanol in blood during inhalation of ethyl acetate vapor. O, one rat breathing 10,000 ppm; ●, one rate breathing 10,000 ppm; △, four rats breathing 5000 ppm. Reproduced with permission from Gallaher and Loomis, 1975, Figure 3.

**(b)** Propose a reasonable kinetic mechanism that would account for the observed behavior of EtOH and show how it would do so.

**14** In a special report on the principles governing the accumulation of toxic metals, the Task Group on Metal Accumulation of the Permanent Commission and International Association on Occupational Health stated (1973),

> The critical organ accumulates metal when uptake exceeds elimination. A steady state is reached when uptake and elimination are equal. Provided that the metal movement is determined by concentration gradients, a slow uptake will result in a longer time for reaching steady state. With a low elimination rate the metal will be retained for a long time even if uptake is stopped.

Comment on this passage.

**15** Moubry et al. (1968) considered the possibility that pesticide residues in the milk of dairy cows might be used as indices of the quantity of pesticide residues in the back fat. To determine whether a correlation exists between milk and back fat pesticide residues, they collected samples of milk and back fat periodically from four cows isolated from a herd that had been eating silage contaminated with DDT. During the 3-month observation period, and for about 3 weeks before it, the four cows were fed DDT-free silage. The authors concluded that there was no correlation between pesticide residues in milk and in back fat, and that

"...it was impossible to predict with accuracy the residue present in the back fat on the basis of the residue present in the butterfat."

Briefly discuss the following:

(a)  The authors' experimental design and kinetic model.

(b)  The reason(s) for the inappropriateness of this kinetic model to their stated purpose.

(c)  The kinetic model you would have used, had you been charged with the conduct of this experiment, and why you would have chosen it.

## REFERENCES

Arthur, L. J. H. and W. L. Burland. "Transfer of cephaloridine from mother to fetus." *Arch. Dis. Child.*, **44**, 82–83 (1969).

Atkinson, A. J., Jr. and J. M. Shaw. "Pharmacokinetic study of a patient with diphenylhydantoin toxicity." *Clin. Pharmacol. Ther.*, **14**, 521–528 (1973).

Blake, D. A. and G. W. Mergner. "Inhalation studies on the biotransformation and elimination of ($^{14}$C) trichlorofluoromethane and ($^{14}$C) dichlorodifluoromethane in beagles." *Toxicol. Appl. Pharmacol.*, **30**, 396–407 (1974).

Bochner, F., W. D. Hooper, J. H. Tyrer, and M. J. Eadie. "Effect of dosage increments on blood phenytoin concentrations." *J. Neurol. Neurosurg. Psych.*, **35**, 873–876 (1972).

Böhlen, P., U. P. Schlunegger, and E. Läuppi. "Uptake and distribution of hexane in rat tissues." *Toxicol. Appl. Pharmacol.*, **25**, 242–249 (1973).

Bray, R. E., R. W. Boe, and W. L. Johnson. "Transfer of ampicillin into fetus and amniotic fluid from maternal plasma in late pregnancy." *Am. J. Obstet. Gynecol.*, **96**, 938–942 (1966).

Buchanan, R. A., A. W. Kinkel, J. L. Turner, and J. C. Heffelfinger. "Ethosuximide dosage regimens." *Clin. Pharmacol. Ther.*, **19**, 143–147 (1976).

Conney, A. H., B. Carver, R. Kuntzman, and E. J. Pantuck. "Drug metabolism in normal and disease states." In *Proceedings of a Conference on Pharmacology and Pharmacokinetics: Problems and Perspectives*, T. Teorell, R. L. Dedrick, and P. G. Condliffe, Eds., Bethesda, Md., October 30–November 1, 1972; publ. Fogarty International Center Proceedings No. 20, Plenum Press, New York, 1974, pp. 147–162.

Curley, A., V. W. Burse, M. E. Grim, R. W. Jennings, and R. E. Linder. "Polychlorinated biphenyls: Distribution and storage in body fluids and tissues of Sherman rats." *Environ. Res.*, **4**, 481–495 (1971).

Davison, K. L., J. H. Cox, and C. K. Graham. "The effect of Mirex on reproduction of Japanese quail and on characteristics of eggs from Japanese quail and chickens." *Arch. Environ. Contam. Toxicol.*, **3**, 84–95 (1975).

Dettli, L. C. "Drug dosage in patients with renal disease." *Clin. Pharmacol. Ther.*, **16**, 274–280 (1974).

DiVincenzo, G. D., F. J. Yanno, and B. D. Astill. "Human and canine exposures to methylene chloride vapor." *Am. Ind. Hyg. Assoc. J.*, **33**, 125–135 (1972).

Dixon, R., M. A. Brooks, E. Postma, M. R. Hackman, S. Spector, J. D. Moore, and M. A. Schwartz. "*N*-Desmethyldiazepam: A new metabolite of chlordiazepoxide in man." *Clin. Pharmacol. Ther.*, **20**, 450–457 (1976).

Eadie, M. J. "Plasma level monitoring of anticonvulsants." *Clin. Pharmacokinet.*, 1, 52–66 (1976).

*The Effect of Disease States on Drug Pharmacokinetics*, L. Z. Benet, Ed., American Pharmacology Association–Academy of Pharmacological Science, Washington, D.C., 1976.

Gallaher, E. J. and T. A. Loomis. "Metabolism of ethyl acetate in the rat: Hydrolysis to ethyl alcohol *in vitro* and *in vivo*." *Toxicol. Appl. Pharmacol.*, 34, 309–313 (1975).

Gérardin, A. P., F. V. Abadie, J. A. Campestrini, and W. Theobald. "Pharmacokinetics of carbamazepine in normal humans after single and repeated oral doses." *J. Pharmacokinet. Biopharmaceut.*, 4, 521–535 (1976).

Gibaldi, M. "Effect of mode of administration on drug distribution in a two-compartment open system." *J. Pharm. Sci.*, 58, 327–331 (1969a).

Gibaldi, M. "Estimation of the pharmacokinetic parameters of the two-compartment open model from post-infusion plasma concentration data." *J. Pharm. Sci.*, 58, 1133–1135 (1969b).

Gibaldi, M., R. Nagashima, and G. Levy. "Relationship between drug concentration in plasma or serum and amount of drug in the body." *J. Pharm. Sci.*, 58, 193–197 (1969).

Goulet, J. R., A. W. Kinkel, and T. C. Smith. "Metabolism of ethosuximide." *Clin. Pharmacol. Ther.*, 20, 213–218 (1976).

Hoben, H. J., S. A. Ching, and L. J. Casarett. "A study of inhalation of pentachlorophenol by rats. IV. Distribution and excretion of inhaled pentachlorophenol." *Bull. Environ. Contam. Toxicol.*, 15, 466–474 (1976).

Hunter, C. G. and J. Robinson. "Pharmacodynamics of dieldrin (HEOD). I. Ingestion by human subjects for 18 months." *Arch. Environ. Health*, 15, 614–626 (1967).

Isaacs, V. E. and R. D. Schoenwald. "Estimation of pharmacological, biophasic and biological half lives of quinidine in rabbits." *J. Pharm. Sci.*, 63, 1119–1124 (1974).

Joselow, M. M., J. E. Banta, W. Fisher, and J. Valentine. "Environmental contrasts: Blood lead levels of children in Honolulu and Newark." *J. Environ. Health*, 37, 10–12 (1974).

Karim, A., J. Zagarella, T. C. Hutsell, and M. Dooley. "Spironolactone. III. Canrenone maximum steady-state plasma levels." *Clin. Pharmacol. Ther.*, 19, 177–182 (1976).

Kato, R. and J. R. Gillette. "Sex differences in the effects of abnormal physiological states on the metabolism of drugs by rat liver microsomes." *J. Pharmacol. Exp. Ther.*, 150, 285–291 (1965).

Kato, R., E. Chiesara, and G. Frontino. "Influence of sex difference on the pharmacological action and metabolism of some drugs." *Biochem. Pharmacol.*, 11, 221–227 (1962).

Knaus, R. M., F. N. Dost, D. E. Johnson, and C. H. Wang. "Fluoride distribution in rats during and after continuous infusion of $Na^{18}F$." *Toxicol. Appl. Pharmacol.*, 38, 335–343 (1976).

Koirtyohann, S. R., R. Meers, and L. K. Graham. "Mercury levels in fishes from some Missouri lakes with and without known mercury pollution." *Environ. Res.*, 8, 1–11 (1974).

Kostial, K., T. Maljković, and S. Jugo. "Lead acetate toxicity in rats in relation to age and sex." *Arch. Toxikol.*, 31, 265–269 (1974).

Kowarski. C. R., C. Giancatarino, R. Kreamer, D. Brecht, and A. Kowarski. "Measurement of sulfamethizole clearance rate by nonthrombogenic constant blood-withdrawal system." *J. Pharm. Sci.*, 65, 450–452 (1976).

Krowke, R. and D. Neubert. "Embryonic intermediary metabolism under normal and pathological conditions." In *Handbook of Teratology*, Vol. 2, *Mechanisms and Pathogenesis*, J. G. Wilson and F. C. Fraser, Eds., Plenum Press, New York, 1977, p. 120.

Krüger-Thiemer, E. "Formal theory of drug dosage regimens. I." *J. Theo. Biol.*, 13, 212–235 (1966).

La Du, B. N. "Pharmacogenetics: Single gene effects." In *Proceedings of a Conference on Pharmacology and Pharmacokinetics: Problems and Perspectives*, T. Teorell, R. L. Dedrick, and P. G. Condliffe, Eds., Bethesda, Md., October 30–November 1, 1972; publ. Fogarty International Center Proceedings No. 20, Plenum Press, New York, 1974, pp. 253–260.

Levy G. "Pharmacokinetic control and clinical interpretation of steady state blood levels of drugs." *Clin. Pharmacol. Ther.*, **16**, 130–134 (1974).

Lindstrom, F. T., J. W. Gillett, and S. E. Rodecap. "Distribution of HEOD (dieldrin) in mammals. I. Preliminary model." *Arch. Environ. Contam. Toxicol.*, **2**, 9–42 (1974).

Loo, J. C. K. and S. Riegelman. "Assessment of pharmacokinetic constants from post-infusion blood curves obtained after i.v. infusion." *J. Pharm. Sci.*, **59**, 53–55 (1970).

MacAulay, M. A., M. Abou-Sabe, and D. Charles. "Placental transfer of ampicillin." *Am. J. Obstet. Gynecol.*, **96**, 943–950 (1966).

Macdonald, H., R. G. Kelly, E. S. Allen, J. F. Noble, and L. A. Kanegis. "Pharmacokinetic studies on minocycline in man." *Clin. Pharmacol. Ther.*, **14**, 852–861 (1973).

Mitenko, P. A. and R. I. Ogilvie. "Pharmacokinetics of intravenous theophylline." *Clin. Pharmacol. Ther.*, **14**, 509–513 (1973).

Moubry, R. J., G. R. Myrdal, and W. E. Lyle. "Investigation to determine the respective amounts of DDT and its analogues in the milk and back fat of selected dairy animals." *Pestic. Monit. J.*, **2**, 47–50 (1968).

Murphy, S. D. and K. P. DuBois. "The influence of various factors on the enzymatic conversion of organic thiophosphates to anticholinesterase agents." *J. Pharmacol. Exp. Ther.*, **124**, 194–202 (1958).

Notari, R. E. *Biopharmaceutics and Pharmacokinetics. An Introduction*, Dekker, New York, 1975.

Pence, D. H., T. S. Miya, and R. C. Schnell. "Cadmium alteration of hexobarbital action: Sex related differences in the rat." *Toxicol. Appl. Pharmacol.*, **39**, 89–96 (1977).

Perrier, D. and M. Gibaldi. "Relationship between plasma or serum drug concentration and amount of drug in the body at steady state upon multiple dosing." *J. Pharmacokinet. Biopharmaceut.*, **1**, 17–22 (1973).

Pitlick, W. H. and R. H. Levy. "Time-dependent kinetics. I. Exponential autoinduction of carbamazepine in monkeys." *J. Pharm. Sci.*, **66**, 647–649 (1977).

Quinn, G. P., J. Axelrod, and B. B. Brodie. "Species, strain and sex differences in metabolism of hexobarbitone, amidopyrine, antipyrine and aniline." *Biochem. Pharmacol.*, **1**, 152–159 (1958).

Remmer, H., J. Hirschmann, and I. Greiner. "Die Bedeutung von Kumulation und Elimination für die Dosierung von Phenytoin (Diphenylhydantoin)." *Dtsch. Med. Wochenschr.* **94**, 1265–1272 (1969).

Rosenblatt, J. E., A. C. Kind, J. L. Brodie, and W. M. M. Kirby. "Mechanisms responsible for the blood level differences of isoxazolyl penicillins." *Arch. Intern. Med.*, **121**, 345–348 (1968).

Rowland, M. "Kinetics of drug-drug interactions." In *Proceedings of a Conference on Pharmacology and Pharmacokinetics: Problems and Perspectives*, T. Teorell, R. L. Dedrick, and P. G. Condliffe, Eds., Bethesda, Md., October 30–November 1, 1972; publ. Fogarty International Center Proceedings No. 20, Plenum Press, New York, 1974, pp. 321–337.

Sardemann, H., H. Colding, J. Hendel, J. P. Kampmann, E. F. Hvidberg, and R. Vejlsgaard. "Kinetics and dose calculations of amikacin in the newborn." *Clin. Pharmacol. Ther.*, **20**, 59–66 (1976).

Schnelle, K. and E. R. Garrett. "Pharmacokinetics of the $\beta$-adrenergic blocker sotalol in dogs." *J. Pharm. Sci.*, **62**, 362–375 (1973).

Shoulson, I., G. A. Glaubiger, and T. N. Chase. "On-off response: Clinical and biochemical correlations during oral and intravenous levodopa administration in Parkinsonian patients." *Neurology*, **25**, 1144–1148 (1975).

Task Group on Metal Accumulation of the Permanent Commission and International Association on Occupational Health. "Accumulation of toxic metals with special reference to their absorption, excretion and biological half-times." *Environ. Physiol. Biochem.*, **3**, 65–107 (1973), pp. 89–90.

Triggs, E. J. and R. L. Nation. "Pharmacokinetics in the aged: A review." *J. Pharmacokinet. Biopharmaceut.*, **3**, 387–418 (1975).

Van Rossum, J. M. "Pharmacokinetics of accumulation." *J. Pharm. Sci.*, **57**, 2162–2164 (1968).

Van Rossum, J. M. and A. H. M. Tomey. "Rate of accumulation and plateau plasma concentration of drugs after chronic medication." *J. Pharm. Pharmacol.*, **20**, 390–392 (1968).

Vesell, E. S. "Application of pharmacokinetic principles to the elucidation of polygenically controlled differences in drug response." *J. Pharmacokinet. Biopharmaceut.*, **1**, 521–540 (1973).

Wagner, J. G., J. I. Northam, C. D. Alway, and O. S. Carpenter. "Blood levels of drug at the equilibrium state after multiple dosing." *Nature* (*London*), **307**, 1301–1302 (1965).

Widmark, E. and J. Tandberg. "Über die Bedingungen für die Akkumulation indifferenter Narkotika. Theoretische Berechnungen." *Biochem. Z.*, **147**, 358–369 (1924).

# 6

# *Dose, Effect Relationships: Receptor Theory*

**6.1** Introduction and background

**6.2** Development of receptor theory

**6.3** Estimation of $\theta_m$ and $K_d$ from experimental data

**6.4** The effect of antagonists

    6.4.1 Competitive antagonism

    6.4.2 Noncompetitive antagonism

**6.5** The relationship between receptor theory and log dose, effect curves

**6.6** Log dose, effect curves in the presence of an antagonist

    6.6.1 Competitive antagonism

    6.6.2 Noncompetitive antagonism

    6.6.3 More complex antagonisms

**6.7** An example of the experimental use of ln dose, effect curves

**Appendix** The slope of the theoretical ln dose, effect curve

## 6.1 INTRODUCTION AND BACKGROUND

Our ultimate concern is not the concentration of drug or toxicant in peripheral tissues and plasma, but rather the effect of its presence in these tissues. In general, biologic effect is a consequence of the physicochemical combination of the drug or toxicant with metabolically or functionally important molecules. Association with receptor molecules may be chemical, as covalent bonding; physical, as hydrogen or Van der Waals bonding or electrostatic interactions; or combinations of the two. The compound (drug or toxicant) eliciting the response is called the effector or the agonist; endogenous messenger and regulator compounds such as neurotransmitters and other hormones are natural agonists. The agonist binds to the receptor molecule at the receptor site.

The concept of agonist combination with receptor site was advanced by Langley (1906) and quantitated in a simple form by Clark (1926). Clark assumed that the percentage of the maximum possible effect produced by a particular concentration of agonist was equal to the percentage of receptor sites occupied by the agonist at that concentration. Percentage occupancy was dictated by the affinity of the agonist for the receptor site. Receptor site occupancy was presumed to trigger identical effects irrespective of the identity of the agonist.

That the nature of the agonist does make a difference, however, is illustrated by the data in Figure 6.1. One of the most convenient tissue functional characteristics to use for the study of agonist dose, effect relationships *in vitro* is muscle contractility. Muscle contractility may be exploited in various ways. One of the simplest is measurement of the contractile force of an isolated muscle preparation in the presence of an agonist. Certain muscles, such as cardiac and visceral muscles, will continue to contract even in the absence of nerve (electrical) stimulation, although cardiac muscle *in vitro* is often paced by the application of an external electrical pulse. The increase in contractile force of a strip of muscle tissue suspended in a complete incubation medium such as Ringer's or Tyrode's solution is measured at a known concentration of agonist dissolved in the medium. Then the suspending solution is washed out of the bath and replaced by another containing a different concentration of agonist. In this way the contractile effects of a series of agonist concentrations can be measured and a curve relating concentration to effect can be constructed.

When the procedure just described was carried out for each of a series of alkyltrimethylammonium ions, Stephenson obtained the results shown in Figure 6.1. The isolated contractile tissue was guinea pig ileum. The relative contractions produced by the series of related agonists are shown as percentages of the maximum contraction produced by amyltrimethylammonium (amyl-TMA) ion, the most active ion of the series. It is apparent that as chain length increases, the TMA ion progressively loses its ability to elicit the maximum effect from the muscle tissue.

Stephenson proposed therefore that agonist potency is determined by two factors: affinity, and intrinsic activity or efficacy. According to Stephenson, an agonist with low efficacy must occupy a greater number of receptor sites than an agonist with high efficacy to produce the same effect. These two concepts, of agonist affinity and agonist efficacy, are now well established. An agonist that can elicit only effects of limited magnitude (i.e., one that has low efficacy) is called a partial agonist.

Other compounds may combine with the receptor molecule either at or away from the receptor site and inhibit the action of an agonist. Such compounds are called antagonists. Antagonism is not necessarily absolute. Although many antagonists elicit no effect themselves, others are partial agonists. In this case antagonism is expressed in relation to the effect of

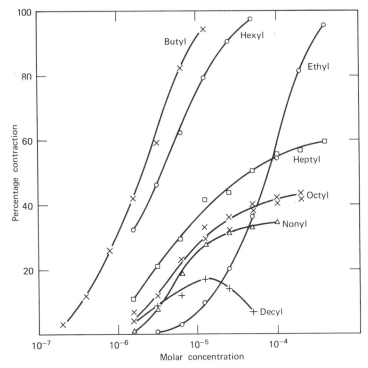

**Figure 6.1** Concentration, effect curves for several alkyltrimethylammonium ions acting on guinea pig ileum. The contractions were produced by additions to the bath to give the final concentrations indicated; each concentration was left in contact with the ileum for about 15 sec before being washed away. Reproduced with permission from Stephenson, 1956, Figure 1.

another agonist of greater efficacy. In the presence of a stronger agonist acting at the same receptor site the partial agonist becomes an antagonist with respect to the action of the second effector molecule.

The receptor site is part of a macromolecule, frequently of a protein or a nucleic acid, with a specific chemical and physical structure. Therefore combination with the active site of a receptor molecule is not different in principle from combination with the active site of an enzyme. In fact, enzymes may be receptors for drug or toxicant action. There are, however, two important quantitative differences between enzymes as receptors and regulatory macromolecules as receptors.

First, receptors involved in essential physiological regulatory mechanisms are usually highly specific for their natural agonists. This specificity reduces the likelihood that the effect will be triggered inappropriately; that is, by a "wrong" stimulus or effector molecule. Both the chemical structure and the physical attributes, such as charge distribution and surface configuration, which derive from the receptor's chemical structure and from its surrounding molecules, are critical factors determining the degree of specificity of a receptor site for potential agonist molecules.

Second, high affinity of natural agonist for receptor site achieves economy of effector molecules by insuring sensitivity of effect. Affinity is expressed in terms of the dissociation constant $K_d$ for the effector-receptor complex, where (provided the agonist binds reversibly)

$$R + X \underset{k_2}{\overset{k_1}{\rightleftharpoons}} RX \quad \text{and} \quad \frac{(R)(X)}{(RX)} = \frac{k_2}{k_1} = K_d. \tag{6.1}$$

Here R represents the number of free receptor sites, X the number of free effector molecules, and RX the number of receptor sites occupied by effector. Accordingly a small $K_d$ value represents rapid association and slow dissociation, or high affinity, whereas a large $K_d$ value represents slow association and rapid dissociation, or low affinity. Differences among affinity constants of groups of compounds for enzyme or other binding sites have been used to suggest the identity of the natural substrate (Kuntzman et al., 1965).

Characteristically, $K_d$ values for the binding of natural agonists to regulatory receptor sites are 5–7 orders of magnitude smaller than $K_m$ values for enzyme-substrate complexes. This observation is consistent with the very small quantities of neurotransmitters and other hormones present in the body compared with the large amounts of metabolic intermediates. The combination of high affinity with high specificity allows critical physiological mechanisms to be regulated by very small quantities of very highly specialized compounds.

The structures of many receptor sites have been characterized fairly completely *in situ*, and several receptors have been isolated from the tissues of which they are a part.

A receptor site is characterized *in situ* by exploiting the biologic effect associated with its occupancy. The potencies of a series of agonists that elicit this characteristic effect are correlated with their chemical and physical characteristics. The probe molecules are systematically designed by incorporating a graded series of modifications into a basic structure, whenever possible that of the natural agonist if the natural agonist is known. These modifications may be either in the chemical structure or in the conformation of the probes. From such structure-activity relationships it has been possible to deduce the essential characteristics of a number of receptor sites. Needless to say, structure-activity studies are tedious and can required sophisticated synthetic techniques. The results must also be interpreted with caution, since there can be no assurance that the probe molecule is in fact acting at the receptor site for effect rather than, for example, at a receptor site for metabolism or excretion. The example given in Chapter 2 (Section 2.8.4) is a good illustration of this point. The insect juvenile hormone analogue (JHA) studied was found to interfere competitively with metabolism of the natural hormone, thereby increasing the half-life of the natural hormone and prolonging its action. Whether JHA also bound to the receptor site for effect was not determined.

Additional information about the receptor site is available if it can be studied *in vitro*. Isolation and partial purification of a receptor allows its binding characteristics as well as its specificity to be defined. $K_d$ and $n$, the number of binding sites per receptor molecule or other unit of receptor quantity, can be determined in isolated receptor preparations by means of the Scatchard plot.

In Chapter 4 the kinetics of combination of drugs and toxicants with binding sites on plasma or tissue proteins were discussed in some detail. There we were concerned primarily with the unbound fraction of drug or toxicant because the kinetic behavior of the majority of compounds, at least at steady state, is determined by the amount unbound in the plasma. Here we are more concerned with the amount of effector-receptor complex formed, since effector action is presumed to be a consequence of association with receptor molecules.

If $X \approx X_{total} = RX + X$, and if $RX + R = R_{total}$, then from Equation 6.1

$$\frac{(RX)}{(X)} = \frac{(R)}{K_d} = \frac{R_{total} - (RX)}{K_d},$$

and

$$\frac{(RX)}{(X)} \frac{R_t}{K_d} - \frac{(RX)}{K_d}. \tag{6.2}$$

Equation 6.2 states that when the ratio of bound to free (or total) agonist is graphed as the dependent variable against the amount of bound agonist, the graph should be a straight line with ordinate intercept $R_t/K_d$ and slope $-(K_d)^{-1}$. This is the Scatchard plot introduced in Chapter 4. Note that when $(RX)/(X) = 0$, $(RX) = R_t$; that is, the abscissa intercept of a Scatchard plot gives the total number of receptor sites $R_t$ and the slope is determined only by the dissociation constant $K_d$. During purification procedures the specificity and binding properties of the isolated receptor are monitored for their constancy, to ensure identity of the final preparation with the native receptor.

Some receptors are found in the cytoplasm of the cell, whereas some are integrated into membranes. Not surprisingly the first receptors to be isolated from the intracellular milieu were soluble receptors. The steroid hormone receptors of various tissues are examples of this receptor type. They are specific not only for the steroid hormone but also for the tissue, so that the effects of these hormones are manifest only within the appropriate target tissues. For example, the uterus contains only estrogen receptors, and the prostate gland contains only androgen receptors.

The glucocorticoid receptor mechanism is particularly interesting. The initial step in receptor activation is binding of the hormone to a receptor site located in the cytoplasm, apparently as part of a soluble protein. The steroid-receptor complex formed then migrates to the nucleus, where it binds to acceptor sites whose occupancy apparently influences the expression of specific genes. Since migration of the steroid-receptor complex is greatly reduced at low temperatures, it is thought to be not a passive diffusion but a process requiring some form of activation of the steroid-receptor complex. Other hormones may also act through a two-step process; see, for example, R. A. Bradshaw (1978).

Specific binding by cytoplasmic preparations from human fetal lung and liver of dexamethasone, a potent synthetic glucocorticoid hormone, is shown in Figure 6.2. There is an exceptionally large number of glucocorticoid binding sites in fetal lung. This large binding capacity, which declines after birth, is reflected in the much larger quantity of dexamethasone bound per unit weight of lung tissue protein than per unit weight of liver protein at maximum occupancy. The Scatchard plot for the binding of dexamethasone by fetal lung and liver tissue is also shown in Figure 6.2. Since the slopes are the same, the affinity of the hormone agonist for its receptor sites in the two kinds of tissue is the same. Furthermore only one kind of site in each tissue binds dexamethasone over the range of concentrations studied, since both Scatchard plots can be fit by single straight lines. But from the abscissa intercepts it is apparent that there are 4 times as many dexamethasone receptors per unit weight of fetal lung than of fetal liver.

Membrane-bound receptors have also been isolated without significant impairment of their specificity or binding properties, even though the isolation techniques are necessarily vigorous and disruptive of the integrated

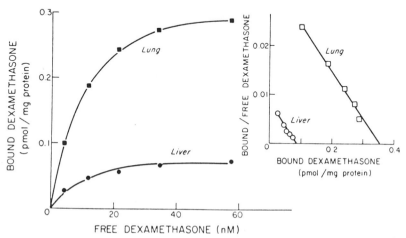

**Figure 6.2** Specific binding of dexamethasone by cytosol of human lung and liver. Cytosol was prepared from lung (5.4 mg protein/ml) and liver (12.6 mg/ml) of a $17\frac{1}{2}$-week gestation fetus and incubated at 2°C for 16 hr. Inset: Scatchard analysis of the binding data. Reproduced with permission from Ballard and Ballard, 1974, Figure 2.

supporting membrane system. A number of important receptors are membrane receptors. Examples are the glucagon and insulin receptors of hepatic and fat cell membranes and the acetylcholine (cholinergic) receptor of nerve cell membranes. All three of these receptors have been solubilized and at least partially purified.

Tsai and Lefkowitz (1978) utilized direct binding of [$^3$H]dihydroergocryptine, an antagonist of $\alpha$-adrenergic agonists, to the $\alpha$-adrenergic receptor site in partially purified canine aortic membrane preparations to identify and study the binding site. As Figure 6.3 shows, binding of the antagonist to the $\alpha$-adrenergic site is saturable with a maximum of $(145 \pm 22.6) \times 10^{-15}$ mole per milligram of protein in this particular membrane preparation. The dissociation constant is $8.8 \pm 2.6$ n$M$.

Scatchard plots for receptor-effector binding are not always linear. When they deviate from linearity, several possibilities are suggested. There may be more than one class of binding site on the receptor molecule. Alternatively even if there is only one class of binding site, occupancy of some of these sites by the agonist may be altering the affinity of the remaining sites for agonist molecules. Such site-site interactions are allosteric; that is, they are mediated from a distance through structural or conformational changes. For example, binding of acetylcholine to its receptor site in cholinergic membranes causes a shift of other binding sites in the membrane from a form having low affinity for acetylcholine to a form having high affinity for acetylcholine (Heidman and Changeux, 1978). This is an example of positive cooperativity. On the other hand, insulin appears to exhibit negative cooperativity, since Scatchard plots for insulin binding to its receptor site suggest a transition from high affinity to low affinity binding as the number of occupied receptor sites increases (Kahn et al., 1974). An alternative explanation for this type of binding behavior, which is demonstrated by a number of hormones in addition to insulin, has also been proposed (Jacobs and Cuatrecasas, 1976). Allosteric interactions are particularly important in connection with membrane receptors, for which induced conformational changes may be integral to the mechanism of action.

In general, high affinity binding is associated with high specificity and low capacity, whereas low affinity binding is associated with lower specificity and greater capacity. At the extreme is nonspecific binding, which in experimental membrane preparations may overwhelm specific binding. Specific receptors occupy only a very small fraction of the membrane surface. Potter (1967) calculated that uptake of the cardioactive drug propranolol by specific receptor sites in guinea pig atrial tissue did not exceed $1.8 \times 10^{-11}$ mole per gram of tissue, or 0.004% of the atrial cell surface. Uptake by nonspecific binding, unsaturable and proportional to the amount of propranolol presented to the membrane surface, was from 5 to 200 times the magnitude of specific uptake in the propranolol concentration range studied. When it occurs, nonspecific binding can obscure specific binding to receptors and complicate the interpretation of experimental results.

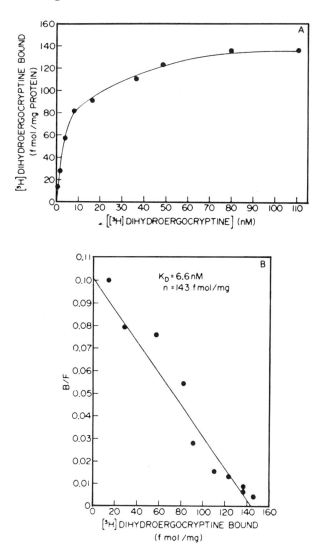

**Figure 6.3** Specific binding of [³H]dihydroergocryptine (DEC) to canine aortic membranes. (*a*) Binding as a function of DEC concentration. Each value is the mean of duplicate determinations. (*b*) Scatchard analysis of DEC binding: B/F is the ratio of bound DEC to free DEC. Reproduced with permission from Tsai and Lefkowitz, 1978, Figure 3, © 1978 by the American Society for Pharmacology and Experimental Therapeutics.

Not all drugs and toxicants act by binding at specific sites on metabolically or functionally critical macromolecules. Those that do not include certain relatively low molecular weight compounds including many of the volatile general anesthetics and probably including alcohol, which appear to interfere with normal membrane function in some nonspecific fashion, and agents that act nonspecifically in other ways as, for example, by altering the pH or the osmolarity of body fluids or by acting as chelating agents. Receptor theory does not apply to these compounds.

Receptor theory as it is developed in this chapter also does not apply to the kinetics of effect of compounds that bind irreversibly (covalently) to macromolecules. This group of compounds includes many of the chemical carcinogens, for which receptor theory must be developed in a way that takes into account irreversibility of binding with consequent potential progressive reduction in the population of available receptor sites, as well as the considerable time lag between exposure and the appearance of an observable effect.

In this context it is worthwhile to distinguish between the action of a compound and its effect. The action of an effector (agonist or antagonist) is the direct and immediate result of its combination with a receptor site. For example, the vitamin K antagonist warfarin acts by inhibiting the synthesis of vitamin K–dependent clotting factors. This action of warfarin occurs promptly upon its penetration to the site of synthesis. It is, however, only one of the effects of warfarin. Because of the intricacies of biochemical interrelationships *in vivo*, all agonists and antagonists generate more than one effect. The other effects are the outcomes of sequences of biochemical steps triggered by the action of the compound. Sometimes the most readily observable effect appears only after a significant time delay. Such effects usually are not observed until after the amount of some biochemical intermediate has decayed below a critical level. The maximum anticoagulant effect of warfarin is not seen until 2 days after peak concentrations of warfarin have appeared in the plasma. This is because the effect of inhibition of clotting factor synthesis is not manifest until natural degradative processes have reduced the available pools of these clotting factors to below a minimum level at which hypoprothrombinemia becomes clinically apparent.

In discussing the theoretical relationship between dose and effect in this chapter, we first take the term "effect" to mean either "action" or some other effect occurring promptly and without a kinetically significant time lag. The reason for this restriction will become apparent in the next section.

## 6.2   DEVELOPMENT OF RECEPTOR THEORY

The qualitative equivalence between reversible enzyme-substrate interaction and reversible receptor-effector interaction has been pointed out. In the case of enzyme catalysis the reaction rate is assumed to be proportional to the number of active sites occupied by substrate:

$$\frac{dP}{dt} = k(\text{ES}),$$

where $dP/dt$ is the rate of appearance of product $P$, (ES) is the concentration of enzyme-substrate complex, and $k$ is a proportionality constant. In the case of receptor occupancy theory the biologic effect is assumed to be proportional to the number of receptor sites occupied by agonist:

$$\theta = k_3(RX), \tag{6.3}$$

where $\theta$ is the magnitude of the effect, (RX) is the number of effector-receptor complexes, and $k_3$ is a proportionality constant.

Note that $k_3$ is not a rate constant; that is, time is not one of its dimensions. It is a proportionality constant relating magnitude of effect to the number of receptor sites occupied. This is equivalent to requiring that the effect occur instantaneously on association of effector with receptor and that it continue throughout the period of receptor occupancy. If the measured effect occurs only after a time delay, it will not be related to the number of receptor sites occupied at the time the effect is observed, as illustrated above for warfarin. Furthermore, depending on the rate-determining step in the mechanistic sequence leading to appearance of the effect, an effect later in the sequence may not be predictably related to the number of receptor sites occupied at any time.

An example is the effect of lead on the hematopoietic system. Lead has many actions. Among them is inhibition of $\delta$-aminolevulinic acid dehydrase (ALAD), an enzyme in the hematopoietic pathway. The activity of ALAD is not ordinarily rate limiting in the sequence of steps leading from succinyl-CoA to heme. At least 90% of ALAD activity can be lost without any observable effect on the rate of heme synthesis. Consequently, although mild to moderate lead exposure is directly related to a measurable inhibition of ALAD activity (Hernberg et al., 1970), the rate of heme synthesis cannot be correlated with lead exposure at these levels. It is for these reasons that we must restrict our consideration to the effects that occur without a kinetically significant time delay.

The analogy between enzyme and receptor molecules can be extended further. In enzyme catalysis the limited total number of enzyme molecules, and hence of enzyme binding sites, imposes a maximum reaction rate on the system. In receptor theory the limited number of receptor sites implies that there is some maximum possible effect that cannot be exceeded. We designate this effect $\theta_m$.

An alternative to the occupancy theory, the rate theory, states that biologic effect is proportional to the rate of combination of effector molecules with receptor sites. The rate theory predicts that the greatest response should occur at the outset, when all receptor sites are available for binding, and that response magnitude should decrease gradually as binding equilibrium is approached, finally reaching a limiting value that is identical to that predicted by the occupancy theory. The rate theory provides an explanation for at least one phenomenon that cannot be accounted for directly by the occupancy theory. This phenomenon is fade, an apparent decrease in receptor site sensitivity with continuing exposure. On the other hand, the rate theory clearly does not apply to the actions of the rather large number of drugs and toxicants that interact directly with enzymes, whose activity is known to be determined by the number of enzyme-substrate complexes formed, not by the rate of their formation. Other experimental observations are consistent with both rate and occupancy theories.

Since, as we have already seen, drugs and toxicants do not all act by the same kind of mechanism, it is entirely possible that the rate assumption applies to the action of some compounds and the occupancy assumption to the action of others. In the end, however, the distinction turns out to be rather an academic one. Penetration of effector into the compartment in which the receptor sites are located is usually the rate-determining step in the sequence from dose to activated (or inhibited) receptor. Therefore the time course of action is controlled by the rate of entry of effector into the receptor compartment. The occupancy and rate theories cannot be distinguished from each other in practice, and the occupancy theory has gained general acceptance as a reasonable and useful description of the most common mechanism of drug and toxicant action.

The assumptions on which the occupancy theory is based are in their general form analogous to those on which enzyme catalysis and membrane transport theories are based. As indicated in the previous section, it is assumed that $R_t = R + RX$ (the conservation of receptor sites) and that $X_t \approx X$ (or that $X \gg RX$). There is an important distinction to be made between receptor and enzyme catalysis or membrane transport theories, however. In receptor theory the biologic effect is considered to be proportional to the number of receptor sites occupied. The receptor-effector complex does not dissociate with generation of the effect as the enzyme-substrate complex does when product is released. Thus the receptor-effector complex does not exist in a pseudo–steady state like the enzyme-substrate complex but rather in a true equilibrium with free effector and receptor so that, as shown above,

$$K_d = \frac{(R)(X)}{(RX)}.$$

Then $\qquad K_d = \frac{(R_t - (RX))(X)}{(RX)} \qquad$ or $\qquad (RX) = \frac{(X)(R_t)}{K_d + X}.$

If it is assumed that effect, or action, is proportional to receptor occupancy,

$$\theta = k_3(RX) \qquad\qquad\qquad\qquad (6.3)$$

$$= \frac{k_3(X)(R_t)}{K_d + X}. \qquad\qquad\qquad (6.4)$$

Now $k_3 R_t$ is the maximum possible effect $\theta_m$ that would be observed if all receptor sites were occupied. (The concept of efficacy implies that $\theta_m$ need not be the same for all agonists acting at the same receptor site.) Therefore

$$\theta = \frac{(\theta_m)(X)}{K_d + X}, \tag{6.5}$$

or, if effect is expressed as a fraction of maximum effect,

$$\frac{\theta}{\theta_m} = \frac{X}{K_d + X}. \tag{6.6}$$

Not surprisingly Equation 6.6 describes a hyperbola that approaches the maximum value $\theta/\theta_m = 1$ as X becomes very large. This hyperbola is illustrated in Figure 6.4*a*. As is to be expected for a saturable process, when

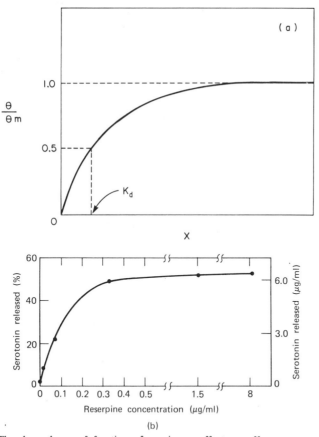

**Figure 6.4** The dependence of fraction of maximum effect on effector concentration. (*a*) Predicted relationship. (*b*) Magnitude of serotonin release from suspensions of rabbit platelets incubated for 4 hr with various concentrations of reserpine. The ordinate represents the percent of total platelet serotonin. Reproduced with permission from Carlsson et al., 1957, Figure 2, © 1957 by the Williams and Wilkins Co., Baltimore.

$\theta/\theta_m = 0.5,$

$$\frac{X}{K_d + X} = 0.5 \quad \text{and} \quad X = K_d.$$

Therefore the concentration of X required for half-maximal response is equal to $K_d$. This point is also illustrated in Figure 6.4a.

Figure 6.4b presents data from a study by Carlsson et al. (1957) of the liberation of serotonin from blood platelets *in vitro* by reserpine, an indole alkaloid with tranquilizing and hypotensive activity. The ordinate represents the percent of total platelet serotonin that was released after a 4-hr incubation with reserpine. The maximum percentage released after 4 hr was about 40–50% in different experiments. Note from Figure 6.4b that 0.1 $\mu$g of reserpine released about 4 $\mu$g of serotonin. Taking into account the difference between the molecular weights of the two compounds (609 for reserpine and 176 for serotonin), the authors calculated that one molecule of reserpine triggered the release of well over 100 molecules of serotonin.

### 6.3  ESTIMATION OF $\theta_m$ AND $K_d$ FROM EXPERIMENTAL DATA

The values of $\theta_m$ and of $K_d$ may be read directly from a graph such as Figure 6.4b, of $\theta$ against X. Alternatively one of the standard linear transforms such as the Lineweaver-Burk or the Eadie transform can be applied to dose, effect data. Use of a linear transform offers the customary advantages: less experimental work is required to define the curve fully, and linear regression techniques may be used.

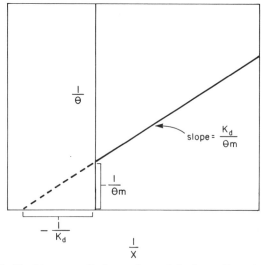

**Figure 6.5**  The Lineweaver-Burk transform of the dose, effect relationship.

The Lineweaver-Burk transform of Equation 6.5 is

$$\frac{1}{\theta} = \frac{1}{\theta_m} + \left(\frac{K_d}{\theta_m}\right)\left(\frac{1}{X}\right). \tag{6.7}$$

Equation 6.7 represents a straight line with ordinate intercept $1/\theta_m$ and slope $K_d/\theta_m$, as shown in Figure 6.5.

The classic example of linear transformation of dose, effect data is the study of Chen and Russell (1950) of the effects of cardiovascular drugs on blood pressure in dogs. In this study a series of doses of each drug was given intravenously. The doses were spaced 5 min apart, and the effect of each dose on the blood pressure was measured. The Lineweaver-Burk line of least slope

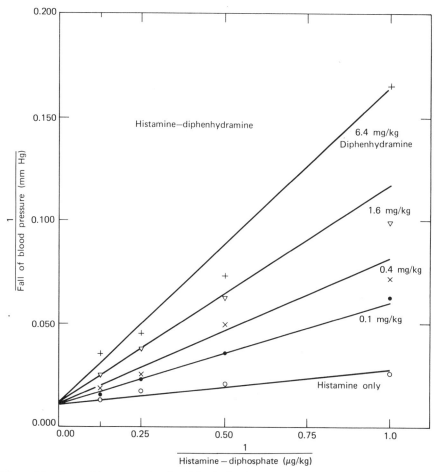

**Figure 6.6** Competitive antagonism by diphenhydramine of the blood pressure drop induced in dogs by histamine. The line of least slope represents the effect of histamine in the absence of antagonist. Reproduced with permission from Chen and Russell, 1950, Figure 4, © 1950 by the Williams and Wilkins Co., Baltimore.

in Figure 6.6 illustrates the relationship between the reciprocal of the histamine dose and the reciprocal of the fall in blood pressure induced by histamine. The maximum blood pressure drop was estimated to be 100 mm of mercury and the estimated $K_d$ value was 0.0068 $\mu$mole of histamine per kilogram of body weight.

Either of the other two linear transforms ($\theta$ as a function of $\theta/X$, or $X/\theta$ as a function of X) could in principle also have been used to analyze these data. However, in practice only the Lineweaver-Burk plot is used to any significant extent in analysis of dose, effect relationships.

## 6.4 THE EFFECT OF ANTAGONISTS

An antagonist was defined as a compound that can combine with the receptor molecule either at or away from the receptor site and by so doing inhibit the action of an agonist. A reversibly acting antagonist that binds at the receptor site is a competitive antagonist; if it binds at a site other than the receptor site, it is a noncompetitive antagonist. As might be anticipated, the standard linear transforms of dose, effect data may be used to classify the type of antagonism as competitive or noncompetitive.

### 6.4.1 Competitive Antagonism

Suppose that the antagonist Y combines reversibly with the receptor site in place of the agonist and elicits no effect (i.e., it is not a partial agonist). The antagonism scheme is shown in Figure 6.7, where $K_y$ is the dissociation constant of the antagonist-receptor complex.

The appropriate conservation equation for receptor sites is

$$R_t = R + RX + RY$$

$$= R\left(1 + \frac{(R)(X)}{K_x} + \frac{(R)(Y)}{K_y}\right);$$

$$R = \frac{R_t}{1 + \dfrac{X}{K_x} + \dfrac{Y}{K_y}}.$$

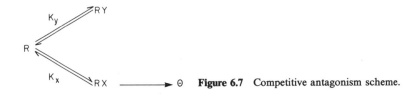

**Figure 6.7** Competitive antagonism scheme.

Now

$$\theta = k_3(\text{RX}) = \frac{k_3(\text{R})(\text{X})}{K_x}$$

$$= \frac{k_3(\text{R}_t)(\text{X})}{K_x\left(1 + \dfrac{\text{X}}{K_x} + \dfrac{\text{Y}}{K_y}\right)} ;$$

therefore

$$\theta = \frac{\theta_m(\text{X})}{\text{X} + K_x\left(1 + \dfrac{\text{Y}}{K_y}\right)} . \qquad (6.8)$$

The Lineweaver-Burk transform of Equation 6.8 is

$$\frac{1}{\theta} = \frac{1}{\theta_m} + \left(\frac{K_x}{\theta_m}\right)\left(1 + \frac{\text{Y}}{K_y}\right)\left(\frac{1}{\text{X}}\right). \qquad (6.9)$$

As expected, therefore, the slope and abscissa intercept but not the ordinate intercept of a Lineweaver-Burk plot are changed by the presence of a competitive antagonist. Figure 6.6 illustrates a competitive antagonism between diphenhydramine and histamine with respect to blood pressure fall in dogs. The antagonist diphenhydramine was given intravenously before the series of four histamine doses of 1–8 μg/kg. Diphenhydramine pretreatment alters the slope of the Lineweaver-Burk plot, but $\theta_m$ is unchanged. Chen and Russell estimated $K_y$ to be 0.84 μmole per kilogram of body weight, from which it can be concluded that diphenhydramine does not bind as tightly to the histamine receptor site as histamine does (Section 6.3).

### 6.4.2  Noncompetitive Antagonism

If the antagonist Y inactivates the receptor by binding reversibly at a site other than the receptor site, the antagonism scheme is as shown in Figure 6.8.

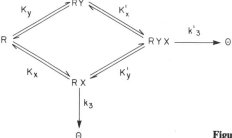

**Figure 6.8**  Noncompetitive antagonism scheme.

For the purpose of this discussion we assume that the complex RYX cannot generate the response $\theta$; that is, that $k'_3 = 0$. We do not assume, however, that the affinity of either effector for its receptor site is independent of the binding of the other; therefore we distinguish between $K_x$ and $K'_x$ and between $K_y$ and $K'_y$. The conservation equation for receptor sites is

$$R_t = R + RX + RY + RYX$$

$$= R\left(1 + \frac{X}{K_x} + \frac{Y}{K_y} + \frac{(X)(Y)}{K'_x K_y}\right).$$

$$R = \frac{R_t}{1 + \dfrac{X}{K_x} + \dfrac{Y}{K_y} + \dfrac{(X)(Y)}{K'_x K_y}}.$$

Now

$$\theta = k_3(RX) = \frac{k_3(R)(X)}{K_x}$$

$$= \frac{k_3(R_t)(X)}{K_x\left(1 + \dfrac{X}{K_x} + \dfrac{Y}{K_y} + \dfrac{(X)(Y)}{K'_x K_y}\right)};$$

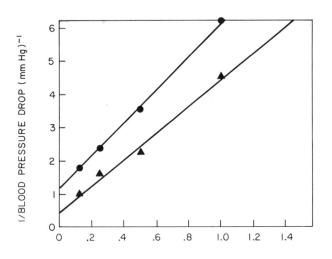

Figure 6.9 Noncompetitive antagonism by ergotamine of the blood pressure drop induced in dogs by histamine: ▲, histamine alone; ●, histamine in the presence of 1 mg ergotamine/kg. Redrawn from Chen and Russell, 1950, Figure 4.

therefore

$$\theta = \frac{\theta_m(X)}{K_x\left(1 + \dfrac{Y}{K_y}\right) + X\left[1 + \left(\dfrac{Y}{K_y}\right)\left(\dfrac{K_x}{K_x'}\right)\right]}.\tag{6.10}$$

The Lineweaver-Burk transform of Equation 6.10, simplified by taking into consideration the fact that $K_x'K_y = K_y'K_x$, is

$$\frac{1}{\theta} = \frac{1}{\theta_m}\left[1 + \frac{Y}{K_y'}\right] + \left(\frac{K_x}{\theta_m}\right)\left(1 + \frac{Y}{K_y}\right)\left(\frac{1}{X}\right).\tag{6.11}$$

Accordingly it is apparent that both the slope and the ordinate intercept of a Lineweaver-Burk plot are changed by the presence of a noncompetitive antagonist. Whether the abscissa intercept is altered depends on whether $K_x = K_x'$, since when $1/\theta = 0$,

$$\frac{1}{X} = -\frac{1 + \left(\dfrac{Y}{K_y}\right)\left(\dfrac{K_x}{K_x'}\right)}{K_x\left(1 + \dfrac{Y}{K_y}\right)}.$$

If $K_x = K_x'$, $(1/X) = -1/K_x$ when $1/\theta = 0$.

The Lineweaver-Burk line representing antagonism of histamine by ergotamine in the study by Chen and Russell is shown in Figure 6.9. The action of ergotamine, unlike that of diphenhydramine, is noncompetitive with respect to histamine.

Note that the slopes of the inhibited and uninhibited lines in Figure 6.9 are not greatly different. Under what conditions is this behavior to be expected? That is, when does the presence of a noncompetitive antagonist have little effect on the slope of a Lineweaver-Burk line?

Consider the form of Equation 6.11. If $K_y$ were very much greater than $K_y'$, there would be a range of antagonist concentrations within which $Y > K_y'$ but $Y \ll K_y$, so that the factor $1 + Y/K_y$ in the second term of the right-hand side of Equation 6.11 would be very small. Y would have little effect on the slope of a Lineweaver-Burk line in this concentration range. Physically this behavior means that the binding of agonist to the receptor site greatly facilitates the binding of the noncompetitive antagonist to the inhibitory site. In its most extreme form, the limiting situation, the antagonist can bind to the receptor *only* if the agonist is already in place on the receptor site. $K_y$ approaches infinity and the slopes of Lineweaver-Burk lines are the same irrespective of the presence or absence of antagonist. This type of noncompetitive antagonism is called uncompetitive antagonism. Chen and Russell interpreted the ergotamine-histamine interaction as an uncompetitive antagonism.

## 6.5   THE RELATIONSHIP BETWEEN RECEPTOR THEORY AND LOG DOSE, EFFECT CURVES

In general we would like to be able to relate the magnitude of an effect, $\theta$, to the amount of effector present in such a way that the expressed relationship is readily interpretable and is amenable to statistical treatment if this is desired. As we have seen, the Lineweaver-Burk plot is one useful form. Another form that is more commonly used than the Lineweaver-Burk plot is the log dose, effect graph.

A word should be said here about the relationship of dose to the amount of effector reaching the receptor site. In the analysis of dose, effect data it is nearly always assumed that the two measures of exposure are equal, or at least proportional. In an isolated experimental setup such as an enzyme assay or an *in vitro* system for measurement of the contractility of a strip of tissue, identity of the amount of effector added to the system with the amount having access to the receptor site is reasonably certain. But the assumption of proportionality is not always justified in whole animal studies, particularly in the case of acute administration. If the receptor site is in a poorly perfused, slowly equilibrating tissue the concentration of effector at the receptor site may not achieve a steady state relationship with that in the plasma. In this case neither dose nor plasma concentration would be proportional to the concentration in the biophase.

For the purposes of this chapter we must assume that the quantity of effector that penetrates to the receptor site is proportional to the dose. In Chapter 7 we consider the relationship between dose and biophase concentration.

When an expression such as

$$\theta = \frac{(\theta_m)(\mathrm{X})}{K_d + \mathrm{X}},\tag{6.5}$$

which is a hyperbola when graphed in a linear coordinate system, is plotted in a semilogarithmic coordinate system (the abscissa being in logarithms in this case), it is a sigmoid curve. This observation is the consequence of applying to the particular convex curvature of the hyperbola the particular distortion associated with the logarithmic transformation of dose. It is perhaps best illustrated by consideration of the behavior of the idealized Equation 6.5 when it is graphed in this coordinate system.

Equation 6.5 can be rewritten in the dimensionless form

$$\frac{\theta}{\theta_m} = \frac{\mathrm{X}/K_d}{1 + \mathrm{X}/K_d}.$$

Figure 6.10 is a graph of the quantity $\theta/\theta_m$ as a function of the logarithm of the experimental variable $\mathrm{X}/K_d$ over the range $0.1 - 10.0$. The data that would

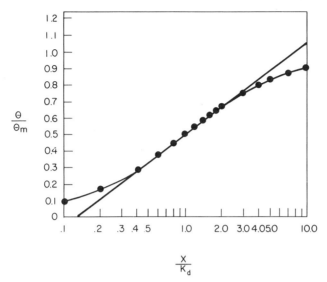

**Figure 6.10** The theoretical log dose, fraction of maximum effect relationship. The slope at the midpoint is also shown.

generate a hyperbola in a linear coordinate system generate a sigmoid curve when the abscissa is scaled in logarithms.

That the sigmoid curve so generated is symmetrical can be demonstrated by calculating its slope. It can be shown (see Appendix) that the theoretical slope of a graph of $\theta/\theta_m$ as a function of $\ln X$ is

$$\frac{d(\theta/\theta_m)}{d\ln X} = \left(\frac{\theta}{\theta_m}\right)\left(1 - \frac{\theta}{\theta_m}\right).$$

In Figure 6.11 this theoretical slope is graphed against $\theta/\theta_m$ for values of $\theta/\theta_m$ from 0.05 to 0.95. It is clear that the ln dose, effect curve is symmetrical and that its inflection point (i.e., the point of its maximum slope) is at half-maximum effect, as Figure 6.10 suggests. Furthermore, the value of this maximum slope is independent of the value of any parameter characterizing either the effector or the receptor, and should be about 0.25 as long as the conditions under which receptor occupancy theory was developed are applicable; that is, as long as one molecule of effector binds reversibly to one receptor site and as long as the number of effector molecules so bound is insignificant compared to the total. Under these conditions ln dose, effect curves for different agonists acting at the same receptor site should be parallel.

Several observations may be made based on Figures 6.10 and 6.11. Although between 30 and 70% of maximum response the theoretical variation in slope is 16% on either side of the maximum slope, Figure 6.10 shows that it is unlikely that these deviations from linearity would be noticeable within the

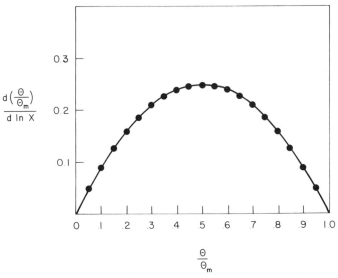

**Figure 6.11**  The slope of the theoretical log dose, effect relationship as a function of the fraction of maximum effect.

experimental variability of a data set, particularly if relatively few observations were made. Careful experimental work might be expected to reveal the greater bending of the ln dose, effect curve predicted at 20 and 80% maximum response. In fact, as examples throughout the rest of this chapter demonstrate, ln dose, effect curves are often quite linear even between 20 and 80% maximum response. Because this transformation tends to linearize the dose, effect relationship in the midrange where effect is usually measured, it has become conventional to graph dose, effect data in this way. Not only can the line segments obtained be analyzed statistically, but also the relationship between magnitude of dose and magnitude of effect is expressed directly rather than reciprocally as in the Lineweaver-Burk plot.

A further advantage of the ln dose, effect graph is that the inflection point occurs at half-maximum effect where $X = K_d$ (Figure 6.10). Therefore $K_d$ can conveniently be read directly from the abscissa of a ln dose, effect plot. But a more important implication of this statement is that the position of a ln dose, effect curve on the ln dose axis is determined by $K_d$; that is, by the affinity of the agonist for its receptor site. Curves for low-affinity agonists, for which $K_d$ is larger, will be displaced to the right of curves for high-affinity agonists.

As an illustration of the transformation of a hyperbola to a sigmoid curve by logarithmic distortion of the abscissa, consider the results of a study of the inhibition of rat hepatic nitroreductase activity by hexachlorophene (Gandolfi et al., 1974). Data for this inhibition are graphed in Figure 6.12, first in a linear coordinate system and then with transformation of the abscissa (dose axis) to a logarithmic scale. A reasonable estimate of the slope at 50%

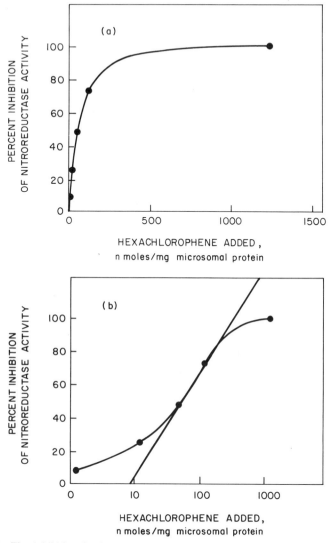

**Figure 6.12** The inhibition by hexachlorophene of rat hepatic nitroreductase activity. (*a*) Graphed in a linear coordinate system. (*b*) Graphed semilogarithmically. Data are taken from Gandolfi et al., 1974.

maximum response is also drawn in Figure 6.12*b*. The slope of the line drawn is 0.62; the theoretical slope at this point, translated from natural logarithms to logarithms to the base 10, would be 0.58. Evidently the assumptions under which the receptor occupancy theory was derived do apply to the inhibition of rat liver nitroreductase by hexachlorophene.

A good example of the use of ln dose, effect curves to assist in the interpretation of dose, effect data is provided by the study by Chan and

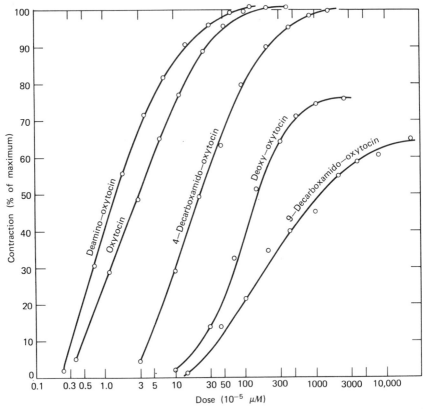

**Figure 6.13** Log dose, effect curves for a series of structural analogues of oxytocin acting on the rat uterine horn. The maximum response to oxytocin itself was taken as 100%. Each curve represents the average value of at least six curves. Reproduced with permission from Chan and Kelley, 1967, Figure 2, © 1967 by the Williams & Wilkins Co., Baltimore.

Kelley (1967) of oxytocin analogues. Figure 6.13 illustrates the relative ability of a series of structural analogues of the hormone oxytocin to induce contractions in the isolated rat uterine horn. The maximum effect of oxytocin itself was taken to represent $\theta_m$. Oxytocin has six functional groups; the authors evaluated the importance of five of these groups to the affinity of oxytocin for its receptor site and to its efficacy. Lowered affinity should result in parallel displacement of the ln dose, effect curves to the right on the ln dose axis, whereas lowered efficacy should result in a reduction in the height of the asymptote that the curve approaches. As Figure 6.13 shows, loss of either of the carboxamide groups or of the hydroxyl group results in lowered affinity for the oxytocin receptor, whereas loss of either the hydroxyl group or the carboxamide group at position 9 results in a reduction in intrinsic activity of the hormone. The 5-decarboxamido analogue was wholly inactive. The amino group has no significant influence on either the affinity or the efficacy of oxytocin. Note that the slope at the midpoint of the oxytocin log dose, effect curve is about 0.52.

Affinity, of course, is determined by the structure and conformation of the receptor site as well as by the nature of the agonist. Any factor operating to alter the receptor site in such a way as to alter its binding properties is to be expected to modify the affinity of agonists for the site. Such alterations may occur during a prolonged experiment with tissue *in vitro*. They are referred to as "aging" of the tissue preparation. The possibility of their occurrence requires that control tissue be maintained and monitored regularly throughout the entire experimental period.

Other examples of the importance of the structure and conformation of the receptor site itself are the genetically determined drug sensitivities. In some cases these are due to the presence in the sensitive person of an abnormal metabolizing enzyme or other key macromolecule whose affinity for the drug is significantly below normal levels. Most persons who are sensitive to succinylcholine, for example, possess two genes for a defective type of cholinesterase with very low affinity for choline esters. As a consequence of its low affinity, the defective esterase is unable to metabolize succinylcholine efficiently, prolonging the half-life and intensifying the effect of the drug (Kalow and Genest, 1957). An example of a low affinity apparently defective regulatory receptor site is the insulin receptor site in persons designated obese-hyperglycemic. These persons are unable to utilize glucose efficiently in spite of the presence of elevated levels of circulating insulin.

## 6.6 LOG DOSE, EFFECT CURVES IN THE PRESENCE OF AN ANTAGONIST

### 6.6.1 Competitive Antagonism

Since competitive antagonism results in general in an increase in the apparent $K_d$ but no change in $\theta_m$, we would predict that in the presence of a competitive antagonist the ln dose, effect curve should be shifted to higher agonist concentrations. In addition it can be shown (see Appendix) that in the case of competitive inhibition the theoretical slope of a ln dose, effect curve is not changed.

Figure 6.14 illustrates an antagonism by lachesine [the benzylate ester of ethyldimethyl (2-hydroxymethyl) ammonium chloride] of the contractile effect of acetyl-$\beta$-methylcholine on isolated pieces of guinea pig ileum (Kuhnen-Clausen, 1972). Increasing concentrations of lachesine cause the ln dose, effect curve to shift successively farther to the right but do not affect either $\theta_m$ or the slopes at the midpoints of the curves. Lachesine is therefore a competitive antagonist of acetyl-$\beta$-methylcholine with respect to its action on guinea pig ileum.

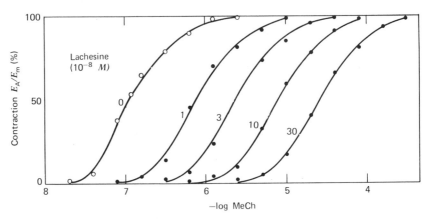

**Figure 6.14** Log dose, effect curves for acetyl-$\beta$-methylcholine (MeCh), acting on the isolated guinea pig ileum, in the presence of various constant concentrations of lachesine: $E_A$ = effect induced by a given agonist concentration; $E_m$ = maximum agonist effect in the absence of lachesine. The symbols are single values; each set of curves was made with one separate piece of the ileum. Reproduced with permission from Kuhnen-Clausen, 1972, Figure 2.

### 6.6.2  Noncompetitive Antagonism

In the presence of a noncompetitive antagonist $\theta_m$ is reduced but $K_d$ may or may not be affected. Accordingly we would predict that in the presence of a noncompetitive antagonist the maximum height achieved by the ln dose, effect curve would be reduced. The Appendix shows that the slope of the theoretical ln dose, effect curve should also be changed, by the factor

$$\frac{1 - B(\theta/\theta_m)}{1 - \theta/\theta_m},$$

where $B$ is $(1 + Y/K_y')$, whenever Y is a noncompetitive inhibitor.

Figure 6.15 shows antagonism of the hypotensive effect of lobeline by two ganglion-blocking agents (Suwandi and Bevan, 1966). The animal model was the anesthetized cat, infused with the ganglion-blocking agents, then injected with the indicated doses of lobeline to obtain the ln dose, effect curve. Measurements were made over a 12-hr period, and the authors monitored the unantagonized lobeline dose, effect curve during this period to ensure that it did not change. As Figure 6.15 shows, the ganglion-blocking agent hexamethonium (C-6) is a competitive antagonist and chlorisondamine is a noncompetitive antagonist.

### 6.6.3  More Complex Antagonisms

The example of uncompetitive antagonism given in Section 6.4.2 demonstrates that antagonism by one drug or toxicant of the effect of another is not

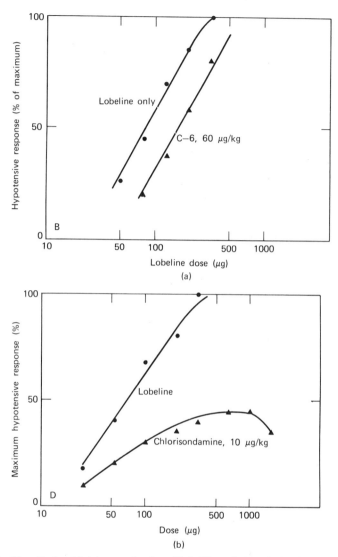

**Figure 6.15** The effects of (*a*) hexamethonium (C-6) (60 μg/kg) and (*b*) chlorisondamine (10 μg/kg) on the reflex hypotensive effect curve of lobeline administered intravenously to cats anesthetized with α-chloralose: ●, controls; ▲, after drug. Adapted with permission from Suwandi and Bevan, 1966, Figure 3, © 1966 by the Williams & Wilkins Co., Baltimore.

always simple competitive or simple noncompetitive. Many antagonisms do fall into one or the other of these two broad categories; the distinction between competitive and noncompetitive antagonism has proved useful because it is based on a fundamental difference in the mechanism of the interaction. However, many antagonisms are not readily classifiable into one category or the other.

Certain antagonists bind irreversibly or essentially irreversibly (i.e., they are not released to any appreciable extent during the period the agonist is in contact with the receptor tissue), either to the receptor site itself or to another site whose occupancy blocks the appearance of an effect. Some irreversible antagonists are alkylating agents; the alkylating agent dibenamine has been used as an experimental tool, as will be shown below.

Irreversible binding can lead to erroneous interpretation of ln dose, effect curves. For example, if irreversible binding at a site other than the receptor site should cause a conformational change altering $K_m$, the antagonist would appear to be acting competitively and reversibly. On the other hand, irreversible binding to the receptor site would appear to be a noncompetitive antagonism, provided maximum effect is associated with full receptor occupancy. When partial receptor occupancy is sufficient to elicit the maximum possible effect, there are said to be spare receptors for the agonist with respect to the effect, and the interpretation of ln dose, effect curves, particularly in the presence of an antagonist, becomes very much more complicated.

The existence of spare receptors was first proposed by Nickerson (1956) to explain the anomalous effect of dibenamine, which appeared to be a reversible competitive antagonist of either adrenaline or histamine except at very high antagonist concentrations, although it was known to bind nearly irreversibly at or near the receptor site. Nickerson pointed out that antagonists binding irreversibly to the receptor site would exhibit anomalous behavior in the presence of spare receptors. Remember that the number RX of receptor sites occupied by a given amount X of agonist is directly proportional to the total number $R_t$ of receptor sites available:

$$(RX) = \frac{(R_t)(X)}{K_d + X}.$$

Now suppose that the maximum effect $\theta_m$ is not $k_3 R_t$ but some fraction thereof, say $\alpha k_3 R_t$. When $R_t$ is reduced to $R_t'$ by a noncompetitive antagonist, X must be increased if the degree of occupancy RX is to be achieved. Since $K_d$ represents the concentration of agonist at which half the maximum effect is observed, it will therefore appear larger when $R_t$ is reduced. Nonetheless $\theta_m$ is still achievable as long as $\alpha R_t$ is less than $R_t'$. Therefore an antagonist that binds irreversibly to the receptor site will appear to be a competitive antagonist until the total number of available receptor sites has been reduced to a critical level below which the maximum possible effect is no longer achievable.

The interpretation of ln dose, effect curves for partial agonists is particularly difficult whenever spare receptors are present. A partial agonist may be capable of eliciting the maximum effect in the presence of spare receptors even though it cannot do so in their absence. Suppose that a potent agonist can elicit the maximum effect by binding to 10% of the existing receptors. Then a partial agonist that produces only 50% of the maximum effect when it is bound to 10% of the receptors will produce the maximum effect when it occupies 20% of the receptors. Therefore the partial agonist will appear to have the same efficacy as the full agonist but a lower affinity, although in fact its efficacy is only half as great as that of the full agonist.

One way to approach the study of partial agonists in systems with spare receptor sites is to block a critical number of those sites. The neurotransmitter acetylcholine provokes the contraction of strips of small intestine. It is a potent agonist and there are spare receptors present with respect to this measure of effect. When the nearly irreversible antagonist dibenamine is added to the tissue incubation medium, the number of receptor sites blocked increases with the length of the incubation period (Furchgott, 1954).

Figure 6.16 shows what happens when strips of rat small intestine suspended in a solution containing dibenamine are tested at intervals for their contractile response to acetylcholine and to the partial agonists ethyltrimethylammonium ion (Et TMA) and butyrylcholine (BuCh) (Takagi et al., 1968). After a 10-min incubation the acetylcholine curve is displaced to the right but is still parallel to the unantagonized curve and achieves the same maximum height. The curves for the two partial agonists, however, are both displaced to the right and reduced in magnitude. With BuCh the slope is also reduced. Ethyltrimethylammonium ion displays intermediate behavior; it is a stronger agonist than butyrylcholine (cf. Figure 6.1). After a 20-min incubation the effect of Et TMA is greatly reduced and that of BuCh has been nearly abolished. After a 30-min incubation the number of receptor sites has been so drastically reduced that even the potent agonist acetylcholine is unable to elicit much more than 50% of the maximum effect. In other words, the number of receptors sensitive to acetylcholine has become limiting.

Like irreversible antagonists that bind to the receptor site, reversible noncompetitive antagonists will appear to be acting competitively in the presence of spare receptors unless the total number of available receptor sites has been reduced to a critical minimum by the presence of antagonist. An irreversible block of spare receptors can be useful also in experimental studies of reversible noncompetitive antagonism. Figure 6.17, taken from the same study as Figure 6.14 (Kuhnen-Clausen, 1972), illustrates antagonism of the contractile effect of acetyl-$\beta$-methylcholine on guinea pig ileum by the noncompetitive antagonist toxogonin, a bisquaternary pyridine, before and after treatment of the tissue with dibenamine for 30 min. Curves obtained before treatment suggest that toxogonin is a competitive inhibitor, but the curves obtained after treatment show that it is in fact a noncompetitive inhibitor. Note also that after reduction of the total number of available receptors by dibenamine treatment, more acetyl-$\beta$-methylcholine is required to elicit a response of a given magnitude, as would be expected. The shapes of the ln dose, effect curves for inhibition by lachesine of the effect of acetyl-$\beta$-methylcholine, shown in Figure 6.14 as an example of competitive inhibition, were not changed by treatment of the tissue with dibenamine, although the curves were shifted to the right on the ln dose axis.

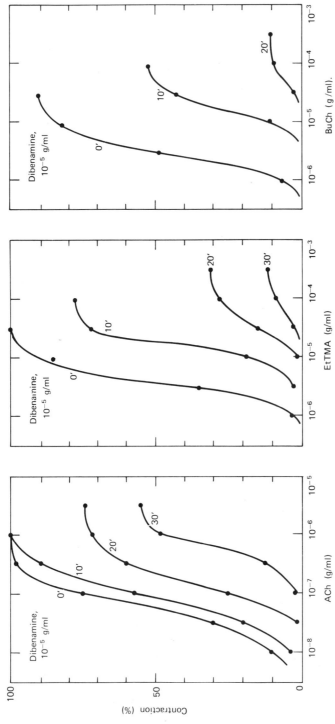

**Figure 6.16** The effects of dibenamine on the log dose, effect curves for acetylcholine (ACh), ethyltrimethylammonium ion (EtTMA), and butyrylcholine (BuCh) acting on rat small intestine: 0′, before incubation; 10′, 20′, and 30′, after 10-, 20-, and 30-min incubations, respectively. Adapted with permission from Takagi et al., 1968, Figure 5.

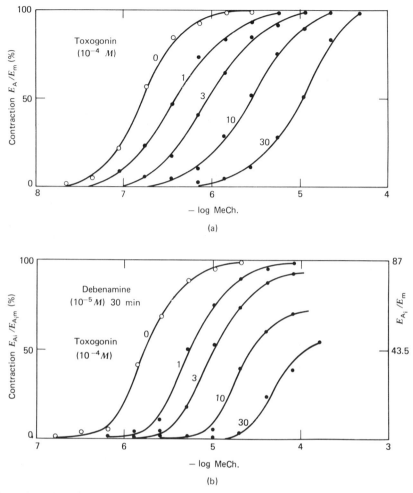

**Figure 6.17** Log dose, effect curves for acetyl-$\beta$-methylcholine (MeCh) in the presence of various constant concentrations of the bisquaternary pyridine toxogonin (*a*) without and (*b*) after treatment of the isolated guinea pig ileum with dibenamine: $E_A$ = effect induced by a given agonist concentration; $E_m$ = maximum agonist effect; $E_{A_i}$ and $E_{A_i m}$ = effects of the agonist after dibenamine blockade of the receptor reserve. Reproduced with permission from Kuhnen-Clausen, 1972, Figure 4.

## 6.7   AN EXAMPLE OF THE EXPERIMENTAL USE OF LN DOSE, EFFECT CURVES

It has been suggested that the externally located cellular membrane enzyme $Na^+$-$K^+$-ATPase is the pharmacologic receptor for the cardiac glycoside digitalis. Caldwell and Nash (1978) studied the *in vitro* behavior of two amino sugar cardiac glycosides that appeared to be highly potent pharmacological agents *in vivo*. The two amino sugar glycosides were 3-$\beta$-$O$-(4-amino-4,6-

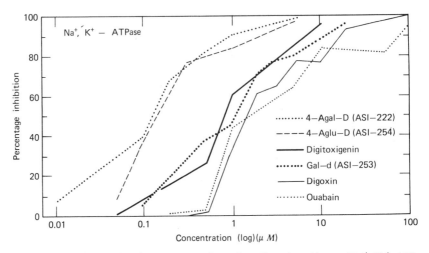

**Figure 6.18** The effects of various concentrations of cardiac glycosides on Na$^+$-K$^+$-ATPase activity. Each observation is the mean of five to eight determinations. Reproduced with permission from Caldwell and Nash, 1978, Figure 1, © 1978 by the American Society for Pharmacology and Experimental Therapeutics.

dideoxy-$\beta$-D-galactopyranosyl) digitoxigenin (ASI-222) and 3-$\beta$-$O$-(4-amino-4,6-dideoxy-$\beta$-D-glucopyranosyl) digitoxigenin (ASI-254). Two effects were studied: inhibition of swine brain Na$^+$-K$^+$-ATPase activity, and stimulation of the contractile force of isolated rabbit atrium. The results were compared with the effects of digoxin, ouabain, and the structurally related nonamino, nondeoxy sugar cardiac glycoside 3-$\beta$-$O$-($\beta$-D-galactopyranosyl) digitoxigenin (ASI-253).

Figure 6.18 shows the effects of the different cardiac glycosides on Na$^+$-K$^+$-ATPase activity. The $K_I$ value; that is, the inhibitor concentration

**Table 6.1** $K_I$ values for inhibition of Na$^+$-K$^+$-ATPase activity and for stimulation of atrial contractile force by various cardiac glycosides

| Cardiac Glycoside | $K_I$ ($\mu M$) | |
|---|---|---|
| | Na$^+$-K$^+$-ATPase Inhibition | Atrial Con-tractile Force |
| ASI-222 | 0.13 | 0.152 |
| ASI-254 | 0.145 | 0.097 |
| ASI-253 | 1.15 | 0.88 |
| Digoxin | 1.6 | 1.20 |
| Ouabain | 1.75 | 0.84 |

Data of Caldwell and Nash, 1978.

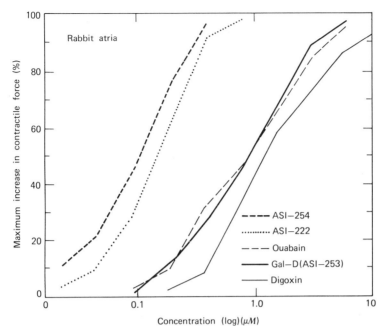

**Figure 6.19** The effects of various concentrations of cardiac glycosides on contractile force of isolated rabbit atria electrically driven at 1 Hz. Each point represents the mean of five to seven observations. Reproduced with permission from Caldwell and Nash, 1978, Figure 2, © 1978 by the American Society for Pharmacology and Experimental Therapeutics.

at which the enzyme activity is 50% inhibited, is given in Table 6.1 for each glycoside. ASI-222 and ASI-254 are about equally potent, and about 10 times as effective as the other glycosides shown.

Figure 6.19 shows the effects of the different cardiac glycosides on atrial contractile force. The concentration at which 50% of the maximum increase in contractile force was observed is also given for each glycoside in Table 6.1. Again, ASI-222 and ASI-254 are 5–10 times as potent as the other glycosides. All elicited about the same maximum increase in contractile force, $243 \pm 23$ to $275 \pm 28\%$; and all ln dose, effect curves were roughly parallel.

It can be concluded that incorporation of a 4-amino group into the sugar moiety of a cardiac glycoside greatly increases the potency of the glycoside in these two test systems. Furthermore, the excellent correlation between $Na^{+}$-$K^{+}$-ATPase inhibitory ability and contractile force stimulatory ability, as expressed in the $K_I$ values, supports the concept that the inhibitory action of the glycosides on $Na^{+}$-$K^{+}$-ATPase is the rate-limiting step in the production of the increase in cardiac contractile force that is the characteristic effect of the cardiac glycosides.

### APPENDIX   THE SLOPE OF THE THEORETICAL LN DOSE, EFFECT CURVE

**Agonist Only**

$$\frac{\theta}{\theta_m} = \frac{X}{K_x + X} .$$

Taking natural logarithms of both sides,

$$\ln\left(\frac{\theta}{\theta_m}\right) = \ln X - \ln(K_x + X);$$

and differentiating both sides of this equation,

$$d\ln\left(\frac{\theta}{\theta_m}\right) = d\ln X - d\ln(K_x + X).$$

$$\frac{d(\theta/\theta_m)}{\theta/\theta_m} = d\ln X - \frac{dX}{K_x + X} .$$

$$\frac{d(\theta/\theta_m)}{d\ln X} = \left(\frac{\theta}{\theta_m}\right)\left(1 - \frac{dX}{(d\ln X)(K_x + X)}\right)$$

$$= \left(\frac{\theta}{\theta_m}\right)\left(1 - \frac{X}{K_x + X}\right)$$

$$= \left(\frac{\theta}{\theta_m}\right)\left(1 - \frac{\theta}{\theta_m}\right).$$

**Agonist with Competitive Antagonist**

$$\frac{\theta}{\theta_m} = \frac{X}{AK_x + X} ,$$

where $A = 1 + Y/K_y$.

Taking natural logarithms and differentiating,

$$d\ln\left(\frac{\theta}{\theta_m}\right) = d\ln X - d\ln(AK_x + X).$$

$$\frac{d(\theta/\theta_m)}{\theta/\theta_m} = d\ln X - \frac{dX}{AK_x + X}$$

$$\frac{d(\theta/\theta_m)}{d\ln X} = \left(\frac{\theta}{\theta_m}\right)\left(1 - \frac{dX}{(d\ln X)(AK_x + X)}\right)$$

$$= \left(\frac{\theta}{\theta_m}\right)\left(1 - \frac{X}{AK_x + X}\right)$$

$$= \left(\frac{\theta}{\theta_m}\right)\left(1 - \frac{\theta}{\theta_m}\right).$$

*Agonist with Noncompetitive Antagonist*

$$\frac{\theta}{\theta_m} = \frac{X}{AK_x + BX},$$

where $A = (1 + Y/K_y)$ and $B = (1 + Y/K_y')$.
Taking natural logarithms and differentiating,

$$d\ln\left(\frac{\theta}{\theta_m}\right) = d\ln X - d\ln(K_x A + BX)$$

$$\frac{d(\theta/\theta_m)}{\theta/\theta_m} = d\ln X - \frac{BdX}{K_x A + BX}$$

$$\frac{d(\theta/\theta_m)}{d\ln X} = \left(\frac{\theta}{\theta_m}\right)\left(1 - \frac{BdX}{(d\ln X)(K_x A + BX)}\right)$$

$$= \left(\frac{\theta}{\theta_m}\right)\left(1 - \frac{BX}{K_x A + BX}\right)$$

$$= \left(\frac{\theta}{\theta_m}\right)\left(1 - B\left(\frac{\theta}{\theta_m}\right)\right).$$

## PROBLEMS

1  Given the scheme in Figure 6.20, where R is the receptor site, X the natural agonist, Y a partial agonist that competitively inhibits the action of X, and Z a reversible noncompetitive antagonist that does not completely block the action of X (e.g., $k_3 < k_2$):

(a)  Would Lineweaver-Burk lines for antagonism of X by Y be straight?
(b)  Would Lineweaver-Burk lines for antagonism of X by Z be straight?

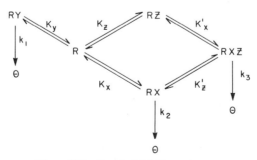

**Figure 6.20**  Sample inhibition scheme.

**2** The antihypertensive drug diazoxide appears to be a more potent hypotensive agent in hypertensive rats than in normal rats. Wohl et al. (1968) undertook an *in vitro* study to investigate the effect of diazoxide on barium-induced contraction of aortic segments taken from normotensive and hypertensive rats. Are their data (Figure 6.21) consistent with the increased potency of diazoxide in hypertensive animals *in vivo*?

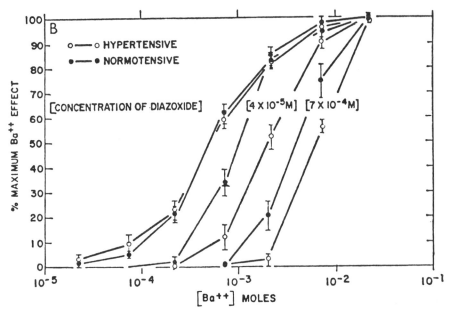

**Figure 6.21** The effect of diazoxide on log dose, effect curves for barium ion acting on aortic segments from normotensive and hypertensive rats. Each point is the mean of at least four observations. Brackets indicate ± standard error. Reproduced with permission from Wohl et al., 1968, Figure 1, © 1968 by the Williams & Wilkins Co., Baltimore.

**3** One of the agents used by Chen and Russell (1950) in their study of the effects of cardiovascular drugs on blood pressure in dogs was epinephrine, which causes a rise in blood pressure. From their data (Table 6.2), determine whether yohimbine is a competitive or a noncompetitive antagonist of epinephrine, and estimate $\theta_m$, $K_x$ (for epinephrine) and $K_y$ (for yohimbine). (Estimate the two dissociation constants in units of $\mu$g/kg.)

**4** Glenn et al. (1967) studied the pharmacologic effect of the antiinflammatory drug indoxole in rats with experimentally induced hind paw edema. Indoxole, given orally in suspension or in solution in different vehicles, was found to inhibit the development of edema. Some of these results are given in Table 6.3. What is the explanation for the vehicle dependency of the potency of indoxole?

**Table 6.2** Blood pressure rise caused by epinephrine in a dog receiving yohimbine

| Epinephrine ($\mu$g/kg) | yohimbine-HCl ($\mu$g/kg) | | | | | | |
|---|---|---|---|---|---|---|---|
| | 0 | 2 | 8 | 32 | 64 | 128 | 256 |
| 1 | 70[a] | 46[a] | 30[a] | 16[a] | 14[a] | 10[a] | 6[a] |
| 2 | 110 | 74 | 58 | 28 | 20 | 12 | 8 |
| 4 | 148 | 110 | 90 | 58 | 42 | 24 | 14 |
| 8 | 180 | 152 | 132 | 96 | 80 | 58 | 34 |
| 16 | 194 | 188 | 178 | 134 | 116 | 96 | 72 |

Reproduced from Chen and Russell, 1950, Table 1, © 1950 by the Williams & Wilkins Co., Baltimore.
[a] mm mercury

**Table 6.3** Comparison of serum drug concentrations and antiinflammatory activity of indoxole in rats with experimentally induced hind paw edema

| Vehicle | Dose (mg/kg, oral) | Inhibition of Edema (%) | 6-hr Drug Serum Levels ($\mu$g/ml $\pm$ SEM)[a] |
|---|---|---|---|
| CMC (1.0 ml) | | 0 | 0 |
| | 5 | 10 | $0.084 \pm 0.017$[b] |
| | 15 | 22 | $0.160 \pm 0.008$ |
| | 45 | 24 | $0.302 \pm 0.054$ |
| | 135 | 38 | $0.406 \pm 0.092$ |
| Cottonseed oil (1.0 ml) | | 0 | 0 |
| | 5 | 16 | $0.146 \pm 0.015$ |
| | 15 | 29 | $0.729 \pm 0.247$ |
| | 45 | 55 | $1.540 \pm 0.326$ |
| | 135 | 66 | $3.567 \pm 0.640$ |

Adapted from Glenn et al., 1967, Table 2, © 1967 by the Williams and Wilkins Co., Baltimore.
[a] Average blood levels of a separate group of five rats given drug on the same day.
[b] Standard error calculated using standard deviation estimated from range.

5  Acetyliodocholine (AICh) is a structural analogue of acetylcholine (ACh). Chiou (1973) studied the effect of atropine, which binds at the ACh receptor site, on the contractile effect of AICh on guinea pig ileum. At the same time he investigated the effect of AICh on the activity of acetylcholinesterase (AChE), the enzyme that deactivates ACh by hydrolysis. Some of his results are reproduced in Figures 6.22 and 6.23. Where does AICh bind to the receptor? Where does it bind to acetylcholinesterase? Is its behavior qualitatively the same in the two systems?

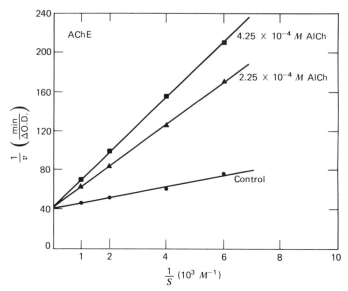

**Figure 6.22** The Lineweaver-Burk plot for inhibition by acetyliodocholine (AICh) of cholinesterase (AChE) activity with acetylthiocholine (ATCh) as the substrate. Each point is the mean of four observations. Reproduced with permission from Chiou, 1973, Figure 4, © 1973 by the Williams & Wilkins Co., Baltimore.

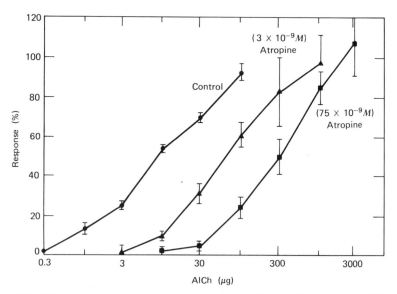

**Figure 6.23** The effect of atropine on the dose, effect curve for acetyliodocholine (AICh) acting on guinea pig ileum. Each point is the mean of four observations. Bars represent ± standard error. Reproduced with permission from Chiou, 1973, Figure 1, © 1973 by the Williams & Wilkins Co., Baltimore.

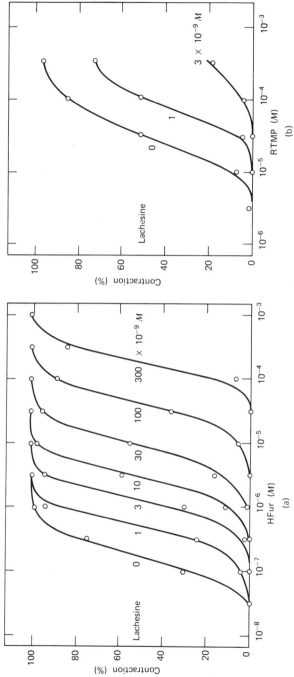

**Figure 6.24** Log dose, effect curves for (*a*) furtrethonium (HFur) and (*b*) a ruthenium chelate (RTMP) acting on guinea pig ileum in the presence of various concentrations of lachesine. Reproduced with permission from Shulman et al., 1970, Figure 5.

6  Certain complexes of ruthenium are cholinomimetic; that is, they are able
   to elicit the effect elicited by acetylcholine itself. Shulman et al. (1970)
   studied the contractile effect of the ruthenium chelate tris(3,5,6,8-
   tetramethyl-1,10-phenanthroline) ruthenium(II) chloride (RTMP) on the
   isolated guinea pig ileum. Inhibitions by lachesine of the effects of RTMP
   and of furtrethonium (HFur) were compared. HFur acts as a direct
   cholinomimetic in this system; in other words, it binds to the acetylcholine
   receptor. Some of the results of this study are reproduced in Figure 6.24.
   Do these data suggest that RTMP acts as a direct cholinomimetic or do
   they suggest that it acts indirectly, by liberating acetylcholine? Give the
   rationale for your answer.

7  Sullivan and Briggs (1968) were interested in determining whether angiotensin stimulates muscle contraction by increasing the permeability of the
   smooth muscle cell membrane to calcium. They studied the effect of
   angiotensin in the presence of various calcium ion concentrations on the
   contraction of rabbit aortic strips. Manganese was added to some of the

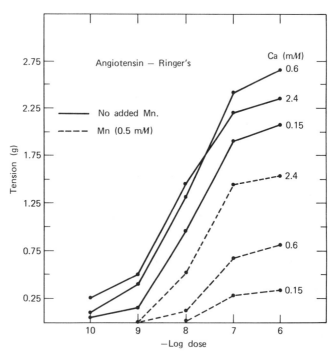

**Figure 6.25**  The effects of manganese ion and various calcium ion concentrations on angioten-
sin-induced aortic contractions in Ringer's solution. Angiotensin concentration is given as the
negative log of the molar concentration. Reproduced with permission from Sullivan and Briggs,
1968, Figure 2, © 1968 by the Williams & Wilkins Co., Baltimore.

bathing solutions because it had been shown to inhibit calcium permeability in certain tissues.

These investigators stated that their results (Figure 6.25) could "be interpreted to suggest that...angiotensin increases the calcium permeability of the smooth muscle cell membrane, and that manganese competes with calcium for the transport sites during activity, producing inhibition." Do you agree? Why or why not?

**8** The insecticide $o,p'$-DDT, like other chlorinated hydrocarbons, elicits some of the same effects as the natural hormone estradiol, including an increase in uterine size and weight. Nelson (1974) correlated this uterotropic effect of chlorinated hydrocarbons with their inhibition of estradiol binding to rat uterine receptor. Some of these results are shown in Figures 6.26 and 6.27. Do these results (*a*) support the hypothesis that the uterotropic effect of $o,p'$-DDT is due to intrinsic estrogenic properties of $o,p'$-DDT, or (*b*) suggest that its effect is due to potentiation of estradiol activity?

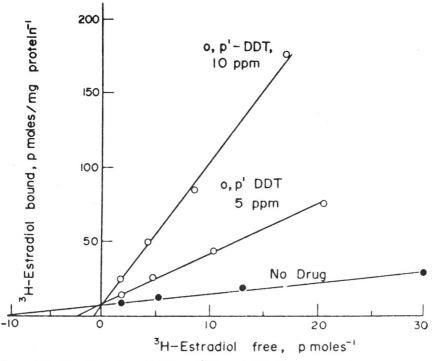

**Figure 6.26** The effect of $o,p'$-DDT on [$^3$H]estradiol binding to rat uterine receptor. Free [$^3$H]estradiol was calculated as the difference between total and bound [$^3$H]estradiol. Reproduced with permission from Nelson, 1974, Figure 3.

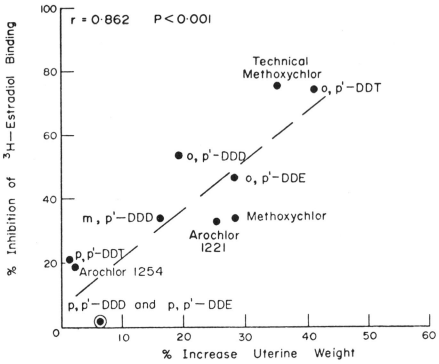

**Figure 6.27** Correlation between inhibition by chlorinated hydrocarbons of [³H]estradiol binding *in vitro* and their uterotropic effect *in vivo*. Mean values for three binding assays and uterine weights from groups of five mice are given. Reproduced with permission from Nelson, 1974, Figure 2.

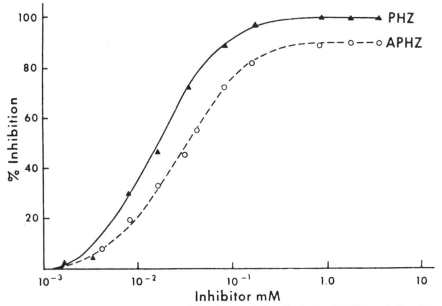

**Figure 6.28** Inhibition of monoamine oxidase by acetylphenylhydrazine (APHZ) and phenylhydrazine (PHZ) *in vitro*. Points represent the means of duplicate determinations. Reproduced with permission from Symes and Sourkes, 1974, Figure 3.

**9** Acetylphenylhydrazine (APHZ) and phenylhydrazine (PHZ) are hemolytic agents that also inhibit rat liver monoamine oxidase (MAO) activity. Symes and Sourkes (1974) studied the mechanism of this inhibition *in vitro* by incubating rat liver mitochondrial preparations with APHZ or PHZ before assaying the mixtures for their MAO activity. Some of their results are given in Figure 6.28 and Tables 6.4 and 6.5.

**(a)** Is this competitive or noncompetitive inhibition? Why?

**(b)** Is it reversible or irreversible? Why?

**Table 6.4** The effects of APHZ and PHZ on kinetic constants of MAO *in vitro*

| Inhibitor | Concentration (m$M$) | Apparent $K_m$ $\times 10^{-5}$ $M$ (mole/l) | $V_{max}$ (units) |
|---|---|---|---|
| APHZ | None | 4.10 | 109.9 |
| APHZ | $5.39 \times 10^{-3}$ | 3.58 | 83.1 |
| APHZ | $1.08 \times 10^{-2}$ | 3.76 | 81.1 |
| APHZ | $4.31 \times 10^{-2}$ | 3.64 | 33.8 |
| PHZ | None | 2.84 | 534.8 |
| PHZ | $1.75 \times 10^{-3}$ | 2.78 | 78.4 |
| PHZ | $8.75 \times 10^{-3}$ | 2.78 | 24.7 |

Reproduced from Symes and Sourkes, 1974, Table 4.

**Table 6.5** The effects of dilution on MAO inhibition by APHZ and PHZ[a]

| Sample | Inhibitor | Concentration ($M$) | Inhibition (%) |
|---|---|---|---|
| Undiluted experimental | APHZ | $4.31 \times 10^{-5}$ | $70.2 \pm 0.83$ (2) |
| Diluted experimental | APHZ | $1.44 \times 10^{-6}$ | $67.51 \pm 0.78$ (3) |
| Diluted experimental with additional APHZ | APHZ | $4.31 \times 10^{-5}$ | $72.06 \pm 1.39$ (3) |
| Undiluted experimental | PHZ | $2.77 \times 10^{-5}$ | $85.14 \pm 0.95$ (4) |
| Diluted experimental | PHZ | $9.23 \times 10^{-7}$ | $83.21 \pm 0.76$ (4) |
| Diluted experimental with additional PHZ | PHZ | $2.77 \times 10^{-5}$ | $84.33 \pm 0.68$ (3) |

Reproduced from Symes and Sourkes, 1974, Table 3.
[a]The enzyme preparation, consisting of washed mitochondria from rat liver, and the inhibitors were incubated together for 20 min at 37°C and pH 7.4. At the end of that interval, aliquots of the mixtures were withdrawn and transferred to vessels containing buffer, 1 m$M$ kynuramine as substrate, and either additional inhibitor to maintain the original concentration or no more inhibitor. The reaction was allowed to proceed for another 20 min. Fluorescence of the reaction product was compared with that of control and undiluted inhibited enzyme preparations. Means $\pm$ SE are shown. The figures in parentheses represent the numbers of determinations made.

## REFERENCES

Ballard, P. L. and R. A. Ballard. "Cytoplasmic receptor for glucocorticoids in lung of the human fetus and neonate." *J. Clin. Invest.*, **53**, 477–486 (1974).

Bradshaw, R. A. "Nerve growth factor." *Annu. Rev. Biochem.*, **47**, 191–216 (1978).

Caldwell, R. W. and C. B. Nash. "Comparison of the effects of amino sugar cardiac glycosides with ouabain and digoxin on Na$^+$,K$^+$-adenosine triphosphatase and cardiac contractile force." *J. Pharmacol. Exp. Ther.*, **204**, 141–148 (1978).

Carlsson, A., P. A. Shore, and B. B. Brodie. "Release of serotonin from blood platelets by reserpine *in vitro*." *J. Pharmacol. Exp. Ther.*, **120**, 334–339 (1957).

Chan, W. Y. and N. Kelley, "A pharmacologic analysis on the significance of the chemical functional groups of oxytocin to its oxytocic activity and on the effect of magnesium on the *in vitro* and *in vivo* oxytocic activity of neurohypophysial hormones." *J. Pharmacol. Exp. Ther.*, **156**, 150–158 (1967).

Chen, G. and D. Russell. "A quantitative study of blood pressure response to cardiovascular drugs and their antagonists." *J. Pharmacol. Exp. Ther.*, **99**, 401–408 (1950).

Chiou, C. Y. "Cholinergic activities and cholinesterase hydrolysis of acetyliodocholine." *J. Pharmacol. Exp. Ther.*, **184**, 47–55 (1973).

Clark, A. J. "The reaction between acetylcholine and muscle cells." *J. Physiol.*, **61**, 530–546 (1926).

Furchgott, R. F. "Dibenamine blockade in strips of rabbit aorta and its use in differentiating receptors." *J. Pharmacol. Exp. Ther.*, **111**, 265–284 (1954).

Gandolfi, A. J., H. S. Nakaue, and D. R. Buhler, "Effect of hexachlorophene on hepatic drug-metabolizing enzymes in the rat." *Biochem. Pharmacol.*, **23**, 1997–2003 (1974).

Glenn, E. M., B. J. Bowman, W. Kooyers, T. Koslowske, and M. L. Myers. "The pharmacology of 2,3-bis-(*p*-methoxyphenyl)-indole (indoxole)." *J. Pharmacol. Exp. Ther.*, **155**, 157–166 (1967).

Heidmann, T. and J.-P. Changeux. "Structural and functional properties of the acetylcholine receptor protein in its purified and membrane-bound states." *Annu. Rev. Biochem.*, **47**, 317–357 (1978).

Hernberg, S., J. Nikkanen, G. Mellin, and H. Lilius. "δ-Aminolevulinic acid dehydrase as a measure of lead exposure." *Arch. Environ. Health*, **21**, 140–145 (1970).

Jacobs, S. and P. Cuatrecasas. "The mobile receptor hypothesis and 'cooperativity' of hormone binding: Application to insulin." *Biochim. Biophys. Acta*, **433**, 482–495 (1976).

Kahn, C. R., P. Freychet, and J. Roth. "Quantitative aspects of the insulin-receptor interaction in liver plasma membranes." *J. Biol. Chem.*, **249**, 2249–2257 (1974).

Kalow, W. and K. Genest. "A method for the detection of atypical forms of human serum cholinesterase. Determination of dibucaine numbers." *Can. J. Biochem. Physiol.*, **35**, 339–346 (1957).

Kuhnen-Clausen, D. "Structure-activity relationship of mono- and bisquaternary pyridines in regard to their parasympatholytic effects." *Toxicol. Appl. Pharmacol.*, **23**, 443–454 (1972).

Kuntzman, R., D. Lawrence, and A. H. Conney. "Michaelis constants for the hydroxylation of steroid hormones and drugs by rat liver microsomes." *Mol. Pharmacol.*, **1**, 163–167 (1965).

Langley, J. N. "On nerve-endings and on special excitable substances in cells" (Croonian Lecture). *Proc. R. Soc. London*, *Ser. B*, **77**, 170–194 (1906).

Nelson, J. A. "Effects of dichlorodiphenyltrichloroethane (DDT) analogs and polychlorinated biphenyl (PCB) mixtures on 17 $\beta$-[$^3$H]estradiol binding to rat uterine receptor." *Biochem. Pharmacol.*, **23**, 447–451 (1974).

Nickerson, M. "Receptor occupancy and tissue response." *Nature (London)*, **178**, 697–698 (1956).

Potter, L. T. "Uptake of propranolol by isolated guinea pig atria." *J. Pharmacol. Exp. Ther.*, **155**, 91–100 (1967).

Shulman, A., G. M. Laycock, E. J. Ariëns, and A. R. H. Wigmans. "The action of selected metal complexes on receptor systems of isolated organs. Part 1. The action of selected ruthenium(II) phenanthroline chelates on the cholinergic mechanism of the rat intestine and guinea pig ileum." *Eur. J. Pharmacol.*, **9**, 347–357 (1970).

Stephenson, R. P. "A modification of receptor theory." *Br. J. Pharmacol.*, **11**, 379–393 (1956).

Sullivan, L. J. and A. H. Briggs. "Effects of manganese on the response of aortic strips to angiotensin and norepinephrine contractions." *J. Pharmacol. Exp. Ther.*, **161**, 205–209 (1968).

Suwandi, I. S. and J. A. Bevan. "Antagonism of lobeline by ganglion-blocking agents at afferent nerve endings." *J. Pharmacol. Exp. Ther.*, **153**, 1–7 (1966).

Symes, A. L. and T. L. Sourkes. "Pharmacological and biochemical actions of the hemolytic agents acetylphenylhydrazine and phenylhydrazine on monoamine oxidase in the rat." *Biochem. Pharmacol.*, **23**, 2045–2056 (1974).

Takagi, K., I. Takayanagi, and Y. Maezima. "An analysis of the sites of action of some partial agonists." *Eur. J. Pharmacol.*, **3**, 52–57 (1968).

Tsai, B. S. and R. J. Lefkowitz. "[$^3$H]Dihydroergocryptine binding to $\alpha$-adrenergic receptors in canine aortic membranes." *J. Pharmacol. Exp. Ther.*, **204**, 606–614 (1978).

Wohl, A. J., L. M. Hausler, and F. E. Roth. "Mechanism of the antihypertensive effect of diazoxide: *In vitro* vascular studies in the hypertensive rat." *J. Pharmacol. Exp. Ther.*, **162**, 109–114 (1968).

# 7

# Dynamics: The Time Course of Effect

**7.1** Correlations between concentration and effect

**7.2** Correlations between dose and duration of effect

    7.2.1 Linear elimination kinetics

    7.2.2 Zero-order elimination kinetics

    7.2.3 Transition between first- and zero-order elimination kinetics

**7.3** Correlations between fraction of maximum effect and time

    7.3.1 First-order elimination kinetics and a linear ln dose, effect range

    7.3.2 Zero-order elimination kinetics and a linear dose, effect range

    7.3.3 Other combinations of elimination kinetics and dose, effect relationships

**7.4** The uses and limitations of temporal effect measurements

In the previous chapter the relationship between concentration at the receptor site and effect was developed in response to the premise that our ultimate concern is not the concentration but the effect of a drug or toxicant. It can be inferred that pharmacokinetic or toxicokinetic analysis is not ordinarily an end in itself. Knowledge of the time course of plasma concentration changes is useful primarily because it provides insight into the magnitude and time course of effect or because it assists in localization of the receptor sites.

Pharmacodynamics and toxicodynamics are the study of the behavior of effect. Although much of the work that has been done in this area is qualitative or semiquantitative, certain quantitative relationships have also been developed. In general, to be amenable to quantitative treatment, effects should be immediate and specific. Delayed effects such as those mediated by a series of biochemical steps, or nonspecific effects such as those associated with alterations in membrane permeability, cannot readily be correlated with effector concentration. But if the drug or toxicant elicits a reasonably prompt effect by combining with a specific receptor site, and if its concentration at the receptor site can be related to its concentration in the plasma, certain simple and useful correlations can be made.

One further point should be made about the dynamics of drug and toxicant action. Experimental evidence suggests that there is much less interindividual variability in the dynamics than in the kinetics of a drug or toxicant. In other words, the receptor site requirement is likely to be more consistent from individual to individual than the amount of effector presented to the receptor site. As an example consider the studies by Kourounakis et al. (1973a, b) of paralysis in rats induced by administration of the muscle relaxant zoxazolamine. Although length of effect varied widely, from 100 to 252 min in rats given 100 mg/kg, plasma levels of zoxazolamine at the moment of recovery were quite consistent, from 24.7 to 28.1 $\mu$g/ml. Concentration of zoxazolamine in the brain, the site of action, correlated closely with plasma concentration.

## 7.1 CORRELATIONS BETWEEN CONCENTRATION AND EFFECT

Most often kinetic studies are carried out by sampling from the blood and blood plasma or by sampling excretion pathways that represent clearance from the plasma. Therefore we are interested primarily in correlation of effect with plasma concentration. The nature of this correlation depends on where the receptor sites are located and on whether the parent compound or a metabolite is the active moiety. All efforts to establish such correlations are based on the assumption that the effect, time curve has the same shape as the concentration, time curve for drug or toxicant in the vicinity of the receptor sites.

If the site of action is part of the central compartment, magnitude of effect should correlate directly with plasma concentration of effector. This is found to be the case for the effect on heart rate of several of the $\beta$-adrenergic blocking drugs. Figure 7.1 illustrates the linear relationship between log dose and effect for one such drug, practolol.

If the effect is due to a metabolite, its magnitude will be correlated with the concentration of metabolite, not parent drug. For example, Lemberger et al. (1972) showed that the peak psychologic "high" from marijuana correlated with peak plasma levels of $\Delta$-9-tetrahydrocannabinol metabolites but not with peak plasma levels of the parent drug, providing evidence that one or more of the metabolites are active while $\Delta$-9-tetrahydrocannabinol itself is not.

Delayed appearance of the maximum measured effect, as in the $\Delta$-9-tetrahydrocannabinol example, suggests either that the effect is due to a metabolite or that the receptor sites are located in a peripheral compartment. In the latter case the initial phase is the result of transfer into the peripheral

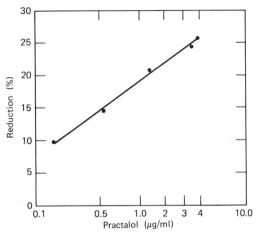

**Figure 7.1** Correlation of the mean reduction of exercise heart rate with the logarithm of the mean blood practolol level. Reproduced with permission from Carruthers et al., 1974, Figure 6.

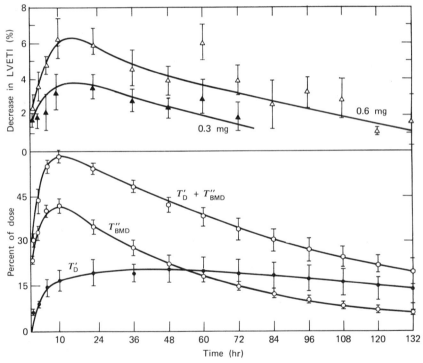

**Figure 7.2** Apparent correlation between the mean percentage left ventricular ejection time (LVETI) decrease at 0.3 (▲) and 0.6 (△) mg of β-methyldigoxin (BMD) and the mean amounts of β-methyldigoxin (○) and (●) in their respective deepest tissues, $T''_{BMD}$ and $T'_{D}$, and in their sum (◯) in percentage of the administered intravenous dose of β-methyldigoxin as a function of time. The LVETI values obtained prior to drug administration served as controls. The vertical bars indicate ±1 SEM of the means. The amounts in the tissues were generated by the analog computer from the best fits of the experimental plasma and urine data for all studies. They are given as percentage of dose. Reproduced with permission from Hinderling and Garrett, 1977, Figure 1.

**324**

tissue instead of metabolic transformation. As an example consider the study by Hinderling and Garrett (1977) of the kinetics and action of the cardiac glycoside $\beta$-methyldigoxin. Two effects were measured: heart rate (HR) decrease and decrease in left ventricular ejection time (LVETI). The time course of these two effects is shown in the upper portions of Figures 7.2 and 7.3 for intravenous administration of 0.3 and 0.6 mg of $\beta$-methyldigoxin in human volunteers. Note that the HR effect peaks at about 80 min, whereas the LVETI effect peaks at about 10 hr. These times coincide with the times of peak concentrations of total $\beta$-methyldigoxin plus its active metabolite digoxin, simulated by analog computer from kinetic constants for both compounds, in "moderately deep" and "deepest" tissue compartments, re-

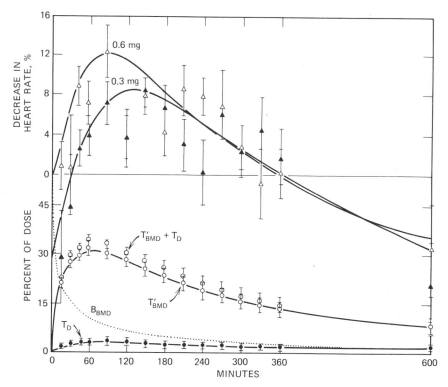

**Figure 7.3** Apparent correlation between the mean percentage heart rate decrease at 0.3 (▲) and 0.6 (△) mg of $\beta$-methyldigoxin and the mean amounts of $\beta$-methyldigoxin (○) and digoxin (●) in their respective moderately deep tissues, $T'_{BMD}$ and $T_D$, and in their sum (⊘) in percentage of the administered intravenous dose of $\beta$-methyldigoxin as a function of time. The heart rate values obtained prior to drug administration served as controls. The vertical bars indicate ±1 SEM of the means. The amounts in the tissues were generated by the analog computer from the best fits of the experimental plasma and urine data for all studies. They are given as percentage of dose. For comparison, the dashed line shows the mean of the analog computer–fitted amounts of $\beta$-methyldigoxin in the central compartment, $B_{BMD}$, in percentage of $\beta$-methyldigoxin administered as a function of time. Reproduced with permission from Hinderling and Garrett, 1977, Figure 3.

spectively. The simulated kinetic behavior of the two active cardiac glycosides is shown in the lower portions of Figures 7.2 and 7.3. On the basis of this analysis it was possible to conclude that the receptor sites for HR action and for LVETI action of digoxin and $\beta$-methyldigoxin are located in kinetically distinguishable compartments.

A related approach to this type of data analysis provides an especially vivid illustration of the exploitation of dose, effect curves to localize receptor sites. The effect associated with a particular concentration of drug or toxicant at the receptor site should be independent of whether concentration in the biophase is rising or falling. Therefore hypothetical log concentration, effect curves may be constructed from measured effects and concentrations simulated as above using an appropriate compartmental model and parameters derived from a separate kinetic study. The shapes of these curves can serve to localize the site of action to a particular kind of kinetic compartment.

A good illustration of this analytical technique is its application by Levy et al. (1969) to data from Aghanajian and Bing (1964). Aghanajian and Bing administered lysergic acid diethylamide (LSD), $2\mu g/kg$, by intravenous injection to five young men. During the following 8 hr the subjects' ability to solve simple addition problems was evaluated periodically. Levy et al. correlated the degree of impairment in this ability with LSD concentration in the tissue

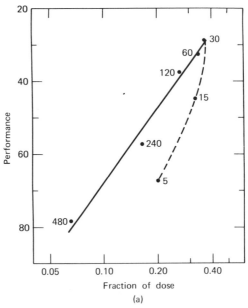

**Figure 7.4** The relationship between the fractional amount of LSD in the biophase and the intensity of the pharmacologic effect. The number next to each symbol represents the time (min) when the measurements were made. ( *a* ) The biophase is part of the tissue compartment of a two-compartment model. ( *b* ) The biophase is part of the deeper compartment of a three-compartment model. Reproduced with permission from Levy et al., 1969, Figures 2 and 4.

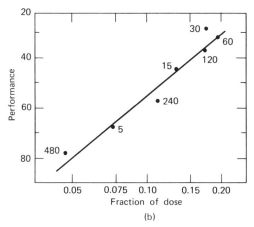

**Figure 7.4** (*continued*)

compartment of a two-compartment model and with LSD concentration in the slowly exchanging or deep compartment of a three-compartment model, using kinetic parameters for LSD determined by analysis of Aghanajian and Bing's plasma concentration data. Figure 7.4 shows that intensity of effect was directly related to the log of the receptor site concentration only in the deeper compartment of the three-compartment model. In this way the site of LSD action was localized to a slowly exchanging compartment.

## 7.2 CORRELATIONS BETWEEN DOSE AND DURATION OF EFFECT

The correlations discussed in this section were originally developed and published by Levy and Nelson (1965) and by Levy (1966). They apply to drugs or toxicants whose intensity of effect can be correlated with plasma concentration. Given intravenous administration and rapid onset of effect, a duration of action $t_d$ can be measured from the time of administration to some time associated with a selected effect end point.* At this time plasma concentration is $C_{th}$, the threshold level. Duration of action is a function both of the distribution characteristics and of the elimination kinetics of a drug or toxicant. The following developments assume a one-compartment body model.

---

*This end point may be zero effect. Sometimes there is a threshold plasma concentration below which no effect is measurable at all. An actual threshold such as this may occur either because there is a range within which the action of the compound is not rate limiting for the effect being measured or because plasma concentration is not an accurate index of concentration in the vicinity of the receptor sites.

### 7.2.1   Linear Elimination Kinetics

If elimination kinetics are first order, the threshold amount $B_{th}$ of drug or toxicant in the plasma is related to $t_d$ by the equation

$$\ln(C_{th}V) = \ln B_{th} = \ln B_0 - k_e t_d, \tag{7.1}$$

as illustrated in Figure 7.5.

Equation 7.1 may be solved for $t_d$:

$$t_d = \frac{\ln D - \ln B_{th}}{k_e}. \tag{7.2}$$

Equation 7.2 states that the duration of action of drugs and toxicants whose elimination kinetics are first order should be linearly related to the log of the dose, the slope of the line being $(k_e)^{-1}$ or $t_{1/2}/\ln_2$. No effect is observed whenever $\ln D \leqslant \ln B_{th}$; that is, when the initial plasma level does not exceed the threshold level. Equation 7.2 can be used to estimate the threshold dose and elimination rate constant of drugs or toxicants whose concentration is not readily measurable in biological fluids but for which an effect is measurable with reasonable accuracy.

This linear relationship between log dose and duration of effect was recognized before it was given a theoretical foundation. An example of its application is the study by Maher et al. (1962) of the duration of acute glutethimide intoxication in a group of 22 patients who had taken an overdose of the sedative. Duration of coma was directly related to the clinical

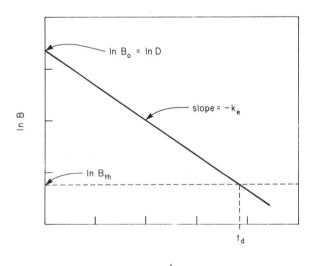

**Figure 7.5**   The relationship between threshold amount of drug or toxicant in the plasma and duration of effect when elimination kinetics are first order.

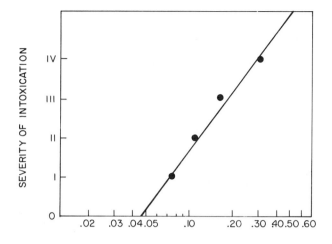

MEAN GLUTETHIMIDE DOSE: g/kg

**Figure 7.6** The mean clinical severity of glutethimide intoxication in groups of patients as a function of the log of the mean glutethimide dose. Data were read from Maher et al., 1962, Figure 2.

severity of the intoxication, the latter being evaluated on the basis of patients' vital and neurologic signs, therapy required, and outcome. Clinical severity, in turn, was a function of the log of the dose, as shown in Figure 7.6. Figure 7.6 suggests that the threshold dose for intoxication should be about 40–50 mg/kg and, indeed, the lowest dose in this patient series was 60 mg/kg.

### 7.2.2 Zero-Order Elimination Kinetics

If

$$B_{\text{th}} = B_0 - k_e t_d, \tag{7.3}$$

then

$$t_d = \frac{D - B_{\text{th}}}{k_e}, \tag{7.4}$$

and duration of action should be directly proportional to the dose rather than to the log of the dose. The classic example of a compound eliminated by zero-order kinetics is ethanol (but see Section 4.3). Sidell and Pless (1971) conducted a systematic study of the temporal correlation of ethanol blood level and selected performance measures in 20 adult males. Three performance measures were used: the number facility test (NF), consisting of simple addition problems; the variable interval time analyzer (VITA), a test of ability to estimate a preset time interval by a series of 25 repetitive estimations with feedback; and the zero-input tracking analyzer (ZITA), a

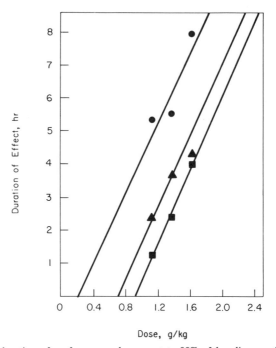

Dose, g/kg

**Figure 7.7** The duration of performance decrement to 80% of baseline on three performance measures: NF (▲), VITA (■), and ZITA (●), in a group of adult male subjects as a function of the log of the ethanol dose. For explanation of performance measures see text. Calculated from equations of best fit given by Sidell and Pless, 1971, for their temporal effect data, Figures 4*a–c*, except for VITA at 1.4 ml/kg (1.12 g/kg), which was read directly from Figure 4*a*.

perceptual motor task requiring eye-hand coordination. Performance decrement was expressed as percentage of baseline. Figure 7.7 shows the duration of performance decrement (calculated from the lines of best fit to temporal effect data) to 80% of baseline as a function of dose for each of the three tasks. The differences in threshold dose could be due to distributional factors or, more probably for ethanol with its high lipid solubility and consequent rapid distribution, to differences in receptor sensitivity. The slopes of the three lines are all about 5.26 hr/g/kg; the ethanol excretion rate constant calculated from effect measurements is therefore 190 mg/kg/hr. The ethanol excretion rate constant calculated from concentration measurements was 140 mg/kg/hr; however, since the apparent volume of distribution used to convert concentration to body burden in this calculation was obtained by extrapolating the dieaway phase of a one-compartment first-order absorption model it is an underestimate of the true volume of distribution (see Section 3.10). Consequently the value 140 mg/kg/hr is also an underestimate, by an indeterminate amount, of the true zero-order rate constant.

### 7.2.3   Transition Between First- and Zero-Order Elimination Kinetics

Transition from first- to zero-order kinetics of elimination will be reflected in the relationship of duration of action to dose, as shown in Figure 7.8 for both methods of graphing.

This is an important point with particularly significant implications for toxicity studies. If metabolism or excretion of a toxicant approaches saturation at the high doses associated with toxicity, duration of effect measurements cannot be extrapolated outside the range of experimental observation.

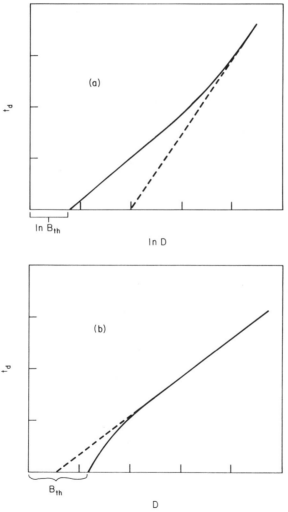

**Figure 7.8**   The appearance of ln dose, duration of action plots (*a*) and dose, duration of action plots (*b*) in the range of a transition from first to zero-order elimination kinetics.

In a lower dose range where natural elimination mechanisms are not overwhelmed, the toxicant will be eliminated from the body much more efficiently relative to the total amount present. It is particularly noteworthy that linear extrapolation of either type of plot out of the saturation range would result in inaccurate estimation of the threshold dose (Figure 7.8). In the case of a plot of $t_d$ versus $\ln D$, the estimate would be too high; in the case of a plot of $t_d$ versus $D$ it would be too low, resulting in an exaggerated estimate of the compound's actual duration of effect.

## 7.3   CORRELATIONS BETWEEN FRACTION OF MAXIMUM EFFECT AND TIME

The correlations between fraction of maximum effect and time are dependent not only on distribution characteristics and elimination kinetics but also on the nature of the dose, effect relationship. Although development of the equations in this section is based on the assumption of instantaneous administration, they may also be applied to first-order absorption models once the absorption phase is complete. This material was first formulated by Levy (1964, 1966).

### 7.3.1   First-Order Elimination Kinetics and a Linear ln Dose, Effect Range

In Chapter 6 the ln dose, effect relationship was developed, and it was shown that for effects mediated through a receptor site this relationship is approximately linear between about 20% and about 80% of maximum effect.*

Let $F$ be the fraction of maximum effect ($\theta/\theta_m$ from Chapter 6). Then in the range of ln dose, effect linearity,

$$F = a + m\ln B = (a + m\ln B_0) - mk_e t, \qquad (7.5)$$

where $m$ is the slope of the ln dose, $F$ line, and $a$ is a constant. Figure 7.9 illustrates this relationship. From measurement of $F$ as a function of time and knowledge of $m$, $k_e$ and $t_{1/2}$ can be calculated. The value of $m$ can be obtained either directly from a ln dose, $F$ curve or indirectly as shown in the example of Figure 7.10.

For many drugs, once the absorptive and distributive phases are over, $F$ does decline linearly with time. A good illustration of this behavior is given in Figure 7.10, taken from a study by Van Rossum et al. (1968) of the kinetics of

*In many populations and for many drugs and toxicants a graph of fraction of maximum response versus ln dose is also linear, although for different reasons, between about 20% and about 80% of maximum response (Chapter 8). Therefore the treatment of effect data described in this section can be applied also to response data. However, it has been in general use only in the context of effect measurements.

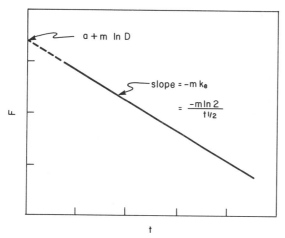

**Figure 7.9** The expected dependence of fraction of maximum effect on time when elimination kinetics are first order and there is a linear relationship between effect and the log of the dose.

D-amphetamine effects in rats. The increase in locomotor activity produced by the drug was measured as the increase in the rate at which the rats' activity interrupted light beams directed through their cages. The rate at which interruptions occurred was recorded as counts per minute (cpm). Figure 7.10 shows the $F, t$ lines for two different doses of D-amphetamine given intramuscularly. To calculate the half-life of D-amphetamine, Van Rossum et al. estimated $m$ from the degree of separation of the two $F, t$ lines. Since the

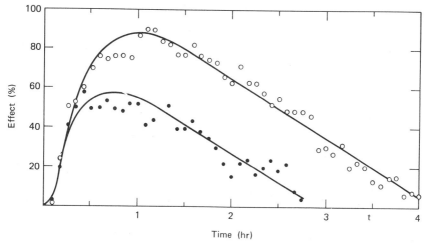

**Figure 7.10** Time, effect curves for doses of 3.12 (●) and 5.62 (○) $\mu$mole/kg of D-amphetamine sulfate given intramuscularly to rats. Each point represents the mean increase in recorded activity, in counts per minute, in seven animals. Reproduced with permission from Van Rossum et al., 1968, Figure 2.

lines are parallel, $m$ may be estimated at any convenient time point:

$$m = \frac{F_{5.62\,\mu mole/kg} - F_{3.12\,\mu mole/kg}}{\ln 5.62 - \ln 3.12}.$$

Estimating $m$ at 2 hr:

$$m = \frac{(65-30)\text{ cpm}}{(1.726-1.13)\text{ ln dose units}}$$

$$= 60 \text{ cpm/ln dose unit}.$$

Then taking the slope between 1.5 and 2.5 hr,

$$t_{1/2} = -\frac{m\ln 2}{\text{slope of } F, t \text{ lines}} = -\frac{(2.5-1.5)(0.693)(60)\text{ (hr-cpm)}}{(12-40)\text{ (cpm)}}$$

$$= 1.5 \text{ hr}.$$

The parallelism of the lines in Figure 7.10 is confirmation of the linearity of D-amphetamine elimination kinetics. It is also possible for $F, t$ lines to be apparently linear but not parallel for different doses (Sturtevant, 1960,

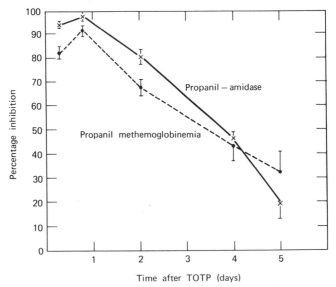

**Figure 7.11** Time course of effect of triorthotolylphosphate (TOTP) on propanil amidase activity and propanil-induced methemoglobin formation. At the indicated times after TOTP (125 mg/kg), mice were either sacrificed for amidase assay or challenged with 400 mg of propanil/kg for methemoglobin determination 1 hr later. Each point represents the mean ± standard error for four mice compared with values obtained from corn oil pretreated controls. Reproduced with permission from Singleton and Murphy, 1973, Figure 4.

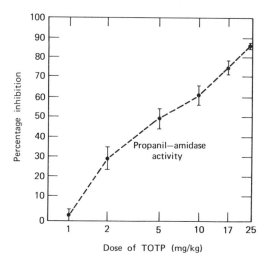

**Figure 7.12**  The linear relationship between percentage inhibition of propanil amidase activity, measured in mice 18 hr after various doses of TOTP, and the log of the TOTP dose (see Figure 7.11). Each point represents the mean ± standard error for four mice compared with values obtained from 12 corn oil pretreated controls. Adapted with permission from Singleton and Murphy, 1973, Figure 3.

discussed by Levy, 1964), suggesting that the apparent first-order elimination constant may vary with dose.

Comparisons may also be made not between the effects of different doses but between different effects of a single dose. From such comparisons inferences may sometimes be drawn about the nature of the receptor sites for different effects. An example is the study by Singleton and Murphy (1973) of the effects of triorthotolyl phosphate (TOTP) on metabolism of, and methemoglobinemia induced by, the herbicide propanil in mice. As shown in Figure 7.11, TOTP inhibits both the activity of mouse liver acetanilide amidase and induction of methemoglobinemia. Percentage inhibition of these effects is calculated by comparing corn oil pretreated controls and TOTP pretreated experimental animals both given propanil intraperitoneally. Since propanil is metabolized by acetanilide amidase, the methemoglobinemia is presumably induced by a propanil metabolite. The two lines in Figure 7.11 are not only parallel but superimposable. The parallelism suggests that the same kind of receptor is rate determining for both effects (barring the unlikely occurrence of different receptors with identical affinity and sensitivity for TOTP). The superimposability suggests that the receptors for both effects are probably located in the same kinetic compartment, since TOTP concentrations at the receptor sites must be identical. The inference is strong that a single receptor is rate determining for both effects. The log TOTP dose, effect curve for inhibition of propanil amidase activity is shown in Figure 7.12.

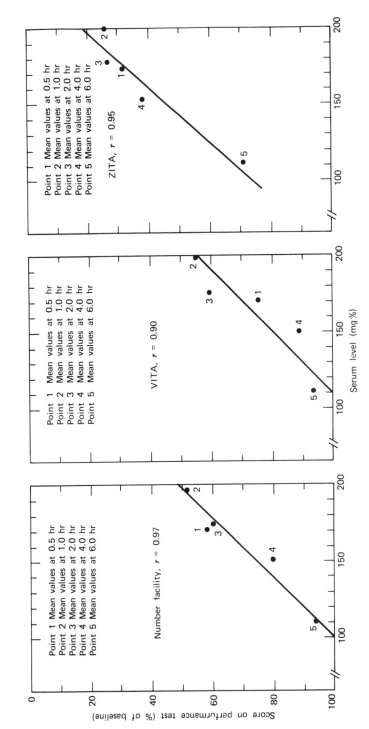

**Figure 7.13** The linear relationship between performance decrement on three performance measures (number facility, VITA, and ZITA) and blood ethanol concentration in adult male subjects during the first 6 hr after ingestion of 2.0 ml of ethanol/kg. See Section 7.2.2 for explanation of performance measures. Reproduced with permission from Sidell and Pless, 1971, Figure 5.

## 7.3.2 Zero-Order Elimination Kinetics and a Linear Dose, Effect Range

Interestingly, for drugs and toxicants whose elimination is zero order,

$$B = B_0 - kt,$$

and whose dose, effect curve is linear, $F = a + mB$, then

$$F = (a + mB_0) - mkt, \tag{7.6}$$

and the relationship between $F$ and $t$ should still be linear. This would be a more or less academic case if it were not for ethanol, many of whose effects are linearly related to dose as shown in Figure 7.13 for the effect measurements discussed in Section 7.2.2 (Sidell and Pless, 1971). Note that dose is here expressed as serum level, the internal dose, since serum levels at times after $t_0$ are not proportional to the dose of ethanol administered. The temporal behavior of the decline in performance decrements and serum levels of ethanol is given for the 1.7-ml/kg dose in Figure 7.14. The ordinate scales are chosen so that concentration and effect lines appear to be parallel. However, the actual slope of the concentration line should be $-k$ and of the effect lines $-mk$. $k$ was calculated to be 19 mg %/hr. The slope of the performance lines is about $-8\%$ decrement/hr, suggesting that $m$ should be about 0.42% decrement/mg %. $m$ can be calculated directly from Figure 7.13; it is about 0.5% decrement/mg %.

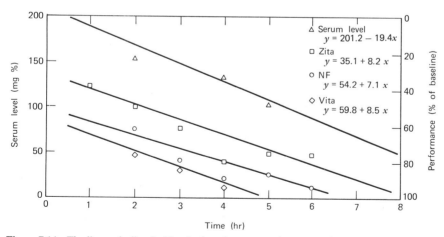

**Figure 7.14** The linear decline in blood ethanol concentration ($\triangle$) and in performance decrement for three performance measures (ZITA, NF, and VITA), in six adult male subjects given 1.7 ml ethanol/kg. Each point is the mean of six values. For explanation of performance measures, see Section 7.2.2. Reproduced with permission from Sidell and Pless, 1971, Figure 4b.

### 7.3.3   Other Combinations of Elimination Kinetics and Dose, Effect Relationships

For a drug or toxicant having a linear log dose, effect curve but exhibiting zero-order elimination kinetics, there is no simple linear relationship of $F$ to $t$:

$$F = a + m\ln(B_0 - kt).$$

For the less likely combination of a linear dose, effect curve and first-order elimination kinetics, however, we would predict a linear relationship of $\ln F$ to $t$, provided no threshold exists:

$$\ln F = \ln(mB_0) - k_e t.$$

## 7.4   THE USES AND LIMITATIONS OF TEMPORAL EFFECT MEASUREMENTS

Equations 7.2 to 7.6 are appealingly simple. Unfortunately they were developed from particularly restrictive kinetic and mechanistic assumptions. What would be the impact of relaxing these assumptions, and of what use are temporal effect measurements for compounds that do not meet these rigid requirements? We examine the assumptions separately.

1   The measured effect occurs without a kinetically significant delay.

This is perhaps the least troublesome restriction. For most drugs and toxicants it is possible to identify a measurable effect that occurs sufficiently rapidly on penetration of the drug to the receptor site that it meets the criterion of immediate onset. For some, however, it is not. Nonetheless even delayed effects may be amenable to kinetic treatment. An example is the effect of warfarin (see Section 6.1).

Warfarin inhibits the synthesis of clotting factors, but a direct correlation between plasma warfarin concentration and the usual measured effect, anticoagulant activity, does not exist, as shown in Figure 7.15. The delay in appearance of maximum warfarin effect is due to the time required for normal catabolic processes to reduce body stores of clotting factors (prothrombin complex, P) to levels associated with a measurable lengthening of clotting time. Nagashima et al. (1969), using data from O'Reilly and Aggeler (1968), estimated the overall rate constant for P catabolism by measuring the first-order decline of P activity as a function of time in 13 adult human subjects administered a dose of warfarin sufficient to block clotting factor synthesis (Figure 7.16). From this value together with net P activity data in six adult human subjects given various doses of warfarin, the authors were able to determine the rate of synthesis of P activity as a function of time following administration of the drug. The relationship between log plasma

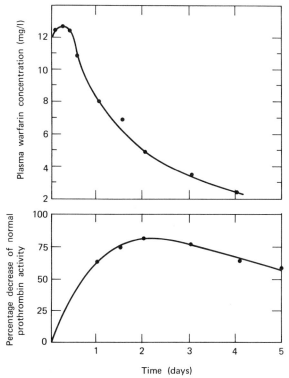

**Figure 7.15** Plasma warfarin concentration and depression of prothrombin complex activity as functions of time after oral administration of 1.5 mg warfarin sodium/kg. Points are the means of data from five normal subjects. Reproduced with permission from Nagashima et al., 1969, Figure 1.

warfarin concentration and simultaneously determined P activity synthesis rate is shown in Figure 7.17. It is a classic log dose, intensity of action relationship within the therapeutic dose range of the anticoagulant. With the help of this relationship the authors were able further to predict accurately the temporal effect of warfarin on clotting time. Therefore, even delayed effects of drugs and toxicants can be analyzed, explained, and predicted using basic pharmacokinetic principles.

2 The compound is distributed instantaneously throughout its volume of distribution.

As stated above, the equations for $F$ as a function of time developed in Section 7.3 may be applied irrespective of whether entry into the system was zero order or first order, provided the absorptive phase is complete. Duration of action, on the other hand, is dependent on the absorption rate constant. Figure 7.18 shows why this is so.

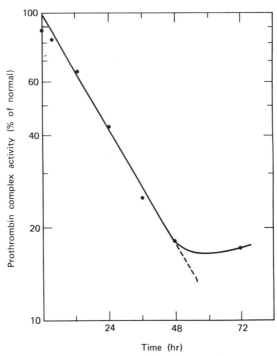

**Figure 7.16** Plasma prothrombin complex activity in a normal subject as a function of time after oral administration of warfarin sodium (1.5 mg/kg). Reproduced with permission from Nagashima et al., 1969, Figure 2.

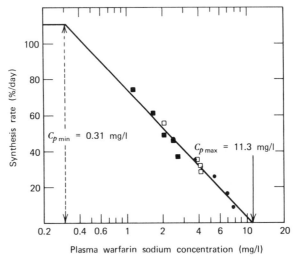

**Figure 7.17** Synthesis rate of prothrombin complex activity as a function of plasma warfarin concentration, based on averaged data from six normal subjects. Dosing schedules of warfarin sodium were: one oral dose, 1.5 mg/kg (●); daily oral doses, 10 mg, for 5 days (■); daily oral doses, 15 mg, for 4 days (□). $C_{p\,min}$ = apparent minimum effective plasma concentration; $C_{p\,max}$ = plasma concentration associated with total suppression of prothrombin complex activity synthesis. Reproduced with permission from Nagashima et al., 1969, Figure 3.

*340*

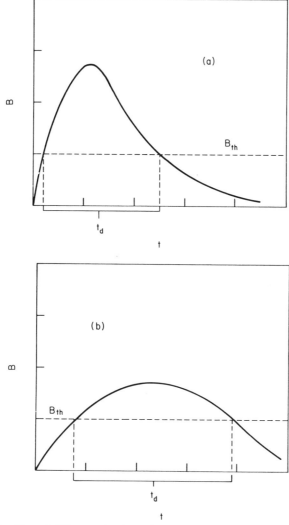

**Figure 7.18** The effect of differences in absorption rate on duration of action. Areas under the curves are equal. (*a*) Large $k_a$; (*b*) small $k_a$.

Duration of effect measurements can be compared only within a single mode of administration and for a single absorption rate constant. For example, the duration of action of a drug cannot be related to the amount given in different oral formulations unless the formulations have identical release rates.

3  The kinetic behavior of the compound is adequately described by a one-compartment body model.

This is the requirement that is least likely to be met by a real drug or toxicant. As a result the impact of multicompartment distribution characteristics on log dose, $t_d$ and $F, t$ relationships has been examined in some detail.

Gibaldi et al. (1971) have shown that compounds with linear multicompartment distribution and linear elimination characteristics will show curvature in the log dose, duration of action graph that may be suggestive (depending on the location of the receptor sites) of a saturable elimination mechanism. For a two-compartment model with receptor sites located in the central compartment, the theoretical relationship between dose and duration of action is illustrated in Figure 7.19. When duration is measured to a very low (10%) intensity end point, the curve in Figure 7.19 should reflect mostly the $\beta$ phase of kinetics and duration should be approximately a linear function of the log of the dose except at very low doses. At the other extreme, when duration is measured to a very high (90%) intensity end point, the duration, log dose relationship should reflect primarily the $\alpha$ or distribution phase of kinetics except at very high doses.

Thiopental is an example of a compound whose duration of action is determined primarily by its distribution kinetics. Thiopental is a rather slowly

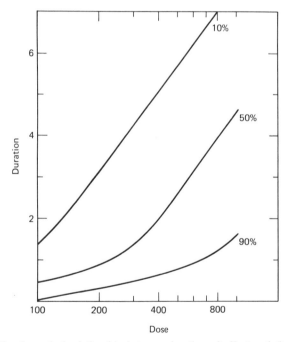

**Figure 7.19** The theoretical relationship between duration of effect and the logarithm of the dose for a compound distributed into one peripheral compartment, assuming that the site of action is in the central compartment. The percentage next to each curve indicates the intensity of the pharmacologic effect used as the end point. Reproduced with permission from Gibaldi et al., 1971, Figure 5.

metabolized barbiturate with rapid but brief action. Thiobarbiturates enter the brain more rapidly than do their oxygen analogues because of their greater lipophilicity. The brain, the site of thiopental action, is kinetically a part of the central compartment. But thiopental also leaves the plasma and brain rapidly to enter peripheral tissues such as muscle and fat. As it does so its concentration drops below the threshold level. Therefore its duration of action is fixed by its kinetic parameters of distribution.

When duration of action is measured to an end point of intermediate intensity, duration, log dose curves are affected by both $\alpha$ and $\beta$ and are not linear anywhere. In this respect they resemble the curves for a compound that is distributed throughout only one compartment but is eliminated by means of a saturable mechanism (compare Figure 7.19 with Figure 7.8$a$).

The neuromuscular blocking agent D-tubocurarine obeys a three-compartment kinetic model; its site of action appears to be in the central compartment (Figure 7.20). Gibaldi et al. (1972) compared duration of action data from Walts and Dillon (1968) with simulated duration, log dose curves to show that D-tubocurarine exhibits the predicted behavior (Figure 7.21). It is also apparent from Figure 7.21 that over different restricted dose ranges (or for different effect intensities) the duration, log dose relationships might have different slopes, though appearing to be essentially linear.

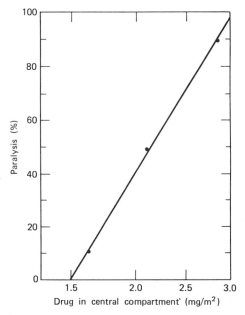

**Figure 7.20** The relationship between amount of D-tubocurarine in the central compartment of a three-compartment model (log scale) and the intensity of its neuromuscular blocking effect. Note that 90% paralysis (or block) is the same as 10% recovery. Reproduced with permission from Gibaldi et al., 1972, Figure 6.

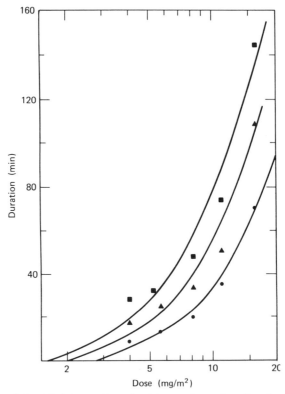

**Figure 7.21**   The relationship between dose of D-tubocurarine and median duration of action in man. The curves are the computer-predicted relationships. The data points are from Walts and Dillon, 1968, and represent the time necessary for recovery of 10% (●), 50% (▲), and 90% (■) of the normal force of contraction of the adductor muscles of the thumb. Reproduced with permission from Gibaldi et al., 1972, Figure 9.

Gibaldi and Levy (1972) showed that $F, t$ plots for D-tubocurarine are approximately linear in the 20–80% effect range but that the slopes of the lines decrease with increasing dose. The rates of decline of the effects of other multicompartment drugs with linear elimination kinetics also appear to be dose dependent, although linear over much of their course.

If the site of action of a drug or toxicant with multicompartment distribution characteristics is in a peripheral compartment, its effect may be not only delayed in onset but also prolonged in duration. The lag in achievement of a dynamic steady state that is characteristic of all kinetically significant peripheral compartments is reflected in the time course of action. This lag is especially pronounced for deep compartments. When the site of action is in a deep compartment, effector may be slow in penetrating to receptor sites but persists in the vicinity of the receptor sites for an extended period of time.

During the $\beta$ phase of plasma dieaway from an acute administration there is no assurance that a dynamic pseudo-steady state has been achieved between plasma concentration and concentrations in peripheral tissues, but only that any distribution still going on is slower than whole body loss. (Recall that the fastest of simultaneous processes dominates.) A compound may continue to accumulate in a deep compartment for some time after its plasma level has entered the $\beta$ phase of dieaway. If the site of action is in a deep compartment the effects of acute and chronic exposures may differ sharply.

On acute exposure there may be no effect at all if threshold levels in the biophase have not been achieved. If there is an effect it will be delayed in onset and persistent; it may even outlast measurable levels of the compound in the plasma. On chronic exposure amounts in deep compartments can become very large as the compound continues to accumulate after plasma concentration appears to have stabilized. Effects may not become manifest until long after the initial exposure and may persist long after cessation of exposure. For this reason toxicants acting in deep compartments may be very difficult to identify; toxicity may not be apparent until well after the occurrence of the initial exposure. Drugs acting in this fashion were at one time called "hit and run" drugs, since the relationship between concentrations in the plasma and at the receptor site was not clearly understood. Many cardioactive drugs appear to act in deep compartments, although they may act by different mechanisms and have different effects. Examples are reserpine, guanethidine (Gibaldi et al., 1972, based on data from Schanker and Morrison, 1965), and digoxin (see Section 7.1).

## PROBLEMS

1 Dollery et al. (1976) measured the effect of the hypotensive drug clonidine on blood pressure in five normotensive adult males. From their results (Figure 7.22), decide whether the site of this action of clonidine is more likely to be in the central or in a peripheral compartment.

2 The $\beta$-adrenergic blocking agent pindolol blocks induced tachycardia. Gugler et al. (1975) correlated the intensity of blockade of exercise-induced tachycardia with plasma pindolol concentrations in eight healthy adults. Intensity of blockade was expressed as percentage of the effect of the exercise load without prior administration of pindolol. From their data (Table 7.1), determine whether the site of action of pindolol is in the central compartment.

3 Paalzow (1975) found that the plasma kinetics of theophylline in rats after intravenous administration of 12.5 mg/kg could best be described by the equation

$$C_p = 35.6e^{-16.4t} + 15.5e^{-0.15t}$$

where $t$ is in hours, $V_1 = 24\%$ of the body weight, and $V_2 = 54\%$ of the

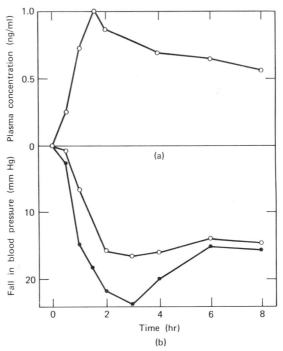

**Figure 7.22**   Mean plasma concentration of clonidine (*a*) in five normal subjects who were given an oral dose of 300 μg of clonidine compared with (*b*) the mean change in their systolic blood pressure (●) and diastolic pressure (O). Reproduced with permission from Dollery et al., 1976, Figure 2.

body weight. A number of effects of theophylline are consequent to its inhibition of cyclic AMP degradation. One of these is reduction in the rat's threshold for pain induced by electrical stimulation. The data in Table 7.2 for the pain threshold reduction effect of a single dose of 12.5 mg theophylline/kg body weight are expressed as percentage of pretreatment pain threshold.

Does theophylline act in the central or in the peripheral compartment?

4   The data in Table 7.3 are taken from Adams and Greene (1964). Is the absence of an anorectic effect at the 0.25-mg/kg dose consistent with your prediction based on the observed duration of effect at the other three doses? Assume that D-amphetamine is eliminated by first-order mechanisms.

5   CI-581 is an ultra-short-acting intravenous general anesthetic that exhibits first-order elimination characteristics. From the sleeping time measurements graphed by Levy (1966) (Figure 7.23), estimate both the rate constant for elimination and the half-life of CI-581 in humans.

**Table 7.1** Pindolol plasma levels and percentage blockade (mean ± SE, $n = 8$) at stated times after the oral administration of 10 mg of pindolol

| Time (hr) | Pindolol Plasma Level (ng/ml) | Percent Blockade |
|---|---|---|
| 0.5 | 18.2 ± 2.9 | 13.8 ± 3.9 |
| 1 | 34.9 ± 7.6 | 32.3 ± 5.2 |
| 2 | 51.9 ± 9.5 | 40.6 ± 4.3 |
| 3 | 45.8 ± 8.5 | 36.4 ± 4.2 |
| 4 | 33.7 ± 7.3 | 31.0 ± 4.6 |
| 6 | 23.2 ± 3.2 | 21.7 ± 5.9 |

Reproduced from Gugler et al., 1975, Table 1.

**Table 7.2** The time course in rats of the pain threshold reduction effect of theophylline, 12.5 mg/kg

| Time (min) | Effect (% of pretreatment threshold) |
|---|---|
| 5 | 60 |
| 15 | 65 |
| 30 | 75 |
| 45 | 78 |
| 60 | 77 |
| 90 | 82 |
| 120 | 82 |
| 180 | 90 |

Data points were read from Figure 5 of Paalzow, 1975.

**Table 7.3** The duration of anorectic action, from the maximum to 50% anorexia, of D-amphetamine sulfate in dogs ($n = 10$; 2–3 trials per dog)

| Dose (mg/kg) | Duration of Action (hr) |
|---|---|
| 0.25 | — |
| 0.40 | 1.5 |
| 0.60 | 3.0 |
| 0.75 | 4.5 |

Reproduced from Adams and Greene, 1964, Table II.

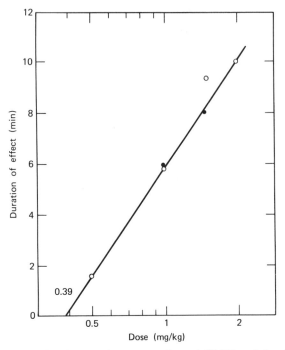

**Figure 7.23** The relationship between intravenous dose of CI-581 and duration of coma in human subjects. Adapted with permission from Levy, 1966, Figure 3, based on data from Domino et al., 1965. (Ignore the distinction between open and closed circles.)

**6** Kuehn et al. (1976) measured the time course of the decrease in rabbits' pupillary diameters caused by single doses of chlorpromazine administered intravenously. Some of their results are given in Table 7.4.

**Table 7.4** Intensity of pupillary diameter decrease in rabbits as a function of intravenous dose of chlorpromazine

| Chlorpromazine Dose (mg/kg) | Maximum Effect[a] | Time to 0.6 of Maximum Effect (min) |
|---|---|---|
| 4.0 | .2561 | 308 |
| 3.0 | .2460 | 277 |
| 2.0 | .2082 | 283 |
| 1.0 | .1703 | 247 |
| 0.5 | .1498 | 176 |

From Kuehn et al., 1976, Table I. Duration of effect data were interpolated.

[a] Effect was calculated as:

$$1 - \frac{\text{pupillary diameter at time } t}{\text{initial pupillary diameter}}.$$

Assuming that the kinetics of chlorpromazine elimination are first order, calculate the elimination rate constant and the half-life of chlor-promazine.

7 McCarthy et al. (1965) measured the duration of anesthesia produced in monkeys by several general anesthetics. Their data for pentobarbital are given in Table 7.5. Do these data support saturability or unsaturability of pentobarbital elimination mechanisms within this dose range?

**Table 7.5** The duration of pentobarbital anesthesia following intravenous administration in monkeys

| Number of Monkeys | Dose (mg/kg) | Mean Duration (min) |
|---|---|---|
| 3 | 34.0 | 263 |
| 3 | 26.0 | 207 |
| 6 | 22.0 | 135 |
| 4 | 20.4 | 110 |
| 6 | 17.0 | 90 |
| 4 | 16.3 | 46 |
| 3 | 13.6 | 9 |

Reproduced from McCarthy et al., 1965, Table II.

8 Quinton (1963) determined the effect of atropine on pupillary diameters in mice. Effect (designated "response" in Figure 7.24) was expressed as the difference between initial pupillary diameter and pupillary diameter at time $t$. From Figure 7.24, estimate the half-life of atropine in mice of this size, assuming that elimination of atropine is first order.

9 Assuming that there is no concentration threshold for the action of a drug with linear one-compartment kinetics and a linear dose, effect relationship with slope $m$, show that following acute administration

$$\ln F = \ln(mD) - k_e t,$$

where $F$ is the fraction of maximum (initial) effect, $D$ the dose, $k_e$ the first-order elimination rate constant, and $t$ time.

10 Levy (1970a) has pointed out that for compounds with linear elimination kinetics and a linear ln dose, effect curve, the product of duration of effect and the slope $-mk_e$ of the $F, t$ line should be independent of $k_e$:

$$(t_d)(-mk_e) = m(\ln B_{th} - \ln D).$$

The data in Table 7.6 on the effects of succinylcholine in infants were

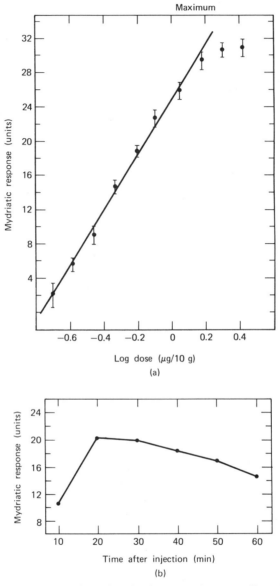

**Figure 7.24** The effect of atropine injected subcutaneously on pupillary diameter in mice weighing 20–25 g. (a) The relationship of mean effect intensity to the log of the atropine dose. The bars indicate standard error. (b) Time course of the effect of atropine, 2 μg/10 g. Reproduced from Quinton, 1962, Figure 1 (with correction of the abscissa units) and Figure 2 (adapted).

Table 7.6  Pharmacokinetic analysis of neuromuscular blocking effects of succinylcholine in nine infants

| Subject Number | Duration of Succinylcholine Action (min) | Rate of Decline of Effect (%/min) |
|---|---|---|
| 11 | 5 | 40 |
| 10 | 6 | 40 |
| 14 | 6 | 40 |
| 15 | 6 | 40 |
| 7 | 7 | 24[a] |
| 4 | 9 | 28[a] |
| 2 | 12 | 28[a] |
| 5 | 14 | 16[a] |
| 8 | 26 | 9 |

Reproduced from Levy, 1970a, Table 1, based on data from Walts and Dillon, 1969.
[a]Average of two values reported.

tabulated by Levy. Three of these infants (subjects 2, 5, and 8) showed an unusually prolonged duration of effect. For which of these three does the prolonged effect appear to be due primarily to the value of $k_e$? For which does it appear that $m$ and/or $B_{th}$ are involved?

11  Levy (1970b) tabulated data from Katz et al. (1969) and from Walts and Dillon (1969) comparing duration and rate of decline of suxamethonium effect in three different human populations. Some of these data are given in Table 7.7. Using the technique introduced in Problem 10, decide whether the prolonged duration of suxamethonium action in the New York population is or is not the consequence of a difference in the mean first-order elimination constant of the drug in this population relative to the other two.

Table 7.7  Neuromuscular blocking effect of suxamethonium in three human populations given the same dose

| Population from | Recovery Time to 10% of Normal (min) | Rate of Decline of Effect (%/min) |
|---|---|---|
| London | 6.3 | 28.6 |
| New York | 10.2 | 18.2 |
| Los Angeles | 7.0 | 26.7 |

Reproduced from Levy, 1970b, Table I, based on data from Katz et al., 1969, and from Walts and Dillon, 1969.

## REFERENCES

Adams, H. J. and L. C. Greene. "Modified method for studying anorexigenic agents in dogs." *J. Pharm. Sci.*, **53**, 1405–1406 (1964).

Aghanajian, G. K. and O. H. L. Bing. "Persistence of lysergic acid diethylamide in the plasma of human subjects." *Clin. Pharmacol. Ther.*, **5**, 611–614 (1964).

Carruthers, S. G., J. G. Kelly, D. G. McDevitt, and R. G. Shanks. "Blood levels of practolol after oral and parenteral administration and their relationship to exercise heart rate." *Clin. Pharmacol. Ther.*, **15**, 497–509 (1974).

Dollery, C. T., D. S. Davies, G. H. Draffan, H. J. Dargie, C. R. Dean, J. L. Reid, R. A. Clare, and S. Murray. "Clinical pharmacology and pharmacokinetics of clonidine." *Clin. Pharmacol. Ther.*, **19**, 11–17 (1976).

Gibaldi, M. and G. Levy. "Dose-dependent decline of pharmacologic effects of drugs with linear pharmacokinetic characteristics." *J. Pharm. Sci.*, **61**, 567–569 (1972).

Gibaldi, M., G. Levy, and W. Hayton. "Kinetics of the elimination and neuromuscular blocking effect of D-tubocurarine in man." *Anesthesiology*, **36**, 213–218 (1972).

Gibaldi, M., G. Levy, and H. Weintraub. "Drug distribution and pharmacologic effects." *Clin. Pharmacol. Ther.*, **12**, 734–742 (1971).

Gugler, R., W. Höbel, G. Bodem, and H. J. Dengler. "The effect of pindolol on exercise-induced cardiac acceleration in relation to plasma levels in man." *Clin. Pharmacol. Ther.*, **17**, 127–133 (1975).

Hinderling, P. H. and E. R. Garrett. "Pharmacokinetics of $\beta$-methyldigoxin in healthy humans. III. Pharmacodynamic correlations." *J. Pharm. Sci.*, **66**, 326–329 (1977).

Katz, R. L., J. Norman, R. F. Seed, and L. Conrad. "A comparison of the effects of suxamethonium and tubocurarine in patients in London and New York." *Br. J. Anaesth.* **41**, 1041–1047 (1969).

Kourounakis, P., S. Szabo, and H. Selye. "Effect of various steroids and ACTH on distribution of zoxazolamine in rats." *J. Pharm. Sci.*, **62**, 1946–1949 (1973a).

Kourounakis, P., S. Szabo, J. Werringloer, and H. Selye. "Effect of various steroids and ACTH on plasma levels of zoxazolamine and dicumarol." *J. Pharm. Sci.*, **62**, 690–692 (1973b).

Kuehn, P. B., A. K. Jhawar, W. A. Weigand, and V. F. Smolen. "Pharmacokinetics of chlorpromazine-induced miotic response in rabbits." *J. Pharm. Sci.*, **65**, 1593–1599 (1976).

Lemberger, L., J. L. Weiss, A. M. Watanabe, I. M. Galanter, R. J. Wyatt, and P. V. Cardon. "Delta-9-tetrahydrocannabinol; temporal correlation of the psychologic effects and blood levels after various routes of administration." *New Engl. J. Med.*, **286**, 685–688 (1972).

Levy, G. "Relationship between elimination rate of drugs and rate of decline of their pharmacologic effects." *J. Pharm. Sci.*, **53**, 342–343 (1964).

Levy, G. "Kinetics of pharmacologic effects." *Clin. Pharmacol. Ther.*, **7**, 362–372 (1966).

Levy, G. "Pharmacokinetics of succinylcholine in newborns." *Anesthesiology*, **32**, 551–552 (1970a).

Levy, G. "Differences in effect of suxamethonium in London, Los Angeles, and New York." *Br. J. Anaesth.*, **42**, 979–980 (1970b).

Levy, G. and E. Nelson. "Theoretical relationships between dose, elimination rate, and duration of pharmacologic effect of drugs." *J. Pharm. Sci.*, **54**, 812 (1965).

Levy, G., M. Gibaldi, and W. J. Jusko. "Multicompartment pharmacokinetic models of pharmacologic effects." *J. Pharm. Sci.*, **58**, 422–424 (1969).

Maher, J. F., G. E. Schreiner, and F. B. Westervelt, Jr. "Acute gluthethimide intoxication. I. Clinical experience (twenty-two patients) compared to acute barbiturate intoxication (sixty-three patients)." *Am. J. Med.*, **33**, 70–82 (1962).

Nagashima, R., R. A. O'Reilly, and G. Levy. "Kinetics of pharmacologic effects in man: The anticoagulant action of warfarin." *Clin. Pharmacol. Ther.*, **10**, 22–35 (1969).

O'Reilly, R. A. and P. M. Aggeler. "Studies on coumarin anticoagulant drugs: Initiation of warfarin therapy without a loading dose." *Circulation*, **38**, 169–177 (1968).

Paalzow, L. K. "Pharmacokinetics of theophylline in relation to increased pain sensitivity in the rat." *J. Pharmacokinet. Biopharmaceut.*, **3**, 25–38 (1975).

Quinton, R. M. "The mydriatic response of mice to atropine." *J. Pharm. Pharmacol.*, **15**, 239–250 (1963).

Schanker, L. S. and A. S. Morrison. "Physiological disposition of guanethidine in the rat and its uptake by heart slices." *Int. J. Neuropharmacol.*, **4**, 27–39 (1965).

Sidell, F. R. and J. E. Pless. "Ethyl alcohol: Blood levels and performance decrements after oral administration to man." *Psychopharmacologia*, **19**, 246–261 (1971).

Singleton, S. D. and S. D. Murphy. "Propanil (3,4-dichloropropionanilide)-induced methemoglobin formation in mice in relation to acylamidase activity." *Toxicol. Appl. Pharmacol.*, **25**, 20–29 (1973).

Sturtevant, F. M. "Mydriatic half-life of a new anticholinergic as affected by dose, route, quaternization." *Proc. Soc. Exp. Biol. Med.*, **104**, 120–123 (1960).

Van Rossum, J. M. and A. T. J. Van Koppen. "Kinetics of psycho-motor stimulant drug action." *Eur. J. Pharmacol.*, **2**, 405–408 (1968).

Walts, L. F. and J. B. Dillon. "Duration of action of D-tubocurarine and gallamine." *Anesthesiology*, **29**, 499–504 (1968).

Walts, L. F. and J. B. Dillon. "The response of newborns to succinylcholine and D-tubocurarine." *Anesthesiology*, **31**, 35–38 (1969).

# 8

# Dose, Response
# Relationships

**8.1** The relationship between effect and response

**8.2** The dose, response curve

**8.3** The probit plot

**8.4** Summary: Comparison of response and effect evaluation

**8.5** The joint action of effectors; synergism

**8.6** The relationship of length of exposure to response

**8.7** Extrapolation of response measurements to very low exposure levels

    8.7.1 The Mantel-Bryan extrapolation

    8.7.2 The linear extrapolation

    8.7.3 Comparison of extrapolation models

The two preceding chapters were concerned with the measurement of continuous variables; that is, variables that can in principle take on any value between zero and some maximum dependent on the number of receptor sites associated with the effect being measured. Although the concept of graded effect is applicable either to an isolated receptor system studied *in vitro* or to that same receptor system in a single individual, it cannot be applied to a population of individuals. Response in a population must be defined in terms of a quantal ("all or none") measurement. In a population an individual either does or does not respond, in terms of some arbitrary criterion, at a fixed drug dose or toxicant exposure. A priori we would expect that there is an exposure sufficiently great that all population members are affected, and that there is likely to be an exposure sufficiently small that no member of the population demonstrates the selected response. We shall define "population response" as the fraction or percentage of the population responding at a particular drug dose or toxicant exposure. Maximum response is then one, or 100%.

Response and effect are qualitatively different measurements. Effect is graded; response is quantal. Effects are measured; responses are counted. Maximum effect is the maximum magnitude or strength of effect; maximum response is 100% of the population.

As will be seen, ln dose, response curves usually resemble ln dose, effect curves. But because their origins, their applications, and the kind and amount of information they contain differ, it is important to distinguish between the two. We will begin by considering the way in which a ln dose, response curve is built up from a population of individual ln dose, effect curves.

## 8.1 THE RELATIONSHIP BETWEEN EFFECT AND RESPONSE

Consider an experimental population of six animals and the log dose, effect curves for the action of a hypothetical toxicant in each of these six animals. The individual log dose, effect curves are drawn in Figure 8.1.

It is apparent that each of the animals 1 to 6 has a different sensitivity to the toxicant, since the six log dose, effect curves are positioned differently along the log dose axis. For simplicity let us choose $\theta_m$ as our criterion of quantal response. Depending on the identity and action of the toxicant, $\theta_m$ could be maximum inhibition of an enzyme system, complete blockage of neuromuscular junctions, or any other maximum effect including death. Then at a dose of 12 units of toxicant (log dose = 1.1), animal 1 should show some signs of toxicity, but none of the animals should have responded in terms of the criterion $\theta_m$. At a dose of 16 units of toxicant (log dose = 1.2), one of the six animals should have responded in terms of $\theta_m$, two more should be

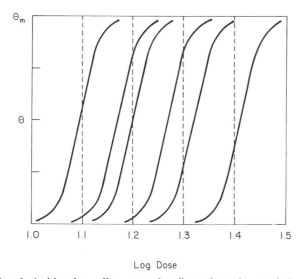

**Figure 8.1** Hypothetical log dose, effect curves for all members of a population of six animals.

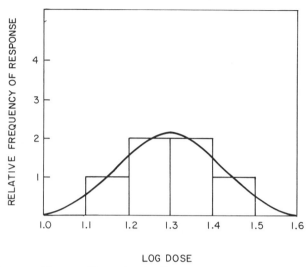

LOG DOSE

**Figure 8.2** Frequency histogram illustrating the distribution of sensitivities of the population of Figure 8.1.

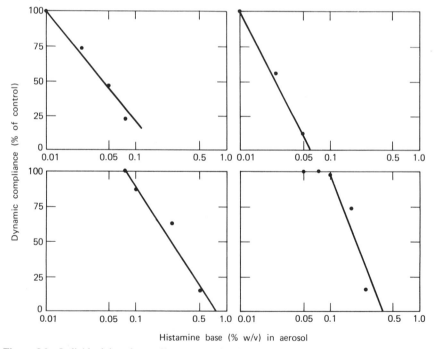

Histamine base (% w/v) in aerosol

**Figure 8.3** Individual log dose, effect curves for four female albino guinea pigs exposed to aerosolized histamine. Adapted with permission from Douglas et al., 1973, Figure 1, © 1973 by the Williams & Wilkins Co., Baltimore.

showing signs of mild to moderate toxicity, and the other three should be unaffected. At a dose of 20 units of toxicant (log dose = 1.3), three animals should have responded, two more should be affected, one of them severely; and one should still be unaffected. At a dose of 25 units of toxicant (log dose = 1.4), all but one animal should have responded in terms of $\theta_m$; and finally, at a dose of 32 units of toxicant (log dose = 1.5), the entire population of six animals should have responded.

This information may be summarized in a frequency histogram (Figure 8.2) that relates the number of new responders at each dose level to the log of the dose.

Figure 8.2 is symmetrical about a mean log dose value of 1.3. A smooth curve drawn through the midpoints of the frequency bars as shown suggests a normal distribution of response frequencies, or a normal distribution of the sensitivities to dose of individual members of the population about a mean log dose value.

We could have chosen the sensitivities of our hypothetical animal population in such a way as to generate any desired frequency distribution. Most often, however, the sensitivities of members of a population are found to be distributed in a Gaussian or normal fashion about a mean log dose value, in this case 1.3. In this example the 20-unit dose is the median effective dose, called the ED50. It is the dose at which half the population responds in terms of the criterion $\theta_m$. Since $\theta_m$ is death, the ED50 in this case is the LD50, the median lethal dose.

Figure 8.3 shows log dose, effect curves for four guinea pigs exposed to aerosols containing different concentrations of histamine (Douglas et al., 1973). The effect measured was the reduction in dynamic lung compliance caused by the constrictive action of histamine. Since effect is here graphed as percentage of control rather than as magnitude of reduction, the effect curves have a negative rather than a positive slope. The four guinea pigs exhibit histamine sensitivities varying over a tenfold dose range.

Similar log dose, effect curves were generated for a total of 131 guinea pigs. These animals were grouped in accordance with their apparent sensitivities, and the ED50 for each group was used to construct the frequency histogram in Figure 8.4. The Gaussian density function derived from the statistical parameters of the observed distribution is also shown in Figure 8.4. Since the predicted frequencies were not significantly different from the observed frequencies, the authors concluded that individual sensitivities to histamine action were log normally distributed.

The "sharpness" of the peak in Figure 8.4 is a reflection of the degree of homogeneity of the population with respect to histamine sensitivity. Population homogeneity is determined not only by the characteristics of the receptor site but also by interindividual variations in absorption, distribution, and excretion kinetics. If the receptor site is located in a poorly accessible or deep compartment, it is to be expected that the population will be more heterogeneous than it would be if the receptor site were in the central compartment,

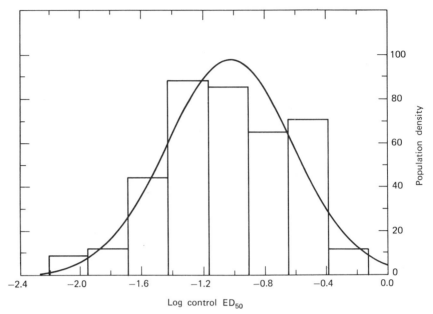

Log control $ED_{50}$

**Figure 8.4** Distribution of ED50 values to histamine aerosols in female albino guinea pigs. Doses of aerosolized histamine that produced a 50% change of dynamic lung compliance from baseline values were determined from control dose, response curves. These data were accumulated into groups and a distribution pattern was constructed by a digital computer. The ordinate is population density. A Gaussian density function derived from the mean and variance of log ED50 values is also plotted. The area under the curve is equal to the area under the blocks. The predicted values were not significantly different from the observed values when tested with the $\chi^2$ test. Reproduced with permission from Douglas et al., 1973, Figure 2, © 1973 by the Williams and Wilkins Co., Baltimore.

since in the former case there are more options for individual differences than in the latter.

The degree of population homogeneity with regard to a normal distribution of sensitivities is expressed by the parameter $\sigma$, the standard deviation. The standard deviation is a measure of the degree of dispersion of incidence frequencies about the mean; in this case, about log ED50. It is defined as

$$\sigma = \sqrt{\frac{\Sigma(\mu - x)^2}{N-1}} \quad ,$$

where $N$ is the number of individuals making up the population, $\mu$ is log ED50, and the various $x$ are the log dose levels used, each log dose level appearing in the calculation a number of times determined by its associated frequency of response. The characteristics of a normal distribution are such that 68% of the population is included within the area bounded by log ED50 $\pm \sigma$ on the frequency histogram, 95.5% within 2 standard deviations on either side of the mean, and 99.7% within 3 standard deviations on either side of the mean. Consequently a small value of $\sigma$ implies a relatively homogeneous population and a large value implies a heterogeneous population.

## 8.2   THE DOSE, RESPONSE CURVE

There is another way to relate response frequency to dose. That is to graph the cumulative number of responders or, more commonly, the cumulative fraction or percentage of the population responding as a function of the log of the dose. For the hypothetical population of six animals in Figures 8.1 and 8.2, the cumulative percentages are listed in Table 8.1 and graphed in Figure 8.5.

The curve in Figure 8.5 is sigmoid. As a result it is sometimes equated to the relationship between $\theta/\theta_m$, the fraction of maximum effect, and the log of the dose. The similarity in the shapes of the two curves is unfortunate, particularly since it may obscure qualitative and quantitative differences between dose, effect and dose, response curves that can provide real and useful information.

Specifically, the "steepness" of the slope at the midpoint of the curve in Figure 8.5, like the "sharpness" of the peak in Figure 8.4, is a measure of the degree of homogeneity of the population. It is entirely unrelated to any mechanism of action of the drug or toxicant. In fact, its value is $\sigma^{-1}$, where $\sigma$ is the standard deviation described in Section 8.1. The more homogeneous the population, the smaller $\sigma$ will be and the steeper the slope of the cumulative distribution function at its midpoint.

This midpoint is, of course, log ED50 (see Figure 8.5). The ED50 is a useful index of population response. It is a measure of median population sensitivity to a drug or toxicant, and as such it can be used as an index of the relative potency of a series of compounds. But it does not give any information about the range of sensitivities within the population. One useful way to do this (other than by giving the value of $\sigma$) is to cite in addition to the ED50 another effective dose such as the ED10 or the ED90. Indeed, it may

**Table 8.1** Cumulative response, as percentage of population responding, for the population of Figures 8.1 and 8.2

| Log Dose | Response (%) |
|----------|--------------|
| 1.1 | 0.0 |
| 1.2 | 16.7 |
| 1.3 | 50.0 |
| 1.4 | 83.3 |
| 1.5 | 100.0 |

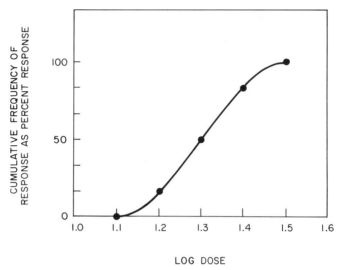

**Figure 8.5** Cumulative frequency of response for the hypothetical animal population of Figure 8.1.

sometimes be more appropriate to use one of these other doses instead of the ED50 in a particular study.

Figure 8.6 is taken from a study of physical dependence on barbiturates in mice and response to withdrawal (Siew and Goldstein, 1978). The measure of hyperexcitability during the withdrawal period was susceptibility to convulsions induced by pentylenetetrazol; the response to pentylenetetrazol of mice not pretreated with barbiturates is shown in Figure 8.6. The ED50 is about 85 mg/kg, administered intraperitoneally. However, since habituation to

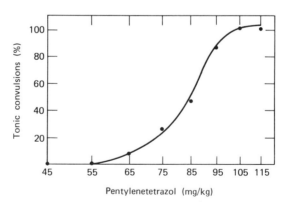

**Figure 8.6** The response of control mice to an intraperitoneal dose of pentylenetetrazol. The ordinate gives the percentage incidence of tonic extensor convulsions within 30 min after injection. Each point represents the response in a group of 12 animals. Reproduced with permission from Siew and Goldstein, 1978, Figure 1, © 1978 by the American Society for Pharmacology and Experimental Therapeutics.

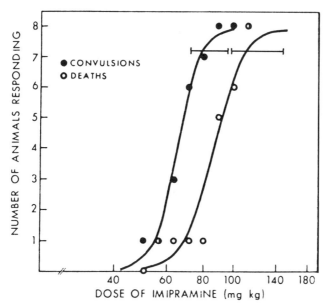

**Figure 8.7** Dose, response curves for imipramine-induced convulsions and death in rats. Each point represents the response in a group of eight animals. Horizontal bars represent the 95% confidence limits of the ED90 for convulsions, and the LD90. Reproduced with permission from Beaubien et al., 1976, Figure 1.

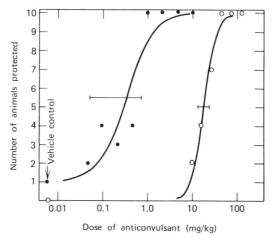

**Figure 8.8** Protection against imipramine-induced convulsions achieved by administration of diazepam (●) or phenobarbital (○) 20 min prior to imipramine (112 mg/kg given intraperitoneally). All data points are calculated for groups of 10 animals. Adapted with permission from Beaubien et al., 1976, Figure 2.

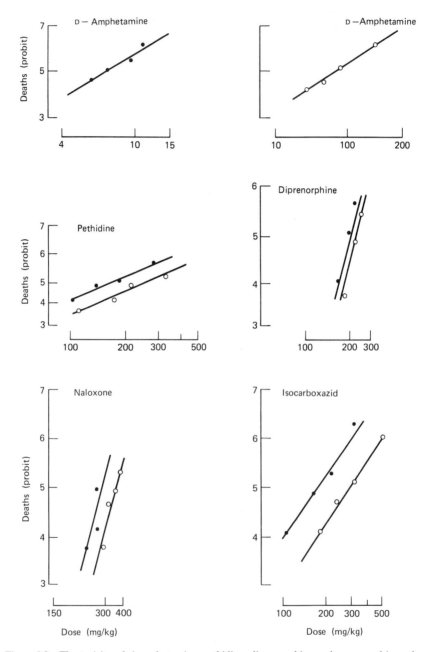

**Figure 8.9** The toxicity of *d*-amphetamine, pethidine, diprenorphine, naloxone, and isocarboxazid in noncrowded (○) and crowded (●) mice showing parallel shifts in the dose, response relationship. All drugs were injected subcutaneously. Each point represents the value obtained from a group of eight animals. Reproduced with permission from Doggett et al., 1977, Figure 2.

barbiturates was expected to increase the sensitivity of the mice to pentylene-tetrazol, the investigators elected to challenge habituated mice with the ED30, 75 mg/kg.

Figure 8.7 gives another example of a log dose, response relationship; here the LD90 was of particular interest. Two responses, convulsions and death, are represented in the same graph; note that the number instead of the fraction of animals responding is given on the ordinate. Because the authors (Beaubien et al., 1976) were interested in the protection afforded against imipramine by several anticonvulsants, they used the LD90, 112 mg of imipramine/kg intraperitoneally, in subsequent studies in which the animals were pretreated with the anticonvulsants and their response to imipramine measured. Figure 8.8 demonstrates that both phenobarbital and diazepam provided significant protection against imipramine-induced convulsions. The ED50 for phenobarbital protection was 17.6 mg/kg and that for diazepam protection was 0.32 mg/kg.

The ED50 of a particular drug or toxicant may also be influenced by factors that affect the sensitivity of a population in a general rather than in a specific way. For example, Doggett et al. (1977) studied the effect of crowding on drug toxicity in mouse populations. Figure 8.9 shows that crowding increased population sensitivity to the five different drugs tested. The effect was most marked with amphetamine, least marked with diprenorphine. Note that the ordinates in Figure 8.9 are all scaled in probit units.

## 8.3 THE PROBIT PLOT

For all the usual reasons it would be advantageous if response data could be transformed to produce a dose, response curve that is linear throughout its entire length. To do this we can take advantage of the presumption that the underlying distribution of population sensitivities is lognormal, and distort the ordinate of a cumulative response plot in such a way that the idealized normal distribution would give a straight line. This distortion can be produced by expressing response in terms of units of standard deviation. Provided the distribution of sensitivities is indeed lognormal, then at a dose 3 standard deviations below the mean, 0.14% of the population will respond; at a dose 2 standard deviations below the mean, 2%; at a dose 1 standard deviation below the mean, 16%;, at the ED50, 50%; at $+\sigma$, 84%, and so on. When the ordinate is scaled in units of standard deviation (these are called normal equivalent deviates in this context) and the abscissa in units of log dose, the cumulative lognormal distribution is linearized throughout.

To avoid the use of negative numbers ($-3\sigma$, $-2\sigma$, etc.), by convention the number 5 is added to each normal equivalent deviate. Accordingly $-3\sigma$ becomes 2, $-\sigma$ becomes 4, $+2\sigma$ becomes 7, and so on. These new units are called probit units. Graph paper is available with the abscissa scaled in logs and the ordinate *scaled* in probits but *printed* as percentage response. This paper is convenient to use. Data graphed directly as percentage response are automatically transformed into probit units by the distortion of the ordinate built into the graph paper. Alternatively, the probit unit corresponding to each observed percentage response may be found and plotted directly. Tables are available for this purpose.

Fitting of a probit line cannot be done by simple linear regression. Proper curve-fitting procedures must reflect awareness that the most reliable data points are those for sample populations exposed to doses near the ED50. Data points at either dose extreme are unreliable. Rosiello et al. (1977) review the history of probit analysis and outline a computer program for estimating the ED50 together with its error. A simplified approach to the tedious but accurate technique on which the computer program was based has been in common use for some time. This, the method of Litchfield and Wilcoxon (1949), combines graphical analysis with the use of nomograms. The slope of the probit line is $1/\sigma$.

Probit analysis is used primarily by toxicologists; response data expressed in this form are usually toxicity data. It is a useful analytical technique. It is important, however, not to forget that probit transformation of toxicity response data is founded on the assumption that the underlying distribution of population sensitivities is lognormal. Significant systematic deviation of data points from a probit line may suggest significant deviation from a lognormal sensitivity distribution, in which case probit transformation may not be the most appropriate analytical technique to use.

## 8.4  SUMMARY: COMPARISON OF RESPONSE AND EFFECT EVALUATION

Both the log dose, fraction of maximum effect and the log dose, cumulative fraction of response relationships are sigmoid. In all other respects they differ. The important features of dose, effect and dose, response curves are summarized and compared in Table 8.2.

**Table 8.2**  A comparison of dose, effect and dose, response relationships

| Curve | Application | Basis | Slope at Inflection Point | Position on Log Dose Axis |
|---|---|---|---|---|
| Log dose, graded effect (fraction of maximum effect) | To an individual or to an isolated receptor system | Receptor theory | Related to molecularity of mechanism of action; should be similar for all similar mechanisms | Reflection of sensitivity of individual to agonist; $K_m$ in isolated receptor system |
| Log dose, quantal response (cumulative fraction of response) | To a population | Observation; empirical | $\sigma^{-1}$, where $\sigma$ is the standard deviation of the distribution of sensitivities within the population | Reflection of median sensitivity of population to drug or toxicant; ED50 |

## 8.5 THE JOINT ACTION OF EFFECTORS; SYNERGISM

McKay et al. (1971) investigated potentiation of the effect of soman, a cholinesterase inhibitor, by 2-(*O*-cresyl)-4*H*-1 : 3 : 2-benzodioxaphosphorin-2-oxide (CBDP), a metabolite of a known potentiator of anticholinesterase toxicity. Their results in Figure 8.10 are presented as graphed on probit paper. The distortion built into the percentage response scale is clearly illustrated. The probit lines are linear and parallel and demonstrate potentiation by CBDP of the effect of soman.

CBDP is not itself lethal even at these relatively large doses. Therefore it is acting solely as a potentiator of soman toxicity. However, there are many instances in which two drugs or toxicants that separately exert the same effect are present in the body at the same time. Their interactions are now considered.

Substances that produce the same measured effect may do so either by means of identical or closely related mechanisms or by means of different mechanisms. Bliss (1939) was the first to discuss the possible relationships among dose, response curves for similarly acting substances administered separately and as mixtures. He defined the combined action of toxicants

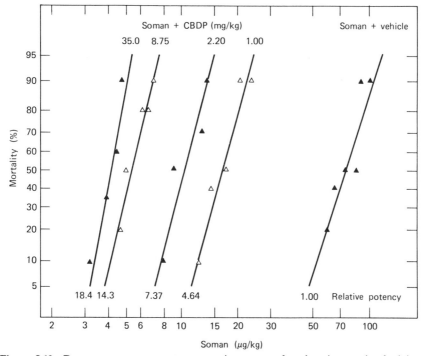

**Figure 8.10** Dose, response curves to soman in groups of male mice previously injected subcutaneously either with propylene glycol alone (controls) or with various doses of 2-(*O*-cresyl) -4*H*-1 : 3 : 2-benzodioxaphosphorin-2-oxide (CBDP) in propylene glycol. Reproduced with permission from McKay et al., 1971, Figure 1.

acting by the same mechanism as similar joint action, and that of toxicants acting by unrelated mechanisms as independent joint action. In the case of independent joint action, susceptibility to one toxicant may or may not be correlated with susceptibility to the other. In the case of similar joint action, complete correlation is usually assumed. Therefore log dose, response curves for toxicants having similar joint action, and for mixtures of such toxicants, should all be parallel.

Synergism is a deviation of the observed effect of mixtures of two (or more) components from the effect predicted on the basis of either independent or similar joint action. Synergism may be either positive or negative, negative synergism being more commonly called antagonism. Often the word synergism is used alone to mean positive synergism.

To identify synergism it is necessary to be able to predict the joint action of mixtures. Finney (1952) synthesized a number of previous analytical approaches to questions surrounding the joint action of toxicants, and developed and presented statistical treatments for all possible cases. The predicted behavior of mixtures of toxicants acting by independent joint action is complex and its mathematical treatment is correspondingly difficult. In general, a mixture whose components act by similar joint action can be expected to have a greater effect than a comparable mixture whose components act by independent joint action. Therefore to test for positive synergism, observed responses to mixtures are compared with the responses to be expected based on knowledge of the log dose, response curves for the components of the mixtures together with the principles of similar joint action. The statistical methods are given by Finney (1952). An illuminating discussion of joint action and a simpler but less rigorous graphical approach to the identification of positive synergism were published by Wadley (1945, 1949).

Suppose that the ED50 values for two toxicants having similar joint action have been separately determined. Then the potency of either of the toxicants relative to that of the other may be expressed as the ratio of the two ED50 values. (Since the log dose, response curves are presumably parallel, any other effective dose could be used as well—e.g., the ED30 or the ED90.) The potency of mixtures of the two toxicants may be calculated in terms of the concentration of one toxicant alone, and the predicted joint action of each mixture read directly from the log dose, response curve for the reference toxicant. In principle it would be desirable to compare the observed with the predicted response to several mixtures of different composition, but in practice it is more usual to compare the observed with the predicted ED50 of a single mixture.

Consider two toxicants, 1 and 2. With 1 as the reference toxicant, the relative potency $p$ is expressed as

$$p = \frac{ED50(1)}{ED50(2)}, \tag{8.1}$$

so that dose $D_2$ of toxicant 2 may be converted to equipotent dose $D_1$ of toxicant 1 where

$$D_1 = pD_2. \tag{8.2}$$

We will write the log dose, response curve for the reference toxicant as

$$\text{response probit} = a + b\log D_1, \tag{8.3}$$

where $a$ and $b$ are constants. Then if the two toxicants have similar joint action, the log dose, response curve of a mixture should be the same as that of an equipotent amount of toxicant 1, or

$$\text{response probit} = a + b\log(D_1 + pD_2)$$
$$= a + b\log[(f_1 + pf_2)D], \tag{8.4}$$

where $D$ is the total dose of toxicant and $f_1$ and $f_2$ are the proportions of the two toxicants present in the mixture.

For a 50% response (probit = 5), from Equations 8.3 and 8.4,

$$a + b\log[\text{ED50}(1)] = a + b\log[(f_1 + pf_2)(\text{ED50}(\text{mix}))],$$

or

$$\text{ED50}(1) = (f_1 + pf_2)(\text{ED50}(\text{mix}));$$

$$\text{ED50}(\text{mix}) = \frac{\text{ED50}(1)}{f_1 + pf_2}. \tag{8.5}$$

The reciprocal of Equation 8.5 is

$$\frac{1}{\text{ED50 (mix)}} = \frac{f_1}{\text{ED50}(1)} + \frac{f_2}{\text{ED50}(2)}. \tag{8.6}$$

Either Equation 8.5 or Equation 8.6 may be used to predict the ED50 of a mixture from knowledge of the individual ED50s and the makeup of the mixture. Selected examples will be taken from a study by Kulkarni (1976) of the joint action of organochlorine insecticides on female houseflies.

Table 8.3 lists the LC50s, or concentrations lethal to half the experimental housefly population, of several of the insecticides studied. Based on the

**Table 8.3**  Relative toxicity of different insecticides to female houseflies

| Insecticide | LC50 (% w/v) | p | |
|---|---|---|---|
| DDT | 0.091730 | 1.000 ⎫ | |
| Lindane | 0.017220 | 5.3269 ⎬ | Relative to DDT |
| Isobenzan | 0.002523 | 36.3575 ⎭ | |
| Carbaryl | 0.151700 | 1.0000 ⎫ | Relative to carbaryl |
| Thiometon | 0.010050 | 15.0945 ⎭ | |

From Kulkarni, 1976, Table 1.

**Table 8.4**  Toxicity to female houseflies of different mixtures of insecticides

| Mixture | Expected LC50(% w/v) | Observed LC50(% w/v) |
|---|---|---|
| 97.3% DDT + 2.7% isobenzan | 0.04689 | 0.02533 |
| 84.2% DDT + 15.8% lindane | 0.05444 | 0.05406 |
| 93.8% carbaryl + 6.2% thiometon | 0.08096 | 0.1111 |

From Kulkarni, 1976, Table 3.

relative potencies of the individual insecticides, a series of mixtures was formulated, each containing equipotent concentrations of two insecticides. Table 8.4 gives three of these mixtures together with the observed LC50 of each mixture and the LC50 calculated using Equation 8.6.

Visual comparison of observed with expected LC50s suggests that DDT and lindane are simply additive, DDT and isobenzan exhibit positive synergism, and carbaryl and thiometon are antagonistic. By use of the appropriate statistical methods (Finney, 1952) the author confirmed these relationships.

A related graphical approach to the identification of synergism is particularly simple. Since

$$f_1 + f_2 = 1,$$

then

$$f_1(\text{EC50}(2)) + f_2(\text{EC50}(2)) = \text{EC50}(2);$$

$$f_2(\text{EC50}(2)) = \text{EC50}(2) - \frac{f_1(\text{EC50}(2))(\text{EC50}(1))}{\text{EC50}(1)},$$

or

$$f_2(\text{EC50}(2)) = \text{EC50}(2) - \frac{f_1(\text{EC50}(1))}{p}, \qquad (8.7)$$

where $p = \text{EC50}(1)/\text{EC50}(2)$ as before. Equation 8.7 states that for the case of similar joint action without synergism, a straight line drawn between the value of EC50(1) (on the abscissa) and the value of EC50(2) (on the ordinate) (line $A$ in Figure 8.11$a$) has a slope of $-p^{-1}$, and that each point on this line is associated with a mixture that should produce the stipulated effect in half the test population. Points lying below the line represent mixtures that should produce the stipulated effect in less than half the test population. If, however, the two components of the mixture are positively synergistic, points associated with the EC50(mix) will determine a curve lying below line $A$ (line $B$ in Figure 8.11$a$). Note that the points on this curve represent mixtures containing less than the amounts of the two components calculated to produce a 50%

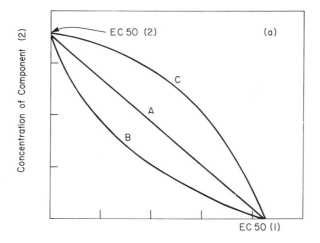

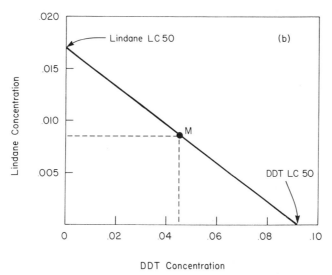

**Figure 8.11** Graphical determination of synergism. (*a*) Principle of the technique: line *A*, additive effects; line *B*, positive synergism; line *C*, negative synergism. See text for complete explanation. (*b*) Application to mixtures of lindane and DDT. Point *M* is the equipotent mixture of Table 8.4.

response. Conversely line *C* in Figure 8.11*a* represents antagonism. In either case the degree of curvature reflects the magnitude of the synergism.

As an example consider again the data on DDT and lindane from Tables 8.3 and 8.4. The line in Figure 8.11*b* is drawn between 0.092%(w/v), the LC50 for DDT, and 0.017%(w/v), the LC50 for lindane. The slope of this line is $-0.017/0.092$, or $-p^{-1}$. Point *M* on this line represents the equipotent mixture of Table 8.4, containing 0.046%(w/v) DDT and 0.0086%(w/v) lindane, calculated and found to be lethal to half the test population of houseflies.


## 8.6   THE RELATIONSHIP OF LENGTH OF EXPOSURE TO RESPONSE

The foregoing discussion has dealt with response to a known dose administered at a single time point or, at the very least, over a short time period. Often, however, exposure to a drug or toxicant is chronic or subchronic (90 days or less). When this is the case it is possible to calculate a kind of "integrated total dose" as

$$\text{total dose} = (\text{dose rate})(\text{length of exposure}).$$

Then we ask: is a given total dose administered at a low rate over a long period of time equivalent to the same total dose administered at a high rate over a short time period?

If total dose is the sole determinant of response, then for 50% response

$$(DR)(\text{T50}) = \text{LD50}, \tag{8.8}$$

where T50 is the time to 50% incidence or median time to incidence of the measured effect in the test population. So-called mean survival times or mean time to incidence of a nonlethal effect are often measured in inhalation and aquatic toxicology studies. In these studies $DR$ is replaced by the concentration $C$ of the toxicant in air or water. Since $DR$ is proportional to $C$, this substitution is straightforward:

$$(C)(\text{T50}) = K, \tag{8.9}$$

where $K$ is a constant proportional to the total dose.

Very often the simple relationships stated by Equations 8.8 and 8.9 are found not to be accurate representations of mean survival time data. A typical relationship is shown in Figure 8.12, taken from Gardner et al. (1977). These investigators found that continuous inhalation of benzene vapor resulted in a reduction in the number of leukocytes in peripheral blood of rodents. When 25–30% leukopenia was used as the response criterion, the relationship between T50 and the concentration of benzene in the atmosphere was observed to be linear on a log, log scale:

$$\log \text{T50} = \log K - \alpha \log C,$$

or

$$(\text{T50})(C^{\alpha}) = K. \tag{8.10}$$

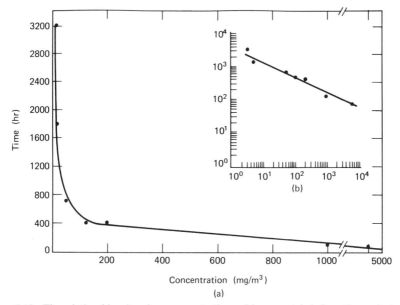

**Figure 8.12** The relationship of various concentrations of benzene inhaled continuously to the time of onset of leukopenia in peripheral blood of rodents. (*a*) Arithmetic coordinate system; (*b*) Logarithmic coordinate system. Reproduced with permission from Gardner et al., Figure 3, *J. Toxicol. Environ. Health*, **3**, 811–820, © 1977 by Hemisphere Publ. Corp., Washington, D.C.

The slope $\alpha$ in this case was less than 1, indicating that time was more important than concentration to the determination of response. In other cases concentration is found to be more significant than time.

Gardner et al. found that several concentration, time relationships for continuous inhalation exposures could be represented by straight lines on a log, log scale. Other representations have also been used, however, in particular by aquatic toxicologists (Sprague, 1969). In general these techniques are not grounded in biological theory but are simply efforts to linearize data sets by employing arbitrary transformations. One simple modification of Equation 8.9 that is biologically reasonable takes into account the probability that kinetic and biochemical time lags result in a minimum median survival time $T50_{min}$, and the possibility that there is a minimum or threshold concentration $C_{th}$ below which no response is observed. The modified equation is

$$(C - C_{th})(T50 - T50_{min}) = K'. \qquad (8.11)$$

Andersen et al. (1977) found that the aerosol concentration of the solvent sulfolane was related to the mean survival time of exposed rats by Equation 8.11, as shown in Figure 8.13.

Equation 8.11 will apply only over time periods that are short relative to the half-life of the toxicant. Over longer time periods processes of metabolism and excretion must be taken into account, since they affect the relationship

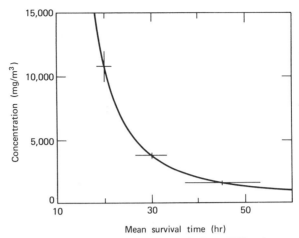

**Figure 8.13** The relationship between mean survival time (T50) of rats and the aerosol concentration of sulfolane to which the animals were exposed. Data points are mean ± standard error for both time to death and concentration. The smooth curve is the curve of best fit based on an equation of the form $(T50\text{-}T50_0)\,(C\text{-}C_{th})=K$ where $T50_0$ and $C_{th}$ represent minimum T50 and threshold concentration, respectively. Reproduced with permission from Andersen et al., 1977, Figure 2.

between length of exposure and body burden. This is true whether exposure is continuous, as in the example above, or intermittent. It will be illustrated here only for intermittent exposure.

When exposure occurs repeatedly, the toxicant is subjected to elimination processes during the intervals between doses. The total amount present in the tissues after $n$ doses therefore is not $n$ times the amount present after one dose. The ratio of the amount $BB(n)$ in the body after $n$ doses to the amount $BB(1)$ in the body after one dose for a one compartment model is (see Section 5.2.1):

$$\frac{BB(n)}{BB(1)} = \frac{1-e^{-nk_e\Delta t}}{1-e^{-k_e\Delta t}}.$$

The dependence of this ratio on $k_e\Delta t$ is graphed in Figure 8.14 for values of $n$ from 1 to 7. It is apparent that as $k_e$ increases with the interval between doses remaining constant, the number of doses required to achieve a given body burden increases. This, of course, is intuitively reasonable, since compounds with short half-lives are eliminated efficiently during the intervals between doses. The practical consequence of this observation is that larger total doses of a toxicant can be tolerated when the compound is given in divided doses than when the total dose is given at one time. For compounds with a very large $k_e$ (short half-life), the difference between the acute LD50 and the chronic LD50 may be very large indeed.

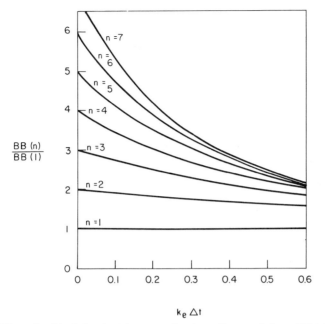

**Figure 8.14** The ratio of body burden after $n$ equal and equally spaced doses ($BB(n)$) to body burden after one dose ($BB(1)$) as a function of $k_e \Delta t$, for values of $n$ from 1 to 7, in the one-compartment body model.

Hayes (1972) tabulated acute and 90-dose LD50s for a number of toxicants. Selected examples are listed in Table 8.5.

Many other factors may affect the relationships among dose rate, length of exposure, and response. Most of these are specific to particular drugs or toxicants. For example, metabolism or excretion mechanisms may be saturable at high doses but not at the low levels characteristic of chronic industrial

**Table 8.5** The ratio of 90-dose LD50 to 1-dose LD50 for compounds with different half-lives

| Compound (in rough order of decreasing $t_{1/2}$) | A: The 1-Dose LD50 (mg/kg) | The 90-Dose LD50 | | |
|---|---|---|---|---|
| | | B (mg/kg/day) | C (mg/kg) | C/A |
| Mirex | 365 | 6 | 540 | 1.5 |
| DDT | 250 | 46 | 4,140 | 16.6 |
| Benzylpenicillin | 6700 | 4140 | 372,600 | 55.6 |
| Sodium chloride | 3750 | 2690 | 242,100 | 64.6 |
| Potassium cyanide | 10 | >250[a] | >2,250 | >225 |

LD50 data from Hayes, 1972, Table II, based in part on data from Boyd and Selby, 1962, Boyd and Shanas, 1963, and Boyd et al., 1966.

[a] 250 mg/kg/day was the largest dose rate. No mortalities were observed.

or environmental exposure. With chronic exposure there is the possibility of either sensitization or tolerance development or of age-related changes in susceptibility. Induction of metabolizing enzymes may occur. And deep compartments, which may not even be kinetically demonstrable after an acute exposure, may control the response to chronic exposure. Consequently the response to a series of repeated small doses may be qualitatively as well as quantitatively different from the response to a single large dose.

There is no reason to suppose that a single theory should explain all the observed deviations from the simple concept of total dose. Undoubtedly a number of different reinforcing and opposing influences contribute to the production of a net dominance of either time or dose rate in determination of response during chronic exposure.

One of the most important groups of environmental agents for which $(DR)(T50)$ is not a constant is the group of chemical carcinogens. Both in human (Whittemore and Altshuler, 1976) and in experimental animal (Druckrey, 1967) populations, it has been established that the effect of time is dominant over the effect of dose, so that response to low levels of environmental carcinogens occurs disproportionately early. For many chemical carcinogens $\alpha$ in Equation 8.10 is from $\frac{1}{3}$ to $\frac{1}{4}$. For a discussion of the significance of these relationships in carcinogenesis, see Albert and Altshuler (1973).

## 8.7 EXTRAPOLATION OF RESPONSE MEASUREMENTS TO VERY LOW EXPOSURE LEVELS

The design of experimental dose, response studies is limited by two important practical considerations. First, the researcher is restricted to the study of animal populations of manageable size, usually 100 to 1000 animals. Second, he is limited to the use of exposures that will produce a measurable response in a test population of the size studied. What would the response be in a larger population exposed to a lower dose of the toxicant? This question can be approached only by extrapolation out of the range of observation into a range where the true dose, response relationship is not known. Such extrapolations are fundamental to risk assessment for chemicals whose effects are so serious that only a very low incidence of these effects can be tolerated. In general these include the carcinogens and the mutagens, both of which are thought to act by irreversible mechanisms.

It is necessary to distinguish between irreversibility of a response—that is, death is an irreversible response; the appearance of a malignant tumor is in most cases an irreversible response—and irreversibility of the process that leads to the response. Conventional dose, effect mechanistic models are based on the assumption that binding of the toxicant to its receptor site is reversible and that the receptor site, once freed of toxicant, has not been permanently altered by its presence (Chapter 6). Irreversible models of toxicity, on the other hand, are based on the assumption that once the receptor site has been occupied it cannot be regenerated unchanged. It is permanently altered, either because the toxicant is covalently and permanently bound or because self-replication of the altered site occurs.

One molecule of any agonist, whether it acts by a reversible or an irreversible mechanism, is potentially capable (i.e., has a finite probability) of combining with one of its receptor sites and thereby exerting an action. Whether the action of a single molecule is significant is determined by whether the resulting effects are significant to the health and well-being of the whole organism.

For reversibly acting toxicants in general, the biochemical decrement associated with the action of a single molecule is not only insignificant but also temporary; therefore one molecule has zero probability of causing an unacceptable or even a measurable effect. For such toxicants it is generally agreed that an exposure threshold usually exists and dose, response data are not ordinarily extrapolated to very low exposure levels. Instead an arbitrary safety factor, commonly 100–1000, is applied to the lowest exposure that produced a measurable response in an animal test population to obtain an estimated safe dose for humans. Sometimes the safety factor includes a correction relating dose to body surface area, since effective dose is more closely related to body surface area than to weight in different species.

For carcinogens, mutagens, and perhaps teratogens, however, the action of one molecule has a finite probability of resulting in an unacceptable effect. In theory therefore no exposure threshold should exist for such substances, although in practical terms if the probability of one molecule producing a measurable effect is very low, no response may be observed in a population of finite size. This leads to the concept of the "no-effect level," an operational "threshold" that is dependent on population size. Repair mechanisms alter the slope of the dose, response curve by decreasing the probability that one molecule can cause an unacceptable effect. They may thereby raise the no-effect level, but they do not create an absolute threshold.

For risk assessment purposes, experimental dose, response data for carcinogens must be extrapolated into a very low exposure range where the true dose, response relationship is not known. There is no general agreement as to the best procedure to use in extrapolating; historically, different procedures have been advocated at different times and for different purposes. There is a vast original literature on the broad subject of extrapolation procedures and their relationship to experimental dose, response curves and to theoretical mechanistic models of carcinogenesis. We discuss several rather general guidelines that are used in the design and development of extrapolation techniques and outline briefly the two procedures that have been most heavily relied on. Lucid descriptions and comparisons of these and other extrapolation procedures have been provided by Hoel et al. (1975) and by

Chand and Hoel (1974). The latter article includes consideration of time to tumor. An excellent review of the state of the extrapolation art has also appeared recently (Maugh, 1978).

Interspecies conversion of extrapolated results is not discussed here. This necessary step in standard setting involves the application of a safety factor with or without adjustment for body surface area. Some of the considerations that should go into selection of an appropriate species conversion factor are discussed by Hoel et al. (1975).

The purpose of extrapolation is to estimate the exposure that is associated with an acceptable incremental risk. The definition of "acceptable" incremental risk is largely arbitrary. It is arrived at by considerations of benefit (better quality of life) versus cost (excess cancer incidence), and may also be influenced by practical limitations in ability to remove the carcinogen completely from the environment.

Sometimes in low dose extrapolation, an effort is made to be conservative; that is, to be reasonably certain that the line of extrapolation lies above the probable true dose, response curve. The reason for this is illustrated in Figure 8.15. As long as the line of extrapolation lies above the true line, the actual incremental risk (response corrected for background) associated with a given exposure will not exceed the predicted risk.

Risks are expressed as lifetime risks. An incremental risk of $10^{-6}$ represents an excess incidence of 1 in $10^6$ or 1 in 1,000,000. This incidence corresponds to 200 excess occurrences over a lifetime in a population of 200 million or about 3 excess occurrences per year in the United States. Several years ago $10^{-6}$ and $10^{-8}$ were widely proposed as acceptable incremental

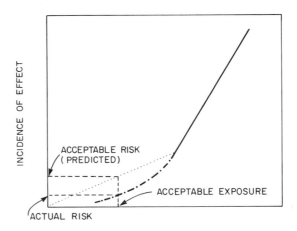

EXPOSURE

**Figure 8.15** Conservatism in extrapolation into the low dose range: solid curve, observed dose, response relationship in experimental animal population; dot-dash curve, true dose, response relationship below observable response range; dotted curve, conservative extrapolation.

risks. More recently an incremental risk of $10^{-5}$ has been used in conjunction with a particularly conservative extrapolation procedure (see Section 8.7.2).

Every extrapolation originates at a point. Figure 8.15 shows an extrapolation from the lowest experimental exposure that resulted in a positive response. But an extrapolation may also be made from a no-effect level by taking into account the uncertainty attendant on using measured response in a randomly selected small test population to represent response in a larger population. Suppose that none of 100 test animals was affected by the toxicant chosen at the dose level used. With what assurance can the researcher state that none of 1000 animals, or none of 10,000 animals, would have been affected by the same exposure?

The upper confidence limits $P$ for possible response when none of a population of $N$ animals has been affected by an experimental exposure are given by the expression

$$1 - \text{level of assurance} = (1 - P)^N. \tag{8.12}$$

The values of a number of upper confidence limits for zero observed response are given in Table 8.6 as fractions. That is, if no animals from a test population of 1000 were affected, the researcher can state with 99% assurance that not more than 45 out of 10,000 animals ($0.0045 \times 10,000$) would have been affected by the same exposure. As is to be expected, the larger the test population, the smaller the confidence interval.

Use of an upper confidence limit as a starting point for extrapolation permits extrapolation from an experimental no effect level. Alternatively it provides a more conservative starting point for extrapolation from the lowest experimental dose associated with a measurable response. Extrapolation from an upper confidence limit is used in the first of the two procedures to be described below.

### 8.7.1 The Mantel-Bryan Extrapolation

If it can be assumed that the distribution of sensitivities within the test population is lognormal, then a log dose, probit response graph should be linear throughout its length. Mantel and Bryan (1961) observed that the

**Table 8.6** Upper confidence limit on proportional risk when no response was observed in a study population of *n* animals

| *n* | 95 | 99 | 99.9 |
|---|---|---|---|
| | \multicolumn{3}{c}{Level of Assurance (%)} | |
| 10 | 0.26 | 0.37 | 0.50 |
| 100 | 0.03 | 0.045 | 0.067 |
| 500 | 0.006 | 0.0092 | 0.014 |
| 1000 | 0.003 | 0.0045 | 0.0069 |

slopes of log dose, probit response relationships were generally greater than 1 in animal carcinogenesis studies. They therefore set a conservative lower bound of 1 probit unit of response per tenfold dose increment (a "probit slope of 1") and extrapolated with this slope from the 99% upper confidence limit of the lowest observed response. The Mantel-Bryan procedure has been modified to allow for combination of data at different dose rates and refined with respect to the correction for spontaneous tumor incidence (Mantel et al., 1975). It was in general use for many years.

Two major problems are associated with the Mantel-Bryan procedure. First, the log dose, probit response relationships for a number of carcinogens including hormones and tobacco smoke have been found to have slopes near and even less than 1. Although this problem can be circumvented by choosing a slope for extrapolation that is less than the observed slope, the degree of conservatism built into the procedure is then reduced to the level of personal choice. Second, the Mantel-Bryan procedure is based on the assumption that the lognormal distribution of sensitivities assumed for all carcinogens extends for some distance below the experimental range. This assumption may not be justified and certainly cannot be verified. As a result, an extrapolation that avoids these difficulties and is based at least to some extent on biological considerations is gradually supplanting the Mantel-Bryan procedure.

### 8.7.2  The Linear Extrapolation

Since carcinogenesis is an irreversible process, it "uses up" receptor sites rather than regenerating them. The number $R$ of unaffected receptors decreases at the rate

$$\frac{dR}{dt} = -k_1(R)(X),$$

or

$$\frac{dR}{R} = -k_1(X)\,dt \tag{8.13}$$

where $X$ is the concentration of carcinogen at the receptor site and $k_1$ is a rate constant. Integrated over the time period of exposure

$$\int_{t=0}^{t=t} \frac{dR}{R} = -k_1 \int_{t=0}^{t=t} X\,dt$$

where $\int X\,dt$ represents the total amount of carcinogen passing through the biophase. If $\int X\,dt$ can be related to dose, the fractions of affected and unaffected receptors at time $t$ can be related to dose. For the case of $\int X\,dt$

proportional to total dose $D$,

$$\int_{t=0}^{t=t} \frac{dR}{R} = \Big|_{t=0}^{t=t} \ln R = \ln R - \ln R_0$$

$$= -\int_{t=0}^{t=t} k_1 X \, dt = -aD$$

where $a$ is a constant and $R_0$ is the total number of receptors available at $t=0$. Therefore

$$\frac{R}{R_0} = e^{-aD} = f_u, \tag{8.14}$$

the unaffected fraction of receptor sites. If the probability $P$ of an effect is equal to the affected fraction $f_a$ of receptor sites, then

$$P = f_a = 1 - f_u = 1 - e^{-aD}. \tag{8.15}$$

For very small values of the exponent $(aD)$ this expression can be approximated by

$$P = aD. \tag{8.16}$$

This is the one-hit carcinogenesis model. It states that at very low exposure levels the risk is linearly related to dose without threshold. Therefore it represents an attempt to provide a "best estimate" of the true risk rather than a conservative upper bound to the true risk. If the slope is sufficiently low (that is, if $aD$ is sufficiently small), the line of extrapolation is simply drawn from the origin in an arithmetic coordinate system either to the lowest experimental point or to its upper confidence limit; the latter, of course, is the more conservative approach. Otherwise Equation 8.15 is used.

Other biologically plausible models, the multistage (sequential) models, also reduce to a linear form at very low exposure levels. In fact almost all mechanistic models of carcinogenesis do become linear at very low dose (Crump et al., 1976). Therefore linear extrapolation is a biologically reasonable and relatively model-independent approach to estimating the risk of carcinogenesis at very low exposures.

The linear models have weaknesses also. Each implies a mechanism of action that is by no means universally accepted. Furthermore, they are all based on the assumption that $P$ for a population is the same as $P$ for each of the individuals making up the population; that is, that all population members have identical susceptibility to the carcinogen. If this is not the case, the true population dose, response relationship at very low dose rates will be concave upward even though no absolute threshold for the carcinogen exists.

Such a population dose, response relationship would be indistinguishable in practice from one predicted by a multihit mechanistic model that does imply the existence of an absolute threshold.

### 8.7.3   Comparison of Extrapolation Models

Interestingly, although the Mantel-Bryan procedure was specifically designed to be conservative, linear extrapolation without threshold is actually the more conservative of the two for risks less than about $10^{-4}$.

Suppose that at a particular experimental dose none of a group of 100 animals was affected. The upper 99% confidence limit on this point would be a fractional response of 0.045 (Table 8.6). Table 8.7 gives the results of extrapolating from this upper confidence limit by both the Mantel-Bryan and the linear procedures, for selected levels of risk. Results are expressed as ratio of acceptable dose, or dose associated with each risk level, to the experimental no effect dose. It is apparent that the estimates of acceptable dose diverge markedly at very low risk levels.

All plausible dose, response models of carcinogenesis, whether mechanistic or empirical, are essentially in agreement with each other and with experimental data in the observable range. This point has been clearly illustrated for several models including the Mantel-Bryan and the linear models (Food and Drug Advisory Committee, 1971). The models diverge widely only at very low exposures, where goodness of fit to the true dose, response relationship cannot be tested experimentally. The linear extrapolation without threshold is the most conservative of the available models for very low risk—so conservative, in fact, that for acceptable incremental risks of $10^{-6}$ or less the allowable exposure would be practically zero. Currently, the linear extrapolation without threshold is being used together with an acceptable risk of $10^{-5}$. The use of this relatively large acceptable risk in conjunction with an ultraconservative extrapolation procedure may be justifiable on pragmatic grounds.

In the long run verification of the accuracy of any extrapolation procedure will have to await the accumulation and analysis of epidemiologic data. Already there is evidence that linear extrapolation without threshold may be too conservative for some carcinogens (Gehring et al., 1978, 1979; Ramsey et

**Table 8.7**   The ratio of acceptable to experimental dose for two different extrapolation models

| Risk Level | Mantel-Bryan | Linear without Threshold |
|---|---|---|
| $10^{-2}$ | $2.3 \times 10^{-1}$ | $2.2 \times 10^{-1}$ |
| $10^{-4}$ | $9.5 \times 10^{-3}$ | $2.2 \times 10^{-3}$ |
| $10^{-6}$ | $8.8 \times 10^{-4}$ | $2.2 \times 10^{-5}$ |
| $10^{-8}$ | $1.2 \times 10^{-4}$ | $2.2 \times 10^{-7}$ |

al., 1979). Modifications and adjustments in extrapolation procedures are made continuously. The approach to risk evaluation at low doses will continue to evolve as our epidemiologic information base on cancer incidence rates continues to broaden.

### PROBLEMS

**1** Maynert (1960) administered various anesthetics intravenously to dogs and estimated the intensity of neurological derangement on a scale of 0–V, level 0 representing freedom from any central nervous system symptoms and level V representing the most severe involvement (deepest level of anesthesia). Some of Maynert's results are reproduced in Figure 8.16.

Is this a dose, response or a dose, effect curve?

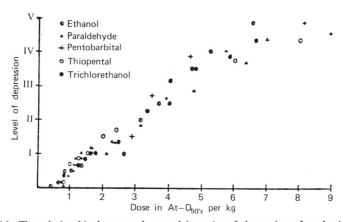

**Figure 8.16** The relationship between dose and intensity of depression after the intravenous administration of selected anesthetics to dogs. Each point represents a group of six dogs given the same dose. Doses are expressed in units of the median ataxic dose At-D50 (the dose that produced a response level of I) for the same drug in the same group of dogs. Reproduced with permission from Maynert et al., 1960, Figure 2, © 1960 by the Williams & Wilkins Co., Baltimore.

**2** Fuhremann and Lichtenstein (1972) were interested in the effect of polychlorinated biphenyls (e.g., Aroclor 1248) on the toxicity of house flies to organophosphorus insecticides (e.g., paraoxon). They presented the dose, response curves in Figure 8.17.

What effect does Aroclor 1248 have on the toxicity of paraoxon?

**3** Lampreys have reduced the rainbow trout population in many areas. The lampricidal agent 3-trifluoromethyl-4-nitrophenol (TFM) is relatively non-toxic to the trout themselves and is excreted by them largely as the

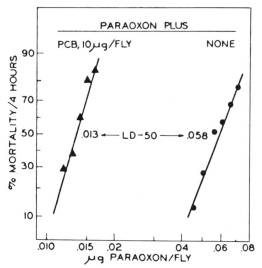

**Figure 8.17** Response of houseflies to paraoxon with and without prior exposure to the polychlorinated biphenyl Aroclor 1248 (PCB). Reproduced with permission from Fuhremann and Lichtenstein, 1972, Figure 1.

glucuronide conjugate. In an effort to determine whether conjugation of TFM serves to protect the trout from its acute toxic effect, Lech et al. (1973) studied the effects of novobiocin, which interferes with conjugation of TFM, on the acute toxicity and disposition of TFM in rainbow trout. Certain of their results are shown in Figures 8.18 and 8.19.

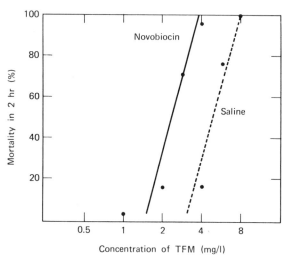

**Figure 8.18** The effect of novobiocin on the acute toxicity of 3-trifluoromethyl-4-nitrophenol (TFM) to rainbow trout: dotted curve, saline injected; solid curve, 200 mg novobiocin/kg. Reproduced with permission from Lech et al., 1973, Figure 1.

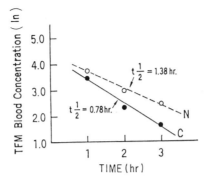

**Figure 8.19** The disappearance of unconjugated TFM from blood of control and novobiocin-treated trout injected intraperitoneally with 0.25 mg [$^{14}$C]TFM/100 g. Abscissa, time after injection. Solid curve, saline injected; dashed curve, novobiocin pretreated. Each point represents the mean of a minimum of three fish. Reproduced with permission from Lech et al., 1973, Figure 10.

Do you believe that the trout's ability to conjugate TFM is an important protective mechanism? Why?

4   A continuation of the study of Problem 3 (Lech and Statham, 1975) was directed at determining whether the lamprey is unable to glucuronidate TFM and, if so, whether such inability is responsible for the lamprey's sensitivity to TFM. The relationships shown in Figures 8.20 and 8.21 were reported. In addition, the effect of salicylamide, which inhibits glucuronide formation, was studied (Figures 8.22).

Is the lamprey unable to form TFM glucuronide? If so, is the inability responsible for its sensitivity? If not, do the data suggest another mechanism that might be responsible?

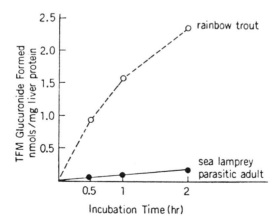

**Figure 8.20** *In vitro* glucuronidation of TFM by liver extracts from rainbow trout and parasitic adult sea lamprey. Each point represents the mean of three separate determinations. Reproduced with permission from Lech and Statham, 1975, Figure 3.

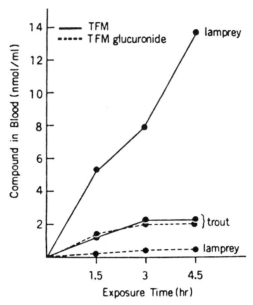

**Figure 8.21** Blood concentrations of TFM and TFM glucuronide in rainbow trout and parasitic adult sea lamprey exposed to [$^{14}$C]TFM. Each point represents the mean of three separate determinations. Reproduced with permission from Lech and Statham, 1975, Figure 4.

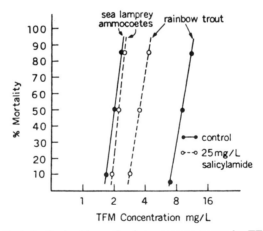

**Figure 8.22** The effect of salicylamide on the dose, response curves for TFM in rainbow trout and sea lamprey ammocoetes (larva). Plots are derived from Litchfield-Wilcoxon methods using a minimum of eight fish at each point. Reproduced with permission from Lech and Statham, 1975, Figure 6.

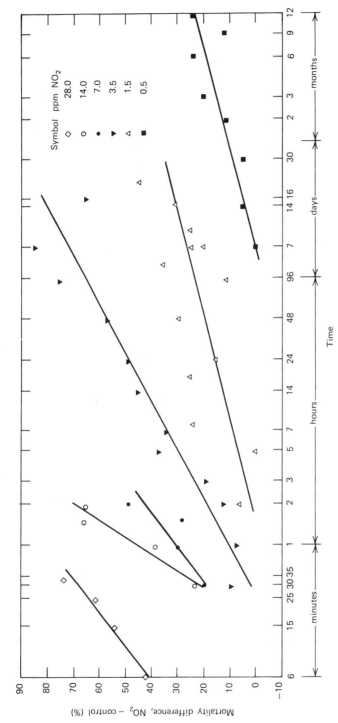

**Figure 8.23** Percentage mortality of mice as a function of continuous exposure to various $NO_2$ concentrations prior to challenge with streptococci. Reproduced with permission from Gardner et al., Figure 5, *J. Toxicol. Environ. Health*, **3**, 811–820, © 1977 by Hemisphere Publ. Corp., Washington, D.C.

**5**  Gardner et al. (1977) expressed their data on the effect of continuous inhalation of $NO_2$ on the outcome of laboratory-induced pulmonary infections in mice as shown in Figure 8.23.

Using 20% increased mortality as the response criterion, determine whether length of exposure or $NO_2$ concentration was more important in determining susceptibility to streptococcal infection in these mice.

**6**  Bernfeld (1975), in a study of the acute toxicity of cigarette smoke, plotted the mean survival time in groups of mice exposed to cigarette smoke against the concentrations of tar (Figure 8.24) and nicotine (Figure 8.25) in the cigarettes.

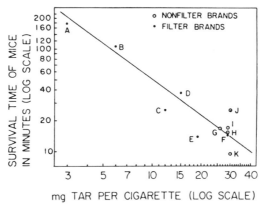

**Figure 8.24**  Mean survival times of mice inhaling smoke from 11 brands of cigarettes, as related to the tar deliveries of the cigarettes. Reproduced with permission from Bernfeld, 1975, Figure 2.

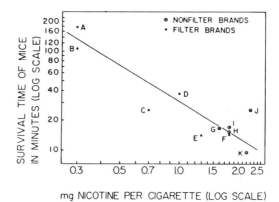

**Figure 8.25**  Mean survival times of mice inhaling smoke from 11 brands of cigarettes, as related to the nicotine deliveries of the cigarettes. Reproduced with permission from Bernfeld, 1975, Figure 3.

Is the concentration of toxic smoke components or the length of time the cigarettes were smoked more important to the toxicity of the total dose of cigarette smoke? Which of the two toxic components (tar or nicotine) is more important? Is this observation consistent with the information contained in Figure 8.26?

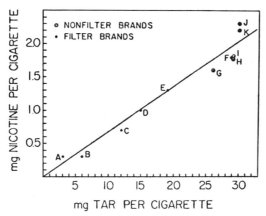

**Figure 8.26** Correlation between tar and nicotine deliveries for the cigarette brands of Figures 8.24 and 8.25. Reproduced with permission from Bernfeld, 1975, Figure 1.

7  By substituting appropriate arbitrary values of $A$ and $k_e$ into Equation 5.19, show graphically that whatever the critical toxic body burden, it is reached earlier during continuous administration of toxicants with small $k_e$ than during continuous administration of toxicants with large $k_e$ for dose rates that represent the same fraction of the ED50 per unit of time.

8  Show mathematically, starting with Equation 5.19, that at times that are very small relative to the half-life, body burden is approximately independent of $k_e$ and is directly proportional to the length of continuous exposure.

9  Graham (1960) studied the interaction of alcohol and a barbiturate, sodium pentabarbitone (PB), in male white mice. Both toxicants were given by stomach intubation. The LD50 of a 40% solution of ethanol in water was found to be 24 ml/kg and that of PB to be 148 mg/kg. When 6 ml/kg of the ethanol solution was given to the mice, the LD50 of PB was 108 mg/kg; when 12 ml/kg of the ethanol solution was given, the LD50 of PB was 66 mg/kg; and when 18 ml/kg of the ethanol solution was given, the LD50 of PB was 31.5 mg/kg. Respiratory failure was the cause of death in all cases.

Are these two toxicants additive, positively synergistic, or antagonistic?

## REFERENCES

Albert, R. E. and B. Altshuler, "Considerations relating to the formulation of limits for unavoidable population exposures to environmental carcinogens." *Radionuclide Carcinogenesis*, AEC Symposium Series, Conf.-72050, National Technical Information Service, 1973, pp. 233–253.

Andersen, M. E., R. A. Jones, R. G. Mehl, T. A. Hill, L. Kurlansik, and L. J. Jenkins, Jr. "The inhalation toxicity of sulfolane (tetrahydrothiophene-1,1-dioxide)." *Toxicol. Appl. Pharmacol.*, **40**, 463–472 (1977).

Beaubien, A. R., D. C. Carpenter, L. F. Mathieu, M. MacConnaill, and P. D. Hrdina. "Antagonism of imipramine poisoning by anticonvulsants in the rat." *Toxicol. Appl. Pharmacol.*, **38**, 1–6 (1976).

Bernfeld, P. "Acute toxicity of smoke from different brands of cigarettes, measured in mice." *Toxicol. Appl. Pharmacol.*, **31**, 413–420 (1975).

Bliss, C. I. "The toxicity of poisons applied jointly." *Ann. Appl. Biol.*, **26**, 585–615 (1939).

Boyd, E. M. and M. J. Selby. "The chronic oral toxicity of benzylpenicillin." *Antibiot. Chemotherapy*, **12**, 249–262 (1962).

Boyd, E. M. and M. N. Shanas. "The acute oral toxicity of sodium chloride." *Arch. Int. Pharmacodyn. Ther.*, **144**, 86–97 (1963).

Boyd, E. M., M. M. Abel, and L. M. Knight. "The chronic oral toxicity of sodium chloride at the range of the LD50 (0.1L)." *Can. J. Physiol. Pharmacol.*, **44**, 157–172 (1966).

Chand, N. and D. G. Hoel. "A comparison of models for determining safe levels of environmental agents." In *Reliability and Biometry*, P. Proschan and R. J. Serfling, Eds., SIAM, Philadelphia, 1974, pp. 681–700.

Crump, K. S., D. G. Hoel, D. H. Langley, and R. Peto. "Fundamental carcinogenic processes and their implications for low dose risk assessment." *Cancer Res.*, **36**, 2973–2979 (1976).

Doggett, N. S., H. Reno, and P. S. J. Spencer. "A comparison of the acute toxicity of some centrally acting drugs measured under crowded and uncrowded conditions." *Toxicol. Appl. Pharmacol.*, **39**, 141–148 (1977).

Douglas, J. S., M. W. Dennis, P. Ridgway, and A. Bouhuys. "Airway constriction in guinea pigs: Interaction of histamine and autonomic drugs." *J. Pharmacol. Exp. Ther.*, **184**, 169–179 (1973).

Druckrey, H. "Quantitative aspects in chemical carcinogenesis." In *Potential Carcinogenic Hazards from Drugs (Evaluation of Risks)*, Réné Truhaut, Ed., UICC Monograph Series, Vol. 7, Springer-Verlag, New York, 1967, pp. 60–78.

Finney, D. J. *Probit Analysis: A Statistical Treatment of the Sigmoid Response Curve*, 2nd ed., Cambridge University Press, New York, 1952, Chapter 8, pp. 122–159.

Food and Drug Administration Advisory Committee on Protocols for Safety Evaluation. "Panel on carcinogenesis report on cancer testing in the safety evaluation of food additives and pesticides." *Toxicol. Appl. Pharmacol.*, **20**, 419–438 (1971).

Fuhremann, T. W. and E. P. Lichtenstein. "Increase in the toxicity of organophosphorus insecticides to house flies due to polychlorinated biphenyl compounds." *Toxicol. Appl. Pharmacol.*, **22**, 628–640 (1972).

Gardner, D. E., D. L. Coffin, M. A. Pinigin, and G. I. Sidorenko. "Role of time as a factor in the toxicity of chemical compounds in intermittent and continuous exposures. Part 1. Effects of continuous exposure." *J. Toxicol. Environ. Health*, **3**, 811–820 (1977).

Gehring, P. J., P. G. Watanabe, and C. N. Park. "Resolution of dose-response toxicity data for chemicals requiring metabolic activation: Example—vinyl chloride." *Toxicol. Appl. Pharmacol.*, **44**, 581–591 (1978).

Gehring, P. J., P. G. Watanabe, and C. N. Park. "Risk of angiosarcoma in workers exposed to vinyl chloride as predicted from studies in rats." *Toxicol. Appl. Pharmacol.*, **49**, 15–21 (1979).

Graham, J. D. P. "Ethanol and the absorption of barbiturate." *Toxicol. Appl. Pharmacol.*, **2**, 14–22 (1960).

Hayes, W. J., Jr. "Tests for detecting and measuring long-term toxicity." In *Essays in Toxicology*, Vol. 3, W. J. Hayes, Jr., Ed., Academic Press, New York, 1972, Chapter 3, pp. 65–77.

Hoel, D. G., D. W. Gaylor, R. L. Kirschstein, U. Saffiotti, and M. Schneiderman. "Estimation of risks of irreversible, delayed toxicity." *J. Toxicol. Environ. Health*, **1**, 133–151 (1975).

Kulkarni, A. P. "Joint action of insecticides against houseflies." *J. Toxicol. Environ. Health*, **1**, 521–530 (1976).

Litchfield, J. T. and F. Wilcoxon. "A simplified method of evaluating dose-effect experiments." *J. Pharmacol. Exp. Ther.*, **96**, 99–113.

McKay, D. H., R. V. Jardine, and P. A. Adie. "The synergistic action of 2-($O$-cresyl)-4$H$-1:3:2-benzodioxaphosphorin-2-oxide with soman and physostigmine." *Toxicol. Appl. Pharmacol.*, **20**, 474–479 (1971).

Mantel, N. and W. R. Bryan. "'Safety' testing of carcinogenic agents." *J. Natl. Cancer Inst.*, **27**, 455–470 (1961).

Mantel, N., N. R. Bohidar, C. C. Brown, J. L. Ciminera, and J. W. Tukey. "An improved Mantel-Bryan procedure for 'safety' testing of carcinogens." *Cancer Res.*, **35**, 865–872 (1975).

Maugh, T. H. "Chemical carcinogens: How dangerous are low doses?" *Science*, **202**, 37–41 (1978).

Ramsey, J. C., C. N. Park, M. G. Ott, and P. J. Gehring. "Carcinogenic risk assessment: Ethylene dibromide." *Toxicol. Appl. Pharmacol.*, **47**, 411–414 (1979).

Rosiello, A. P., J. M. Essigmann, and G. N. Wogan. "Rapid and accurate determination of the median lethal dose (LD50) and its error with a small computer." *J. Toxicol. Environ. Health*, **3**, 797–809 (1977).

Siew, C. and D. B. Goldstein. "Osmotic minipumps for administration of barbital to mice: Demonstration of functional tolerance and physical dependence." *J. Pharmacol. Exp. Ther.*, **204**, 541–546 (1978).

Sprague, J. B. "Measurement of pollutant toxicity to fish. I. Bioassay methods for acute toxicity." *Water Res.*, **3**, 793–821 (1969).

Wadley, F. M. "The evidence required to show synergistic action of insecticides and a short cut in analysis." USDA Bureau Entomology Plant Quarantine Publ. No. ET-223 (1945).

Wadley, F. M. "Short-cut procedure for error estimate in laboratory studies of synergism in insecticides." USDA Bureau Entomology Plant Quarantine Publ. No. ET-275 (1949).

Whittemore, A. and B. Altshuler. "Lung cancer incidence in cigarette smokers: Further analysis of Doll and Hill's data for British physicians." *Biometrics*, **32**, 805–816 (1976).

# Index

Abscissa, defined, 3
Absorption, defined, 21
Absorption phase, 128
N-acetyl-$\alpha$-D-glucosaminidase, 66–67, *2.18*
Acetyl-$\beta$-methylcholine, 301, 305, *6.14, 6.17*
Acetylcholine, 54, 284, 305, 313, *2.10, 6.16*
Acetylcholine receptor, 284
Acetylcholinesterase, 313, *6.22*
Acetyliodocholine, 313, *6.22, 6.23*
N-acetyl para-aminosalicylic acid, 216–217, *4.28*
Acetylphenylhydrazine, 319, *6.28*
Acetylsalicylic acid, 185, 206, 210–213, *4.24, 4.25*
Acetylsulfisoxazole, 213, 215
ACHC; *see* Cyclacillin
Action, of effector, 286
Affinity
  of agonist for receptor, 279, 281
  and agonist structure, 300–301
  and receptor site structure, 301
Age, and kinetics, 260–261
Agonist
  defined, 278
  partial, 279–280
Albumin
  binding to, 182–183, *4.5*
  restricted to capillaries, 91
Alkyltrimethylammonium ions, as agonists, 279, *6.1*
Allosteric interactions, 284
Alpha-adrenergic receptor, 284
Alpha phase; *see* Distribution phase
Amikacin, 245–246
Amino acids
  membrane transport, 34
  uptake into erythrocyte, 41–42
Aminopyrine, 77, *2.27*

Amniotic fluid, as deep compartment, 262
Amobarbital, 191–197, 208, *4.12, 4.13, 4.14, 4.15, 4.16, 4.17*
D-Amphetamine, 332–334, 346, 363, *7.10, 8.9*
Amyltrimethylammonium ion, 279, *6.1*
Androgen receptors, 282
Anesthetics, volatile, 285
Angiotensin, 316–317, *6.25*
Antagonism, of effect
  defined, 279–280
  irreversible, 304–305
  reversible competitive, 292–293, 301
  reversible noncompetitive, 293–295, 302, 305
Antipyrine, 87
  and total body water, 103–104
Arbutin, 63–66, *2.15, 2.16, 2.17*
Area under the curve, 137–140
  calculating, 137–138
  and fraction absorbed by time $t$, 138–139
  relationship to internal dose, 137
Aspirin; *see* Acetylsalicylic acid
Atropine, 313, 349, *6.23, 7.24*
Average concentration in $n$th dose interval ($\bar{C}(n)$), 227–229, 233
  comparison of, with $C(t)$, 241

Barbital, 162–163, *3.46*
Barbiturates, as inducers, 260
Benzathine penicillin G, 134–135, 154, *3.34*
Benzene, 370–371, *8.12*
Benzylpenicillin (penicillin G), 373
Beta-methyldigoxin, 323–326, *7.2, 7.3*
Beta phase, 117, 118–120
  volume of distribution in, 125
Bicarbonate, 61–62, *2.14*
Bile flow rate, effect on kinetics, 205–206
Biological half-life; *see* Half-life

Biscoumacetate, 179, 180
Body burden, 117, 125
Boundary conditions, 5, 8, 18
Bromobenzene, 163-164
Bromsulfalein, 158-159
Butyramide, 87-88, *3.4, 3.5*
Butyrylcholine, 305-306, *6.16*

Cadmium, 33, 210, 260-261, *4.23*
Calcium, 316-317, *6.25*
Canrenone, 270
Capacity-limited processes; *see* Saturable
    processes
Carbamazepine, 132-133, 256-257, 270-272,
    *3.32, 5.12, 5.18*
Carbaryl, 367-368
Carnosine, 69, *2.20*
Catenary models, 148
CBDP; *see* Soman
Central compartment, defined, 21, 26
Cephaloridine, 262
Cephapirin, 148-149, *3.42*
Cephradine, 155
Chemical carcinogens, 286, 374
Chloramphenicol, 260
Chlordiazepoxide, 236, *5.6*
Chloride, 61-62, 103, *2.13, 2.14*
Chlorimipramine, 56, *2.11*
Chlorinated hydrocarbons, 261, 317, *6.27*
    as inducers, 204
Chlorisondamine, 302, *6.15*
Chloroform, 141, 203, *3.38*
Chlorophenothane (DDT), 204, 273-274, 317,
    373, 367-370, *6.26, 8.11*
Chlorpromazine, 348-349
Chronic exposure, 222-274
    and deep compartments, 256, 261-262
    defined, 223
    and saturable elimination, 247, 257
CI-581, 346, *7.23*
Cigarette smoke, 386-387, *8.24, 8.25, 8.26*
Clearance, 140-145, 199-202, 208
    defined, 140
    with filtration plus secretion in the kidney,
        201-202
    with first-order elimination, 141, 199-200
    with saturable elimination, 200-201
Clonazepam, 247-248, *5.8*
Clonidine, 345, *7.22*
Compartment, defined, 21
Competitive antagonism, 292-293, *6.7*
    and the ln dose, effect curve, 301
Competitive inhibition, 50-53

Complex antagonisms, 302-307
Computer fitting of kinetic data, 150-151
Concentration during constant infusion
    ($C(t)$), 233
    comparison of, with $\bar{C}(n)$, 241
Conservation equation, 36
Cooperativity, 284
Creatinine clearance, 215, 260, *4.27*
Cyclacillin, 260-161, 213-214, 160
Cycloleucine, 71, *2.22*
Cytosine arabinoside, 262

DDT; *see* Chlorophenothane
Deep compartment, 117, 147, 121-122, 252
    amniotic fluid as, 262
    bone as, 122
    on chronic exposure, 256, 259, 261-262
    defined, 121-122
    fat as, 121-122
    fetus as, 122-123, 259, 262
Delta-aminolevulinic acid, 50, *2.8*
Delta-aminolevulinic acid dehydras, 287
6-Deoxyglucose, 66, *2.17*
Derivative, 13-17
    defined, 15
    of exponential function, 16, 20
    properties, 16
N-desmethyldiazepam, 236, *5.6*
Deuterium oxide, 103-104
Dexamethasone, 283, *6.2*
Diazepam, 363, *8.8*
Diazoxide, 312, *6.21*
Dibenamine, 304, 305-307, *6.16, 6.17*
Dichlorodifluoromethane, 265-268
Dicumarol, 180
Dieaway
    from acute administration, 98-128, 145-147
    from maximum after absorption is
        complete, 130-132
    from steady state, 247-255, 262
    terminal, 128, 153
Dieldrin, 237-238, *5.7*
Diethylstilbestrol, 159-160, *3.44*
Diffusion; *see* Membrane transport,
    mechanisms; Passive diffusion
Digitalis, 307
Digitoxigenins, 308-309, *6.18, 6.19*
Digoxin, 308-309, 323-326, 345, *6.18, 6.19,
    7.2, 7.3*
Dihydroergocryptine, 284, *6.3*
Dimensions, 22-25
    rules for using, 22-23
    utility, 23

Dimethylsulfoxide, 166-167
2,2-dimethyl valeric acid, 75, *2.25*
Diphenhydramine, 163, 165, 293, *6.6*
Diphenylhydantoin, 33, 179, 243, 247-248, *5.8*
Diprenorphine, 363, *8.9*
Disease states, and kinetics, 243, 244, 246, 260-261
Disopyramide, 145
Distribution, defined, 21
Distribution phase, 116-120, 128
Disulfiram, 260
Dixon plot, 61-62, 77, *2.14*
Dose, effect relationship, 278-309
  effect of log dose transform, 296-301, *6.10, 6.11*
Dose interval, and half-life, 243-245
Dose regimen, 243-246
  in disease states affecting kinetics, 243, 244, 246
Drug-drug interactions, kinetics of, 260-261
Dynamics
  defined, 322
  variability, 323

Eadie (Hofstee) plot
  in competitive inhibition, 50-51, *2.9*
  of effect data, 290, 292
  in noncompetitive inhibition, 56, *2.11*
  for uninhibited process, 43-46, *2.6*
ED50
  defined, 357
  as midpoint of log dose, response curve, 359
Effect
  defined, 286, 354
  maximum, 288-289, 355
Effect, duration of, 327-332
  correlation with dose, 327-332
  when elimination is saturable, 331-332
  and first-order half-life, 328
  restrictions on correlations with dose, 338-345
  and zero-order half-life, 329
Effect, magnitude of, 323-327, 332-338
  concentration in peripheral compartments, correlation with, 323-327
  metabolite, correlation with, 323
  plasma concentration, correlation with, 323
  restrictions on correlation with time, 338-339, 344-345
  time, correlation with, 332-338
Effector, defined, 278

Efficacy, of agonist, 279
  and agonist structure, 300-301
Elimination, defined, 21
Enzyme catalysis, considered as saturable process, 67-68
Epinephrine, 312-313
Ergotamine, 295, *6.9*
Estradiol, 317, *6.26*
Estrogen receptors, 282, 317
Ethanol, 70-71, 89, 203, 260, *2.21*
  duration of effect, 329-330, *7.7*
  effect, 285, 381, *8.16*
  magnitude of effect and time, 336-337, *7.13, 7.14*
  and plateau principle, 272-273, *5.19, 5.20*
  saturable elimination, 33, 180, 187, *4.9*
Ethosuximide, 269
Ethyl acetate, 272-273
Ethyltrimethylammonium ion, 305-306, *6.16*
Evans blue, 103
Excretion, defined, 21
Exponential function
  decaying, 26, *1.6*
  defined, 8
  differentiating and integrating, 20-21
  inverted, 26, *1.6*
  properties, 16
Extraction efficiency, 141-142

Feathering
  and one-compartment model with first-order absorption and elimination, 132, 154, *3.32*
  and three-compartment model, 146, *3.41*
  and two-compartment model, 126-127, *3.28*
Fetus, as deep compartment, 122-123, 259, 262
Fick's first law, 3, 82-83, 99, *3.1*
  as limiting case of saturable kinetics, 38, 82
First-order kinetics; *see also* Linear kinetics
  defined, 21
  descriptive of diffusion, 84-86, *3.3*
First-pass effect, 138
Flip-flop
  for metabolite excretion, 111
  in one-compartment model with first-order absorption, 134-135
  in peripheral compartment of two-compartment model, 252
  in two-compartment model with first-order absorption, 135
Fluoride, 262-263, *5.14*

Formate, 208–209, *4.22*
Functional relationships, 2–11
common kinetic, 26–28, *1.6*
dependent variable, defined, 2
independent variable, defined, 2
linear transforms, 4–11, *1.2*
straight line, 3–4, *1.1*
Furtrethonium, 316, *6.24*

Galactose, 40, 56, 71, *2.3, 2.11, 2.22*
Gamma-aminobutyric acid, 43, 75, *2.5, 2.25*
Glomerular filtration, 197–198
measurement of, 199–200
Glomerulus; *see* Kidney
Glucagon receptor, 284
Glucocorticoid receptor, 282–283
Glucose, 33–34, 40, *2.3*
Glucuronide formation from salicylic acid, 210–212
Glutethimide, 328–329, *7.6*
Guanethidine, 345

Half-life
biological (terminal), 124, 146–147
dose dependent in nonlinear kinetics, 186–191
dose independent in linear kinetics, 174
in one-compartment model ($k_e$), 102
and time to achievement of steady state, 235–237, 256, 258, 262
and time to onset of drug action, 244
in two-compartment model ($\beta$ phase), 124
Half-saturation constant, 39–40
defined, 37
factors influencing, 40–41
Hanes (Woolf) plot, 46, *2.7*
Heme, 50, 287, *2.8*
Hemoglobin, restricted to capillaries, 91
Henderson–Hasselbalch equation, 92
Hexachlorophene, 298–299, *6.12*
Hexamethonium, 302, *6.15*
Hexane, 203, 270–271, *4.19, 5.17*
Histamine, 291–293, 295, 357–358, *6.6, 6.9, 8.3, 8.4*
Hydroxyamobarbital, 192–197, *4.13, 4.14, 4.15, 4.16, 4.17*
5-Hydroxytryptamine, 45, 56, *2.1, 2.6, 2.11*

Ibuprofen, 77, *2.27*
Imipramine, 363, *8.7, 8.8*
Indomethacin, 161, *3.45*
Indoxole, 312–313

Inducing agents, 204, 260
and steady state during chronic exposure, 256–257
Induction, of metabolizing enzymes, 204
Inhibition, of transport or of enzyme action, 47–59
competitive, 50–53
noncompetitive, 53–59
Insect juvenile hormone, 67–68, *2.19*
Insect juvenile hormone analogue, 67–68, 281–282
Insulin, 284
Insulin receptor, 284, 301
Integral, 16–20
as area under curve, 20
defined, 17
definite, 18
of exponential function, 16, 20–21
indefinite, 18
properties, 16
Interactions, drug–drug, 260–261
Inulin, 30
Inulin clearance, 199
Iodipamide, 60, *2.12*
Ionization, and membrane transfer, 91–98, *3.7, 3.8, 3.9, 3.10, 3.11*
Isobenzan, 367–368
Isobutyramide, 87–88, *3.4, 3.5*
Isocarboxazid, 363, *8.9*
Isoniazid, 261
Isovaleramide, 87–88, *3.4, 3.5*

Joint action, of mixtures, 366

Kepone, 205
Ketamine, 54, *2.10*
Kidney
kinetics of excretion from, 197–202
structure, 197–198

Lachesine, 301, 316, *6.14*
LD50, defined, 357
Lead, 260, 261, 287
Levodopa, 163, 165–166, 230–231, *5.3*
Lidocaine, 260
Lindane, 367–370, *8.11*
Linear extrapolation, for carcinogens, 378–380
Linear kinetics
characteristics of, 174–175, *4.1*
defined, 22
use of plateau principle to test for, 247

Lineweaver–Burk plot, 8
in competitive inhibition, 50, *2.8*
of effect data, 290–291, 295, *6.5*
in noncompetitive inhibition, 53–54, *2.10*
in uncompetitive inhibition, 77
for uninhibited process, 43, 46, *2.5*
Lipid, increase in liver, 203–204
Lipid solubility; *see* Partition coefficient
Lipopolysaccharide, 100, 104, 109, *3.15*
Loading dose, 226, 244–246
Lobeline, 302, *6.15*
Log dose, effect relationship, 296–301
comparison with log dose, response, 364
effect of antagonists, 301–307
experimental use, 307–309
Log dose, response relationship, 359–364
comparison with log dose, effect, 364
Logarithmic function, 8–13
common (base 10), 9
defined, 9
graphing, 11–13, *1.3*
natural (base e), 9
properties, 10–11
Loo–Riegelman method
for absorbed drug, 139
LSD; *see* Lysergic acid diethylamide
Lysergic acid diethylamide, 326–327, *7.4*

Maintenance dose, 244–246
Mammillary models, 147
Manganese, 316–317, *6.25*
Mantel–Bryan extrapolation, for carcinogens, 377–378
Marijuana; *see* Δ-9-Tetrahydrocannabinol
Maximum effect, defined, 288–289, 355
Maximum plasma level
attained in one-compartment model with first-order absorption, 154
in $n$th dose interval ($C(n_{oo})$ or $C_{max}$), 227
Maximum rate, in membrane transport, 37, 39
factors influencing, 41–42
Maximum response, 354–355
Medazepam, 111–113, *3.19*
Membrane transport, mechanisms, 34–35
active transport, 35, 59–60, 63–66, 85
considered as saturable process, 35–43
facilitated diffusion, 35, 59–62
Mercury, 261
Metabolism, 21
alterations in, and effect on steady state, 256–257
considered as active process, 186

effect of hepatic blood flow on, 204–205
factors influencing, 260–261
induction of, 204, 260
saturation of, and effect on kinetics, 186–197
Metabolite
excreted, 111
kinetics, 110–111, 129
Methadone, 96–98, 260, *3.11, 3.12*
Methamphetamine, 56–58, *2.11*
Methanol, 89, 208
Methaqualone, 135–137, 156, *3.36*
Methsuximide, 155
Methylene blue, 210–211
Methylene chloride, 264–266, *5.16, 5.17*
Methylmercuric chloride, 122–123, *3.26*
Metoprolol, 167–168, *3.48*
Microconstants, defined, 21, 101–102
dieaway after chronic exposure without steady state, 253–254
dieaway from steady state, calculation for, 252
maximum number calculable, 147
one-compartment acute model, calculation for, 104–115
one-compartment model with first-order absorption, calculation for, 130–134
two-compartment acute model, calculation for, 126
Minimum plasma level in $n$th dose interval ($C_{min}$), 227
Minocycline, 229–230, *5.3*
Mirex, 205, 262, 264, 373, *5.15*
Mixed function oxidases, 204
Models (schematic)
closed two-compartment, *3.2, 3.23*
first-pass effect, *3.37*
one-compartment with first-order absorption and elimination, *3.29, 3.30, 3.31*
open one-compartment, *3.13*
open one-compartment with constant input, *5.1*
open one-compartment with parallel elimination routes, *3.18*
open two-compartment, *3.22*
open two-compartment during dieaway from steady state, *5.9*
two-compartment with first-order absorption and elimination, *3.35*
Molecular size, as determinant of membrane transfer rate, 88–91, *3.5, 3.6*
Monoamine oxidase, 319, *6.28*

Multicompartment models, 145–150

Nafcillin, 165–166, 206, *3.47*
Naloxone, 363, *8.9*
Nephrotoxicity, effect on kinetics, 206
Nitrogen dioxide, 386, *8.23*
Nitroreductase, 298–299, *6.12*
Noncompetitive antagonism, 293–295, *6.8*
  and the ln dose, effect curve, 302
  and spare receptors, 305
Noncompetitive inhibition, 53–59
Nonlinear kinetics
  characteristics of, 175–179, *4.2, 4.3, 4.4*
  defined, 22
  due to capacity-limited processes, 181–202
  due to changes in kinetic parameters,
    202–207
  due to protein binding, 181–186
  due to saturable elimination, 186–197
Novobiocin, 381–383, *8.18, 8.19*

Occupancy theory, 287–288
Ochratoxin A, 71–72, *2.23*
One-compartment model, 98–115
  flip-flop, in, 134–135
  with first-order absorption, 128–135
  maximum concentration in, with first-
    order absorption, 154
  with parallel elimination routes, 109–115
  parameter estimation from cumulative
    excretion data, 105–106, 110
  parameter estimation from excretion rate
    data, 106–109, 110
  parameter estimation from metabolite data,
    110–111
  parameter estimation from plasma data,
    101–105, 110
  parameter estimation in, with first-order
    absorption, 130–135
  parameters, 101–104
  schemes, *3.13, 3.18, 3.29, 3.30, 3.31*
  time at which maximum concentration is
    reached, 132–133
Ordinate, defined, 3, 4
Ouabain, 206, 308–309, *6.18, 6.19*
Oxacillin, 240
Oxyphenbutazone, 204
Oxytocin, 300–301, *6.13*

Pactamycin, 100, *3.15*
Para-aminohippuric acid, 71–72, *2.23*
Para-aminosalicylic acid, 216, 217, *4.28*
Paraldehyde, 381, *8.16*

Paraoxon, 54, 381, *2.10, 8.17*
Parathion, 54, *2.10*
Partial agonist, 279–280
  and spare receptor, 304–305
Partition coefficient
  defined, 86
  as determinant of membrane transfer rate,
    86–88
Passive diffusion, 35
  first-order nature of, 84–86
  ionization and, 91–98
  lipid solubility and, 86–88
  molecular size and, 88–91
Penicillins, 185, 206; *see also* Benzathine
    penicillin G, Cyclacillin, Nafcillin
  dose regimen in renal disease, 244
Pentachlorophenol, 258–259, *5.13*
Pentobarbital, 87, 349
Pentylenetetrazol, 360–363, *8.6*
Peripheral compartment, 21, 128–129, 116,
    118–120, 147
  elimination from, 147
Pethidine, 363, *8.9*
pH, and ionization of drugs, as determinant
    of membrane transfer rate, 91–98, *3.7,
    3.8, 3.9, 3.10, 3.11*
Pharmacogenetics, 261
Phenazone (antipyrine), 204
Phenobarbital, 87, 205–206, 381, 363, *8.16,
    8.8*
  as inducer, 163, 197, 204
Phenol-3,6-dibromphthalein disulfonate, 206
Phenol red, 156–157
Phenylbutazone, 33, 204
Phenylhydrazine, 319, *6.28*
2-Phenylsuccinimide, 155
Phlorizin, 63–66, *2.15, 2.16, 2.17*
5-Phosphoarabinonate, 53, *2.9*
Phosphoglucose, 53, *2.9*
Pindolol, 345
Pinocytosis, 35
  considered as saturable process, 66–67
Piperonyl butoxide, 54, *2.10*
Plasma flow rate, effect on kinetics, 204–205
Plateau level; *see also* Steady state, in chronic
    exposure
  in chronic exposure, 232–235
  in clinical practice, 243–246
  comparison of statements of, 241–243
  defined, 223–224
  demonstration of, 223–225
  development of, 225–235
  experimental applications of, 246–258

Plateau level (Continued)
  in industry, 258-261
  in repeated administration, 226-232
  in toxicology, 261-262
Polybrominated biphenyls, 204
Polychlorinated biphenyls, 126-128, 266, 269, 381, *3.28, 8.17*
Polycyclic aromatic hydrocarbons, as inducers, 204
Population homogeneity, and dose, response relationship, 357-359
Potassium, 89
Potassium cyanide, 373
Potency, of agonist, 279
Potentiation, 365
Practolol, 323, *7.1*
Pregnancy, and kinetics, 260
Probenecid, 179, 206
Probit transform, 363-364
Procaine amide, 87
Procaine amide ethyl bromide, 206
Product inhibition, 204
Propionamide, 88, *3.4, 3.5*
Propranolol, 205, 260, 284, *4.20*
Protein binding
  displacement of drug by metabolite, 257
  and elimination, 185-186
  and kinetic nonlinearity, 183-184
  measurement, 181
  and pharmacologic activity, 184-185
  in plasma, 181-186
  in tissues, 184
Prothrombin complex, 338-339

Quinidine, 240, 254-255, *5.11*

Radiolabel, use of, in kinetic studies, 112-113
Rate constant, defined, 21
Rate theory, 287-288
Receptor
  membrane-bound, 283-284
  purification of, 282-284
  soluble, 282-283
Receptor site
  defined, 278
  enzyme, 280-281
  regulatory, 280-281
  structure and activity, 281-282
Receptor theory, 286-295
  and antagonists, 292-295
  development, 286-290
  estimation of Kd and Θm, 290-292
Reserpine, 290, 345, *6.4*

Residuals, method of; *see* Feathering
Response, quantal, 354-381
  defined, 354
  dependence on half-life in chronic exposure, 371-374
  extrapolation into low dose range, 374-381
  and length of chronic exposure, 370-374
  maximum, 354-355
  relationship to effect, 355-359
Response frequencies, 357-359
  lognormal distribution of, 357-359
  and median effective dose, 357
  standard deviation of, 358
Riboflavin, 206, 215-216, *4.21, 4.27*
Risk assessment, 374-381
  comparison of models, 380-381
  principles of, 374-377
Rose bengal, 175-178, 190, *4.2, 4.3, 4.4*

Salicylamide, 383-384, *8.22*
  area under curve, 139-140
  clearance, 143-145, *3.39*
  elimination, 113-115, *3.20, 3.21*
Salicylic acid, 47, 87, 210-214, *2.7, 4.24, 4.25*
Salicyluric acid, 47, *2.7*
Saturable biliary excretion
  of iodipamide, 60, *2.12*
  of rose bengal, 176, *4.4*
Saturable elimination, 173
  effect on kinetics, 186-202
  and the kidney, 197-202
Saturable metabolism of amobarbital, 191-197
Saturable processes
  competitive inhibition, 50-53
  development of theory, 32-43
  effect on kinetics, 173, 180-202
  in the kidney, 197-202
  noncompetitive inhibition, 53-59
  parameter estimation, 43-47
  uncompetitive inhibition, 77
Scatchard plot, 182, 207, 282, 284, *4.5*
Serotonin, 290, *6.4*
Sex, affecting kinetics, 98, 160, 260, *3.12*
SKF 525 A, 163, 197, 204, 205
Smoking, and kinetics, 260
Sodium, 89, 103
Sodium chloride, 373
Soman, 365, *8.10*
Sotalol, 174-175, 240, *4.1*
Spare receptors, 304-307
  and irreversible antagonists, 304

Spare receptors (Continued)
  and partial agonists, 304–305
  and reversible noncompetitive antagonists,
    305
Specificity, of receptor site, 280–281
Spironolactone, 161, 182, 270, *3.45, 4.5*
Steady state
  of bimolecular complex in saturable
    process, 32, 36–37
  in chronic exposure, 122, 223–235, 237–239
  distributional, 116, 118–121
  dynamic nature of, 98
  estimation of parameters, 235–236
  factors affecting, 257
  first-order nature of approach to, 235–236
  half-life and, 235–236, 256
  related to $V_\beta$, 238
  use of, to infer exposure, 261
*Cis*-Stilbene, 72–73, *2.24*
*Trans*-Stilbenimine, 72–73, *2.24*
Stripping of curve; *see* Feathering
Succinylcholine, 301, 349–351
Sugars
  conformational stability and uptake into
    erythrocyte, 41, *2.4*
  membrane transport, 34
Sulfamethizole, 234–235, *5.5*
Sulfate, 146, *3.41*
Sulfisoxazole, 105–106, 213, 215, 240,
    253–254, 262, *3.16, 5.10*
Sulfolane, 371, *8.13*
Sulfonamides, 185
Superposition, principle of, 174–176, 207,
    *4.3*
Suxamethonium, 351
Synergism, 365–370
  defined, 366
  testing for, 366–370

2,4,5-T; *see* 2,4,5-Trichlorophenoxyacetic
    acid
Terminal dieaway phase, 124, 128, 146–147
Tetraethyl lead, 154–155, *3.43*
  tris (3,5,6,8-tetramethyl-1,10-phenanthro-
    line) ruthenium chloride, 316, *6.24*
Δ-9-Tetrahydrocannabinol, 323
Theophylline, 240, 345
Therapeutic range, 243, 247
Thiometon, 367–368
Thiopental, 120–121, 342–343, 381, *3.25,
    8.16*
Tocainide, 95–96
Toxogonin, 305, *6.17*

Transfer across membranes, 35; *see also*
    Membrane transport, mechanisms;
    Passive diffusion, Pinocytosis
Trapezoidal rule, 137
Trichloroethanol, 381, *8.16*
Trichlorofluoromethane, 265–268
2,4,5-Trichlorophenoxyacetic acid, 189–190,
    *4.10, 4.11*
3-Trifluoromethyl-4-nitrophenol, 381–384,
    *8.18, 8.19, 8.20, 8.21, 8.22*
Triorthotolylphosphate, 334–335, *7.11, 7.12*
Tryptophan, 70–71, 75, *2.21, 2.26*
D-Tubocurarine, 106–109, 343–344, *3.17,
    7.20, 7.21*
Tubular reabsorption, 198, 202
Tubular secretion, 198–199
Two-compartment model, 83, 116–128,
    135–137
  with first-order absorption, 135–137
  kinetic characteristics of, 116–120
  parameter estimation from plasma data,
    126–128
  parameters, 123–126
  schemes, *3.2, 3.22, 3.23, 3.35*
Tylosin, 133–134, *3.33*

Uncompetitive antagonism, 295, 302
Urea, 89
Urine flow rate, effect on kinetics, 205–206

Valeramide, 87–88, *3.4, 3.5*
Valine, 41, 56, 68–69, *2.11*
Volume of distribution, 125–126
  and clearance, 141
  in one-compartment model ($V_D$), 102–104
  relationships among, 238–241
  at steady state ($V_{ss}$), 239
  in two-compartment model during $\beta$ phase
    ($V_\beta$), 125
  in two-compartment model by extrapo-
    lation of $\beta$ phase ($V$ extrap), 124–125
  and values of microconstants, 119

Wagner–Nelson method, for absorbed drug,
    138–139
Warfarin, 286, 287, 338–339, *7.15, 7.16,
    7.17*

Yohimbine, 312–313

Zero-order kinetics, 22, 33, 38; *see also*
    Nonlinear kinetics
Zoxazolamine, 323